THE BODY

VOLUME 2 OF *THE HUMAN GARAGE* TRILOGY

Published by Snazell Publishing

Cromwell House
Wolseley Bridge
Stafford
Staffordshire
ST17 0XS
NickyS@painreliefclinic.co.uk

ISBN: 978-0-9931678-2-9

Paperback Edition June 2016

THE
BODY

VOLUME 2 OF *THE HUMAN GARAGE* TRILOGY

BY

NICKY SNAZELL

Snazell Publishing

To all those scientists and creative thinkers prepared to think outside the box, who gave their time and hearts to this fascinating subject, and to all those entrepreneurs of knowledge mentioned within the covers of this book, whose shoulders I stand on to write this.

My mother's suffering led to my vocational work on back pain relief strategies, so this is also for her, and to my husband, thank you for understanding my need to get these books written.

Thank you to Jessica Coleman and Tanya Back for all their work on these books.

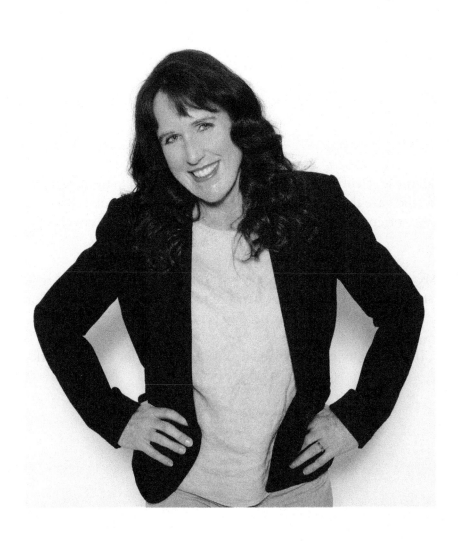

Praise for THE BODY – COLLEAGUES

These are comments from a handful of friends who present and write internationally on holistic physical medicine and health.

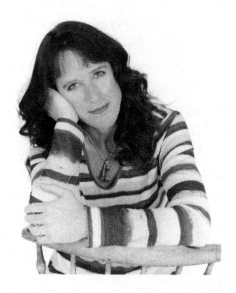

"Congratulations, Nicky, on your second award (AACP Excellence Awards 2016 for Patient Service) and your third book. You deserve the absolute best and I am thrilled for you in your new offering to the world. You are the gift to everyone that has the privilege of learning from you. Well done, Nicky, you are the best."

- Joseph McClendon III, ultimate performance coach, PhD in psychology, founder of Z Factor seminars, and co-presenter with Tony Robbins for the world renowned UPW events.

"I've had the privilege of working with Nicky at several Z Factor health seminars. She's a mesmerising speaker and her life work in pain treatment and management is always on the leading edge. Most of all, I've come to know Nicky's heart. Nobody cares more and wants to help you more than Nicky."

- John Lewis Parker, musician, mentor, and international speaker on the effect of meditation on the mind and body. California, USA.

"One's good health depends on having healthy body cells. In a healthy body, each and every cell must be in contact with another cell. Those cells unable to do so must be touched by a nerve. The healthy body therefore depends on having healthy nerves; yet nerves are the first body cells to suffer damage and degenerate. The most vulnerable nerves are the spinal nerve roots as they exit from the bony spinal column. Regrettably, the medical examination often neglects examination of this peripheral nervous system that regulates and integrates the entire body's function. Fortunately, the body's condition is examined by physiotherapists, especially those who have been trained to examine the spinal nerves. Their examination includes scrutiny of the body's motor function as well as the autonomic system.

"I handed out my first honorary fellowship to you. The Institute for the Study and Treatment of Pain is pleased to award 'Nicky Snazell' an Honorary Fellowship in recognition of extensive knowledge, outstanding contributions, and expert teaching abilities in IMS. Thank you, Nicky."

- *Chan Gunn, MD, CM, OBC, FRCP.*

"Understanding that the human body has an esthetic geometry, which is fractal in nature and is designed as a biotensegrity so that it dissipates stress as opposed to focusing it, changed the way I approached physiotherapy. I was intrigued by the possible implications for our profession that these understandings might represent and have therefore endeavoured to comprehend, integrate and teach new concepts such as these over the past few years. Concurrently, physiotherapy has entered the early stages of a technology-led revolution with our ability to measure and change both the body's physiology and structure developing rapidly.

"Currently innovation is taking place in a haphazard way, yet if we pooled our resources as a profession it would magnify the rate of change and also its impact. Therefore, for physiotherapists to begin raising and directing the flow of money within research might be considered the next logical step, yet it also represents a giant leap of faith for many of us. I hope we have the courage and conviction required when the time comes to take whatever action is required to make this a reality. It is my opinion that an opportunity to create a new destiny for the

profession within which physiotherapy treatments can be clearly demonstrated to deliver significant cost effective benefit is dawning. New understandings about the nature of the human body coupled with advanced technologies and the age-old skills with which to exploit them is a potentially powerful cocktail."
- John Wood, Clinical Director/Specialist Physiotherapist
MCSP, GHEA, DipAc.

"Integrated Dry Needling is a unique system of dry needling involving a broad range and tissue irritability screening process to identify all of the significant abnormal impulse generating sites in the musculoskeletal system contributing to movement dysfunction, pathological processes, and pain sensitivity. Tissue is considered significant and appropriate to treat if it exhibits both movement dysfunction and tissue irritability on palpation. The site of pain is viewed as a result, and not a cause, of a problem.

"One of the great advantages of a tool like Integrated Dry Needling is that in the right hands, movement dysfunction can rapidly be resolved or optimised, and pain treated as a result. The altered load on the wider autonomic central nervous systems often result in other collateral benefits and are recognised though not directly addressed within the scope of the integrated paradigm. The challenge for the movement therapist is to solve the problem of why an individual is initially presented with pain as a result of movement dysfunction and how to ensure that their optimised movement profile not only progresses but is maintained. This extends far beyond the application of dry needling techniques."
- Andrew Hutton, Sports Consultant Physiotherapist, Developer and
International Presenter, Integrated Dry Needling - www.dryneedling.com.au

"Congrats on your award, Nicky! It's great having you present on our show; you are never short of things to talk about and I love the peacefulness of your *Harrogate clinic.*"
- Beth Parsons. Stray FM Radio Presenter and host for the Health and
Well-being show (you can access Nicky's recordings at the Stray FM website).

"As mentioned, you are a brilliant addition to the shows, our listeners will love you, plus this is information that can turn their lives around."

- Joanne Smith, Stray FM.

"I think a lot of physios would benefit from your experience and insight within this book. Nicky is a unique individual; a multifaceted medical professional who is not afraid to draw on knowledge from a broad spectrum of specialities to aid her goal in understanding and treating pain as effectively as possible. Her understanding comes from both ends of the treatment spectrum; the cutting edge of research-based medical sciences and the more intuitive ancient healing arts."

- Jonathan Hobbs, MSc, MCSP, FHEA, AACP.
ATP Ltd Director and tutor, Stoke.

[Note from Nicky: "Jon Hobbs is, in my opinion, one of the top UK lecturers in Chinese Acupuncture to physiotherapists. He teaches precise, easy to follow practicals, backed up by lashings of research. I have written this because he is too humble to say it himself."]

"Good for you regarding the award and the book!"

- James Pinkney, Consultant Physiotherapist & Gunn IMS lecturer, London.

"Well done Nicky with your book and award, you deserve it."

- Joanne McBrinn, International Lecturer in Gunn IMS University of British Columbia, Calgary.

"Nicky, this is absolutely brilliant! I love it! I read it without pausing at all, a fabulous read and very much needed in this day and age: well done and I look forward to reading the rest."

- Mary Fickling, Director Physiopod UK Ltd.

"By writing about her own experience as 'the patient' and beautifully weaving this in with her many years of research, education and experience,

Nicky has produced the most wonderfully insightful, engaging and relatable body book.

"It takes real courage to embrace our personal challenges, and even more to tell everyone about it, yet by writing about it Nicky has given the reader the gift to understand more about their body and how they can avoid certain pitfalls or help themselves out of such situations, putting themselves in a more informed position to thrive."

- Linda Hill, Linda Hill Fitness

Praise for THE BODY — CURRENT PATIENTS

"Nikki was born to relieve or remove our pain or at least keep it at bay. She has developed incredible knowledge, techniques, and skills, which when shared, make life more comfortable for so many. We suspect she was born to heal and has learnt and developed skills and techniques to enhance her innate abilities. She has removed pain for both of us and for the many friends and acquaintances referred on her direction."

- David A, patient at the Pain Relief Clinic

"I first met Nicky Snazell over 22 years ago, when, having been diagnosed with fibromyalgia, I saw an article in the local paper about this young woman who had left a supervisory physio post in the NHS to open a pain relief clinic at her home. I had nothing to lose, as I was in a lot of pain and reluctant to take too much medication. That meeting changed my whole outlook on health and pain control.

"Getting to know the amazing Nicky, I found someone whose outlook and care of the wellbeing of others was imperative to her. Also, her knowledge of the healing powers of the body and musculoskeletal make up were something she shared with all seeking her help. I was one of the first to be treated with IMS, a groundbreaking needling treatment she had studied and perfected.

"From that first meeting, I have controlled pain with diet, exercise, and now occasional visits to Nicky. Her books are my bible if anything is wrong. I have sent many friends to Nicky, who have also found someone who would listen, advise both medically and spiritually, AND help.

"It was 10 years ago when, to me, a miracle happened. My husband found, on standing up, that his left leg had no feeling and was like a swinging pendulum. On admission to hospital and 8 days' stay, they didn't have a diagnosis, but thought it may be a mild stroke. I was sure it wasn't so I phoned Nicky, and she said 'I am sure I can help'. So off we went, with a leg that had no feeling and on crutches. After a short examination, Nicky diagnosed a Lumbar Root Nerve Entrapment, treatment started and, in a very short time, he was walking again.

"Nicky is a superstar in our eyes; she totally believes in all she says and does. Take control of your body and lifestyle, its healing powers are not to be ignored. We wish you success with your latest book, Nicky, and in continuing your groundbreaking work."
                                      - Diana Scott, MBE, patient at the Pain Relief Clinic

---

For those practitioners who don't believe we change people's lives, YOU ARE WRONG:

"Last week I thanked you, Nicky, for your care of me, and your reaction so surprised me that I want to spell out more exactly why I am so thankful. From the very beginning – a few years ago now – I have known that, though I'm one of the many people whom you treat, whilst I am in your presence I have your undivided attention, and healing me occupies you totally and matters to you. This induces in me an almost trance-like state in which I heal in body and mind. Elderly people who have lost their partners spend much more time alone and it is easy for them to slip into negative attitudes about almost every aspect of life, but you give me hope and with that the determination to surmount not just the problem with my back but other things as well. 'Thank you' is much too small a phrase to convey my feelings."
                                      - Daphne Starling, patient at the Pain Relief Clinic

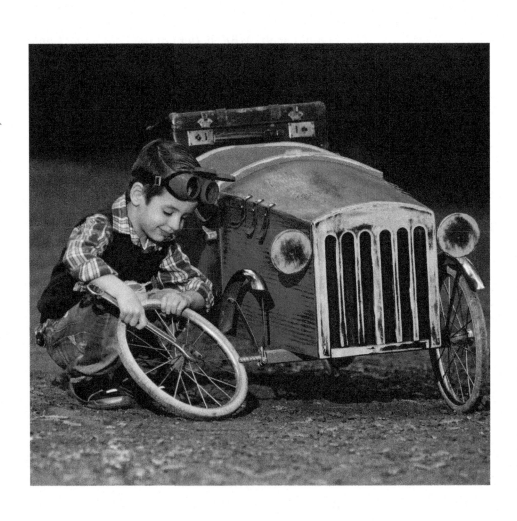

CONTENTS

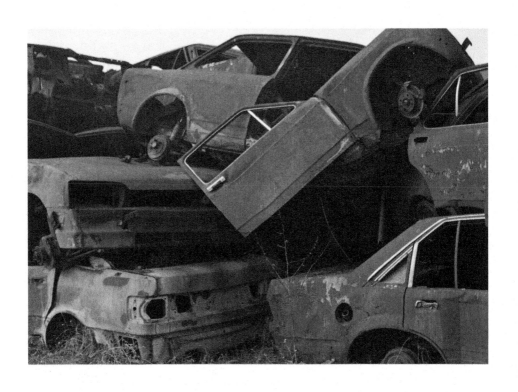

Introduction

"At 50, everyone has the face he deserves."

– George Orwell

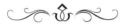

"When you are inspired by some great purpose, some extraordinary project, all your thoughts break their bonds: Your mind transcends limitations, your consciousness expands in every direction, and you find yourself in a new, great and wonderful world. Dormant forces, faculties and talents become alive, and you discover yourself to be a greater person by far than you ever dreamed yourself to be."
- –Patañjali

There is the healer and then there is the mechanic.

My team of friends came to the Human Garage – my clinics – armed with a multitude of 'orthodox' skills and qualifications, including: nursing, physiotherapy, sports therapy, orthopaedic medicine, and surgery. For some of them, however, their skills didn't stop there: they'd also already embraced a more holistic approach, being versed in reiki, nutrition, and spiritual and shamanic training. They were born both mechanics and healers.

Once they started working at my clinic, they began to study and apply my integrative, intuitive, alternative medical approach, soon awakening to a wholistic healing and curing approach – and yes, that's wholistic with a 'w', as it was originally written: as in a 'whole' person. The psychological, neurolinguistics part of me thinks that this change of spelling makes it seem less significant, as we think of holes – and therefore the word 'holistic' – as being empty or dangerous. Based on nearly thirty years of study and treating patients, I've found that combining what I consider the best of both western and eastern medicine is the best, most sensible way forward – isn't it? I ponder for a moment on the way we refer to just two directions of medicine. What happened to the medicine of the northern and southern hemispheres?

So why have I written *The 4 Keys To Health* and now *The Human Garage Trilogy: Mind, Body & Soul*? There isn't a day that doesn't go by without someone – colleagues, patients, friends – asking that very question, and luckily, it's always an easy one for me to answer: to share my life's work, to share my frustrations about working in the *illness* industry, not the *wellness* industry. That's why I wrote *The 4 Keys To Health*, and also why I have integrated it into my patients' physiotherapy treatment programs – although not, I hasten to add, without a lot of resistance from the mechanics within my peers.

WHAT MAKES YOUR CLINIC DIFFERENT?

I get asked this a lot, and I was even asked the question yesterday for a northern radio show I write for (a little plug here for the Health and Wellbeing Show on Stray FM!). It's uncanny that my brother should spend such a large part of his life presenting for the BBC up north and editing radio shows, and that I should – in some small way – be able to follow in his footsteps.

I chose the analogy of a car/human garage for this series for good reason, and this is something I will explain further as I go along. Basically, just like the evolving technology of car performance, I eagerly utilise all the hard work that researchers have put into creating the latest technology for human health. My very own Human Garage – the Nicky Snazell pain relief clinics – are a utopia of pioneering physiotherapy and technology, and my dream is for all of this to be available to everyone on the NHS. After all, healthy, fit bodies need fewer pit stops and therefore receive a smaller repair bill at their health checks/MOTs.

With machines (mainly our magnetic resonance equipment), I am currently exploring the physiotherapy possibilities of going beyond simplistic cell repair and actually regenerating cartilage, tendon, spinal disc, and bone in older people, and even now, the results on a person's quality of life are breath-taking. We can break down calcified nodules with shockwave, and speed up healing with lasers, pulsed shortwave, and ultrasound. We can even scientifically measure how healthy our cells are without resorting to invasive techniques. QuadScan, for example, carries out cellular health analysis, meaning we can measure nutrients, fat, water, bone, and muscle ratios. Using this information, my nutritionists can make tailored healthy eating plans for optimum cellular health and correct hydration levels.

HeartMath is another clever scientific – but fun – tool for observing and self-managing stress. I use this for measuring heart rate variance (HRV), a strong indicator of chronic stress, and this is incredibly important to be aware of as stress can and will hinder healing. This kind of self-help tool improves the ability to create the correct mind state for healing and not stressing. At my clinic/human garage we can assess fitness using cardiovascular tests – this shows us how well our lungs and heart cope with exercise – as well as our flexibility and strength, which allows us to use computer programs to prescribe exercise to our patients. Theraflex – which I call R2-D2 after Star Wars – is a robotic hand that improves spinal flexibility by adjusting facet joint alignment and increasing elasticity.

Gaitscan shows us where pressure moves up through our feet and body as we run and walk, using biomechanical assessments to provide the data. I strongly believe we need to look holistically at how we can improve our posture and reduce joint wear, especially spinal experts. Unfortunately, too often it is only sportsmen or hip/knee/ankle problems that get biomechanically screened. It is useful to check tyre pressure – I mean, foot pressure – in order to prescribe exercises to alleviate future wear issues in your chassis, and if we need to prescribe orthotics, we do. We have all of this equipment and more at my clinics, or 'Batman's cave' as one patient described it last week.

Then we carry out several varied assessments, including: neuromusculoskeletal physiotherapy, neuropathic and psychosocial pain assessments, and arthritic joint and sports injury objective allopathic assessments, all before prescribing our tailor-made treatment plans. My wholistic mechanics – with a w – will then listen to patients, weaving in lifestyle advice and suggestions for improving mind state with stress busters, nutrition, and activity. The treatments we prescribe can include: massage, manipulation, acupuncture, revolutionary IMS for nerve pain, exercise for life, and electrotherapy such as shockwave, laser, and ultrasound healing where appropriate. We also offer Magnetic Resonance Therapy (MRT) for joint repair in terms of sports injuries, disc damage, and osteoarthritis. Hands-on massage, soft tissue work, and reiki all help to soothe the mind and prepare for healing. On top of all this, with our healers' hearts inside our mechanic bodies, we can listen with empathy and work on a patient's energy matrix, whispering to their soul.

The treatment plan is carried out, and once we're happy that we've got our patient as close to optimum health as possible, we can start using our revolutionary technology – magnetic resonance, or MRT – that can actually push back the hands of time. Early on in my career, I used to involve my surgical buddies when it came to osteoarthritis, as I simply didn't have the capability at my fingertips to regrow cartilage and bone cells (that normally would not regenerate due to aging) at an accelerated rate. Never before have we gone this far within physical medicine. That's right, Star Trek-like technology is slowly emerging; it's the new science of today, whether we like it or not. Most importantly, never have I been so aware of the fading disbelief in anything non-surgical or drug-based.

"Man did not weave the web of life – he is merely a strand in it. Whatever he does to the web, he does to himself."
- **Chief Seattle**

With my background in shamanic reiki healing and neurolinguistics programming with psychology, I am very aware of the power of the mind, and I feel privileged to be in the driving seat of the physical medicine of tomorrow. Hence my body book sits in-between these two. I strongly feel that it is of vital importance to analyse and reanalyse any block to a patient getting the healing results they want, before they start overpowering their body with synthetic drugs or surgery. Keeping accurate records and applying both an intuitive and scientific approach will give us a broader understanding as we pave the way forward for healing future generations.

Throughout this series of books, I am going to share with you my recipes of integrated medicine for physical health. Through sharing with you these stories of just a handful of my current patients (while these are true, they are a composite of several stories in order to disguise my patients and protect their privacy), my aim is to allow you to walk in their shoes, feel their pain, and hear their stories and beliefs about suffering. Hopefully you can then relate this information to your own story, getting those light bulb moments – those ah-ha's – and enabling you to get in a good place to heal. I want to open up an awareness in you about the stories you tell yourself and how self-destructive they can be.

If you don't have a specific problem that needs treating, but you would like help on keeping healthy, you may want to come along to one of my talks or seminars, or listen in to the radio shows I'm involved with – why not? It'll cost you nothing, and you might learn something new. My patients are too shy to be on stage, so when I do live shows I came up with the idea of having puppets made. I dress them up to represent my patients, and in this way I can carry these troubled souls into the room, so we can learn from their stories. One of my patients said to me only this week: "if my suffering helps another soul then I can bear it more easily."

Have you got hidden beliefs/tragic memories locked into a place in your body? Then let me help you with them; once you understand with these books how to look after yourself, you are no longer a victim to illness but a student as to what illness teaches us. We all tell ourselves stories about our bodies – I know I certainly do: for every injury or operation I've ever had, I have a story to go with it, and I have to be careful how I replay that story to myself. Memory is fluid; every time we recall something, we mould a new version of it. It isn't like a DVD that plays the exact same story every time, no matter how many times you watch it. So let's rewrite the story of your life, starting today. And how do you do that? Just read on, and remember: you are the author of your life. You can make today a whole new chapter – you just have to decide that you want to end one chapter and start another.

My own life has had all sorts of twists and turns, and yet it always circles back to the same thing: I have spent the majority of my life feeling like a square peg in a round hole. I've had to take on challenges to be qualified in degrees that allowed me to converse with medics and scientists, have walked away from fascinating hobbies and holidays, and have spent little time with friends and family I love in order to fulfil my believed life's purpose. You cannot smash another's beliefs about health, however misled they are – it is not up to us to do this, though it is so damn hard that false beliefs have caused the illness industry to come into being, as well as causing war, unnecessary suffering, cruelty to kids and animals, and the pollution of this planet. And so on. The old memes (verbal viruses) have a lot to answer for.

My physiotherapy degree was a reductionist orthopaedic medical course (another name for this is allopathic) and it's much like the way doctors are taught medicine – in that kind of course, my *4 Keys* book would have been used as toilet paper. This book, on the other hand, is about both the strengths and weaknesses of allopathic (opposite disease) and wholistic medicine.

There may come a day when you get a devastating diagnosis and have to make several important decisions regarding your treatment. While it may not be a very nice thing to think about, it is wise to think through these decisions before this day comes, arming yourself and your family with all the available facts – making an informed decision armed with sound knowledge will really help.

In every culture there are many fixed preconceived beliefs. For instance, in the west we lean heavily towards allopathic medicine. Why? Everyone does it, insurance covers it, and we trust that our GP keeps studying and is up to date on all available treatments. Well, fasten your seat belts, please, because I'm afraid I'm about to upset you. In fact, you might want to put on your crash helmets too.

The third leading cause of death in the USA is doctor-supervised medical errors. Let me repeat that: it's the third leading cause of death, after cancer and heart attacks (JAMA, 1998). Apologies if your air bag just went off. Cultural conditioning means that my patients believe it's their doctor's or therapist's job to keep them healthy, that an entire lifetime of abuse can be fixed with just a pink tablet or a quick manipulation. Well, it's time to get your seat belts on again, and don't forget those helmets!

Here's the thing: my wholistic colleagues think that allopathic physios and doctors are arrogant, close-minded, unhealthy (the life expectancy for a doctor is just 59 years of age), and simply lapdogs to the drugs companies. The doctors then reply, saying that holistic means 'quackery', that it is sub-standard training, dangerous, and incompetent, done using unproven tech-niques. A marriage made in heaven – NOT.

It was interesting to study physiotherapy with both physios and doctors, and I will say this: the allopathic approach has at least moved away from bloodletting and mercury – we've come a long way since then. However, I was trained as a car mechanic, looking at the reductionist view that the body is made of parts. If your car is faulty the mechanic takes it apart, finds the defective part, and takes it out. The mechanic will find it with diagnos-tics, put your body up stationary – not dynamically on the car ramp – and use diagnostic equipment such as human Magnetic Resonance Imaging (MRI), and computerised axial tomography (CAT scans) in order to figure out what's wrong.

The car analogy fits, and this is why so many of my patients take many syn-thetic drugs to treat lots of different problems. It is an overpowering, con-trolling approach, as the body is seen as incapable of healing itself – which, at times, it is. The trouble is that the body then increases its symptoms to try to regain control and thus more synthetic drugs are needed. If this then fails, nutrition isn't even mentioned – they just go straight to surgery.

When in pain, the brain is warning the body that there is danger, and if no danger is perceived – regardless of the tissue damage – we do not feel pain. Hence suffering is so complex. When the brain is fully fired up to kill pain, it is sixty times stronger than any painkilling drug. Now, it is true that synthetic painkillers may give welcome relief in the short-term, but what about the long-term? The chronic suppression of healing responses is unhealthy and can even be deadly; if the subconscious is artificially quelled by drugs, it steps down and does nothing to repair the situation. There are also times where faulty nerves keep firing off inappropriate pain, which can be a damn nuisance. There'll be more about this later on.

So, back to drugs: they oppose illness, hence the anti-inflammatory, biotic, and coagulant properties. In many cases the body reacts violently to being suppressed, and magnifies the symptoms, resulting in death. I grew up on vitamins, herbs, and healthy food, and when I asked schools why they didn't discuss nutrients with children, the answer was something I didn't want to hear: I was told that as you couldn't patent plants, companies could not make money out of it – that was the bottom line. Money. The conditioning was that if a child was ill, they should go to the doc and get a pill, the colour and shape having a different outcome! Yes, really – studies have shown this.

But what about the power of the mind? Or even the power of the soul? Well, heaven forbid we go there! I wasn't allowed to discuss any kind of religion, politics, or sex with patients – though the latter was never a problem! Traditional physio and medical training rejects any influence of a soul over the body; if it is not objectively measurable, it simply does not exist. Interestingly, even deeply religious physios and doctors do not include its importance in healing. However, the ancient shamanic doctors always included prayer, meditation, and soul healing techniques as part of their treatment. There will be more about this in my Soul book.

We are culturally trained to accept the illness industry in the form that it is. Now, it's seat belt time again: the World Health Organization puts aside a staggering 2% of its budget to improve wellness using preventative medicine. Hence I was trained traditionally to aim my treatments at treating illness, effectively chasing the horse after it has bolted. The same World Health Organization ranks the USA as 72nd in the world in overall health. In twenty years of modern medicine they have slid from the 14th position to 72nd, and to think that in the UK we look up to their advanced medical system, research facilities, and teaching hospitals. Something isn't quite right there, wouldn't you say? If your child was 14th in their year and then came out 72nd, I would say that some questions have to be asked.

Just like you, I don't know what the answer is to the contradictions listed above, but I know what I would *like* to happen. I've seen so many patients get sick either through their ignorance of self-help, or their fear of hospitals. Then, as most of our culture believes, all they have to do is dump their health in the lap of a doctor, and a magic pill or surgery will make them healthy again. They only have to turn up, with no effort or responsibility on their part whatsoever. On top of all this, someone else will benefit from the money they've been paying into their pension, as they certainly won't be collecting it! This kind of self-destructive behaviour is spread through memes (verbal viruses), TV adverts, and schools – it's 'copying what everyone else does' syndrome.

Disease management means just that: it manages rather than cures. Before we know it, we'll not only be taking daily synthetic drugs, but we'll also need more drugs to address the disease induced by the former drugs. Then we'll have to undergo surgery to cut bits out, even having false joints and throwing out the diseased ones.

I believe that sound, scientific, objective tests and assessments are very important indeed – in fact, they're essential for severe illness and trauma. My gripe is that if we'd only known about and done all of our own preventative care, we could avoid so much unnecessary suffering, not to mention time and money. Knowledge certainly is power, but we need to learn this knowledge for ourselves, rather than relying solely on our doctors to give it to us.

At times – through no fault of our own – we will become ill. Stress exposure will destabilise us, and our natural defences will be overpowered, just like sea defences in a storm – we can end up capsizing without a paddle. I talk about this within the lifestyle key in my first book. I also go into more detail about stress in my Mind book (the first in this series), but basically put, stress can be caused by poor weather, food, bugs, work deadlines, unpleasant neighbours, bosses, family problems, relationship issues, poor sleep, grief, hard work, driving conditions, accidents, and more. If stressors turn into chronic stressors, the impact on our health mounts up: dying relatives, poor posture, financial worries, and just old age can all have a big impact. When too much stress makes the body break, allopathic medicine comes into its own, aiding survival until you get to the point where the body can heal itself again.

WHOLISTIC

Let's talk a bit more about 'wholistic' medicine, or "candles and sandals" as my colleague Jon calls it. I have both candles and sandals, not to mention all the joss sticks – should I be worried? What it really means is that we see the body as a complex system of interrelated parts, and beyond using all the normal objective assessment skills and scans, we holistic practitioners like to evaluate the body's natural ability to regulate, maintain, and fix itself. Personally, I believe in the need for good nutrition, as well as looking at detoxification and digestive processes. If the self-healing mechanisms are failing and meds are therefore needed, these have to be detoxified in the liver, and the gut may get harmed as they are digested.

So, why consider diet? Well, as echoed by the American Dr. Wallach, our bodies need 91 essential nutrients, though as they are no longer all found in the soil, these aren't all available to us in food. This is exactly like our car analogy: the car needs brake fluid, water, oil, and petrol/diesel, and if it runs out, it's breakdown cover, please. I aim for my tailor-made treatments to act as a catalyst to trigger self-healing, with the idea being that they go on long after my hands and voice have left the side of the patient.

I also believe, where able, that I need to invoke the help of the vital life force/soul/influence of the mind. Without that, when I see defeat or disbelief in a patient, the outcome is rarely good. Traditional teachings led to 5 to 10 minute doctor consultations, where patient utterances were seen as distracting. We were trained to look at and assess, rather than listening to meaningless, timewasting chitter chatter from patients telling us what was wrong with them. In the same way, some mechanics look at and take the engine apart, whereas others listen to its sounds and rumbles. If we don't start questioning this approach soon we will all be in a queue, like sheep, unquestioningly typing our symptoms into a robot that will assimilate the info and give us a diagnosis, tablet, or date for surgery, without wasting valuable human medical time and money! Wake up.

The unconscious mind is constantly attending to our health. We, as practitioners, simply tap into this source and simulate the process where able. Exercise is so needed by the body that it literally cries out for it, and the softer mind-body exercises are also incredibly important in self-awareness and healing. If you want to read more about these, I cover a little about Chi Kong, Tai Chi and Yoga in my book, *The 4 Keys To Health*. I also delve much more into the science behind exercise in this book. The body is biological and you have to stress it for the muscles and bones to strengthen!

At university, science taught me attention to detail, as well as how to measure outcomes in order to put forward a convincing argument for the truth. I developed such a deep fascination with nature, and the deeper I delved into scientific principles, the more my spiritual fascination grew. I studied lots of 'ology's'. Nothing existed unless measured by a machine. The soul was said to be a figment of my imagination and I was ridiculed to suggest that it could impact on a patient's health. I got told that the mind – our consciousness – was just a biochemical electrical phenomenon to be copied into robotic brains. Meridians and ley lines were apparently imaginary, just something that eastern quacks had polluted my mind with. The vital life force that leaves the carbon unit behind at death – that shines through the windows of the soul, our eyes – was simply labelled as an uncategorised biochemical event. Intuitive or psychic gifts were seen as insanity itself. My square peg in a round hole existence – my interest in a holistic approach at university and then when managing hospital departments – was ridiculed. So, I kept it under wraps, getting promotions and awards for expert teaching and outstanding contributions for the stuff my peers could actually understand.

When we were training to practice, we never paid much attention to wellness, only disease where we dissected the hell out of it in order to give labels to the disease process. The body was given synthetic drugs or cut up to heal. There were no other options. Body wisdom, counselling, nutrition, and emotion were all dirty words. You specialised. You were either an organ or limb person, or a mind expert. You chose to be an elbow or knee or chest specialist mechanic, and never the twain should overlap, nor should you stand on the toes of another specialist – that was *his* field, not yours. God forbid you should look at more than one of the patient's problems on the same consult, or even suggest they could be related. That brought down the accounts department to arrest you for f***ing up their monthly figures, as insurance funding and their billings are done with codes for specific parts of the body.

You can imagine what a pain in the arse I was, coming from a background of studying science and healing, teaching about peripheral pain around the world, not to mention my psychology angle. These days my husband processes the clinics' accounts ready for the accountant – he now has white hair!

The 4 Keys to Health has been a useful doorstop, coffee mat, or table leg leveller to my colleagues, as it challenges their programmed beliefs. My hope is that my Human Garage trilogy will challenge them further – if it makes it past the loo paper stage, that is…

So, let's start writing that new chapter in your life – it's time to learn some things you may not know about the body.

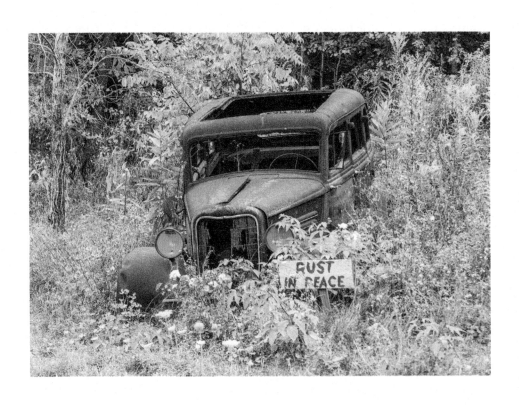

Chapter One

"You don't stop laughing when you grow old,
you grow old when you stop laughing."

– *George Bernard Shaw*

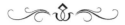

Snazzy's personal journey to healing back strain

"Everyone has a purpose in life, a unique gift or special talent to give to others. And when we blend this unique talent with service to others, we experience the ecstasy and exultation of our own spirit, which is the ultimate goal of all goals."
- Deepak Chopra

WHERE DID THE IDEA FOR THE HUMAN GARAGE COME FROM?

Snazzy's early days working in hospitals

Going back in my time machine to 1991, this was the year I made a pretty important decision: I chose to head in a new direction career-wise, going from an enthusiastic biologist studying the diversity of life to working as an unorthodox/holistic physiotherapist concentrating on human pain. In fact, it was that very word – 'unorthodox' – that would be used to introduce me over the next several years, in terms of both attending and teaching physiotherapy postgraduate courses. I found it amusing yet irritating that after so many years of international lecturing under my belt, the medical fraternity could still be so short-sighted about holistic preventative health.

So yes, I did pass the mechanics exams at the human garage workshops, and while I appreciate from the bottom of my heart my excellent NHS training in the orthodox world, I hungered to embrace a more holistic approach.

Over the years, I slowly learnt – as I shed the immaturity of youth – that I could not change the world from within the culture of hospitals, either national health or private. Back in the 90's, my enthusiasm for changing patients' lives stressed me out; I was youthful and passionately driven to make changes from within the NHS, but I was simultaneously running a hospital physio department, studying for a masters degree, writing rehab programs, and running private sports injury clinics (to help fund acupuncture training for the department). Of course, such a huge, slow-moving institution like the NHS was clearly not going to change their financial status for patient care due to the mutterings of one young lady, and unfortunately, my insanely driven passion to give the care I wanted to my patients led to a suspected heart attack, lots of daffodils, and a few days off to walk in the snow and rethink my goals! I remember being told that if I could only lose my annoying sense of humour I would be promoted, and I nearly did! (That is, lose my sense of humour – I actually did get promoted).

I hated the time constraints with patients and not being able to have any kind of relationship with them. It was like being a car mechanic, one who only takes a brief look under the bonnet before giving a quick estimate of the time it would take to fix the problem. However, there is the other side of the coin here: we give our car keys to the mechanic when we break down, handing the sole responsibility over to them in order to get the vehicle road worthy again, but without any input from ourselves whatsoever. As a driver, we need to take at least some of the responsibility: we have to drive carefully, check the tyre pressure, oil, and water, and give it the correct fuel. That is our part to play, *before* we go running to the mechanics – get my drift?

HOMEWORK:
Think back to when you last had a medical problem or an injury. Did you take any responsibility for your own recovery? Write down what you did (if anything) to help your body recover.

So, my career has suffered a few bumps in the road over the years, but on the brighter side, I liked my white jacket, stethoscope, and pager very much, and whenever I was on call overnight, I felt very important – especially when it went off, and I could rev up the car and zoom off to the hospital in the middle of the night to help someone, such as holding someone's hand as I suctioned disgusting stuff out of their lungs so they didn't drown. I felt a real sense of purpose in being part of someone's recovery, or by helping them have a less distressing death. If the Gods were on my side, and the wind blowing in the right direction, these poor souls would suffer less before passing, and the priest could go home for a nice brew.

Yes, I know; what has this got to do with physiotherapy? Those were my thoughts exactly when a patient handed me their spit in a sputum pot – the very first pot of spit I'd ever received. Well, strangely enough, respiratory medicine is part of our training in the UK, and having suffered with bronchitis in the depths of winter myself, my heart goes out to people struggling to breathe. Having had asthma all through my teens, then as a biologist studying mast cells (the cells that make histamine to cause allergic reactions) under the scanning electron microscope, I was delighted to be able to help; not being able to breathe must be one of the most terrifying experiences one can ever have. If you suffer with chest problems, pay attention to the yoga breathing mentioned later on in this book.

During those early years on call, I couldn't help but think that I should have pursued medicine, but the idea of being a GP left me cold, and I still hankered over the idea of my own healing clinics. I left my job (where I'd been promoted) early on in my career in order to manage a department, and I have mixed feelings about working in NHS hospitals. On the one hand, the learning experience was great, and the social camaraderie was incredibly fun. On the other hand, however, being a manager sucked big time, and making the strategic differences I wanted to make for the patients' care was just not possible for me. I was too little a fish in too big a tank, and I was swimming in the opposite direction. I knew I had to leave in order to grow into a bigger fish, and that I'd only come back when I might be in a better position for someone to actually listen to my ideas.

I then chose to work in a local private hospital, both in order to gain more experience in the business side before going it alone, and in order to gain experience in treatments that could only be carried out by spending more time with patients. Back in those days, the hospitals' sports injuries were looked after by a local private practice, therefore my skills in acute sports injuries were not sought after there. This being the case, and with my being on call seven days a week, I stopped my postgrad courses in manipulation and my masters in sports medicine, and I soon found I could actually concentrate more on my favourite subject – spines and pain management – without stepping on any toes. Most spine patients were getting inadequate treatment, as orthodox physios did not address back and neck pain in a holistic way; instead they ended up on long-term meds, or worse still, surgery, which could do little for chronic pain. My mother's experience still haunted me – when she'd been in pain from a bad back for so long with absolutely nothing working to alleviate that pain – and as there wasn't a masters in holistic spinal treatment, I instead decided to take a more unusual journey, one that would end up taking me abroad several times.

I still worked and studied long hours in those days – mostly seven days a week – and I knew I needed to be brave enough to leave the security blanket of working in hospitals. The long training period knocks out a lot of confidence in your own thinking, and my training period had been pretty long: I'd done three years as an undergraduate biologist studying in the hospital library, three years as a student physiotherapist, then another five in the NHS, going from Junior to Senior Physiotherapist and then on to Billy-no-mates Manager. After that I'd completed another six years as a Physio Manager in a private hospital – this was in a smaller department, enjoying the mix of being on call, treating outpatients, and visiting the ward. However, while I had more time with patients, I had no power to improve holistic patient care.

I even said I would not take a salary if they would like me to teach holistic physiotherapy with pain-relieving IMS (Intramuscular Stimulation) to all the hospital physio departments, and they said NO. So I left. I still remember putting my things in a cardboard box, knowing that I would need to demolish even more of my home to expand the practice from there. That same box actually doubled up as a chair, as my funding wasn't exactly great in the early days. I actually had movie stars and directors sit on that box, waiting for treatment, as I had a commitment at that time to treating the crew on a local film set. It's not all about the glamour if the results speak for themselves.

JUMPING WITHOUT A PARACHUTE

Then I realised that D-day had finally come: I had to go it alone. I'd already done some mental prep with June, my reiki master, and Lin from Australia – who'd taught Brandon Bays 'The Journey' – but I still had a lot of excuses about not giving up my secure job, and not destroying and converting my home into a holistic clinic, especially as there was no guarantee of an income. If I was going to do this, there would be no going back. Can you imagine my return to work interview? "Hello, I resigned to prove I could set up my own clinics with a duty of care second to none, and treatments that could cure incurable patients, but I f***ed up. Can I come back?" There were some great staff at my job, and I had become friends with a lot of them, so while they would have laughed in my face, I'm sure they would have laughed in a nice way.

Anyway, June and my friend Lin knocked every excuse out of me, talking me out of every possible thing that could go wrong. I could feel in my gut and my heart that it was the right thing to do; I just feared failure. Of course, I knew that I could do nothing more with my plans to bring alternative medicine to orthodox care where I currently was, so I bravely left to go it alone.

I left without a parachute, and the rest is history.

HOMEWORK:
Can you remember making a life-changing decision? Did you feel it was the right thing to do? Did you make the decision based on a gut feeling?

SETTING UP A HOME PRACTICE IN A BUILDING SITE

My home – which is next door to my parents – had planning rights for a medical/physio or law practice to operate from it, so I would often be treating patients in the evening when normal people would be resting. Having little in the way of finances to either buy or lease a building, and having spent a fortune on training courses and books, my only option was to make my home into a full-time practice.

It wasn't the most traditional of practices, at least to start with. For instance, if patients arrived on Sundays or early mornings, they could be treated while I was in pyjamas and slippers, or perhaps even when I was covered in painting overalls – I've done both, before you ask. My garages were completely demolished (there's still nothing there even now), and builders took a bulldozer to part of the house. It was like living in a building that had been bombed – several times over. Alan, my husband, left aerospace after 9/11 made his job untenable, and started helping with the renovation of the clinic, not to mention all the paperwork that needed doing. He did qualify in massage and Chinese medicine, but healing people is not his thing – let's just say he has a Doc Martin-type approach to treating patients.

CROMWELL WOULD TURN IN HIS GRAVE

Anyway, then followed four intensive years of treating patients from home, writing articles, and teaching internships. Then – once the bank was happy – I was able to borrow enough to renovate a beautiful and spooky local property called Cromwell House. The history books say that Cromwell's troops were fed and watered at this building whilst resting before the Battle of Hopton Heath in 1643. I would have been burnt at the stake back in those days, but luckily by the time I found the building it was the 21st Century, and I was onto Phase Two.

We worked on the new clinic at Cromwell House in the evenings, drilling and painting and sawing and carrying. I remember muttering to anyone who'd listen that when I'd said I'd wanted to build up a practice, I didn't mean with my own poor hands! We met every problem possible with this Grade 2 listed building: damaged sewers, drains, insulation, height restrictions on floors, ceilings and stairs, windows, signage, wiring, phones, computers, staff… not to mention ghosts. Yes, you read that right. Mother used to help her friend with his lighting shop in Cromwell House, and she would sell healing crystals and do reiki there (like they still do in one of its outbuildings). It was strange, because years before the place was renovated and turned into a clinic, Mum said a psychic had come into the shop and had seen a sign with my name on it hanging outside the building…

Year after year we worked on building up a reputation so we could afford the best friends/therapists available to help me. We then expanded and renovated more of the building, before going on to renovate a second clinic.

In the early days the recession had us on our knees, but we kept to our beliefs and values, rebuilding and following the original plan of a private, one-on-one, healing environment for people not only to recover from an injury, but also to discover a journey to a healthier, happier, and more purposeful life. We were bullied to accept contracts to give short sessions for patients without hands-on treatment or technology for little money. However, we did not succumb to poor quality driven treatment, instead putting our prices up and giving more specialist treatments, swimming against the tide and watching helplessly as other clinics succumbed to insurance blackmail, consequently letting their patients down, hitting the wall, and closing.

Patients intuitively feel the care you offer, and are driven to tell others how quickly they are fixed. Patients, therefore, are your strongest marketers. Changing lives and health care for the better is one hell of a purposeful life, hence the analogy of a body being taken to a garage for an MOT with a careless driver, compared to the car being driven with an informed and careful owner/driver. There's a big difference.

This first chapter is very personal to me, and I'll also be weaving in treatment modalities for my back pain throughout.

IT'S ALL ABOUT HOW YOU FALL FROM GRACE

"The trees in the storm don't try to stand up straight and tall and erect. They allow themselves to bend and be blown with the wind. They understand the power of letting go. Those trees and those branches that try too hard to stand up strong and straight are the ones that break."
- Julia Butterfly Hill

Yes, it's all about how you fall from grace – or rather, in my case, from a gate. It was early one summer's morning in 2015, close to the Yorkshire Dales, when outside my new northern practice, I took a tumble. It was just like any other morning when we'd hurtled up the motorway to arrive, sleep deprived and hungry, at my newest clinic. My daily energy boost lay dormant in my muddy trainers, and after running full tilt across the fields, I came across a locked gate. I nimbly climbed over, then – just as I was putting a foot onto a wet, slippery gate bar – I found myself flying off. It was a rather muddy, gritty, and ungraceful landing to say the least. I felt alright really, but my scheming back had other ideas about my clumsiness, not to mention my overwhelming workload.

SNAZZY'S BACK HEALING JOURNEY IN THE HUMAN GARAGE

A slow, insidious inflammation bubbled away in a bruised, swollen disc, closing the gate on a facet joint hinge that made my running shoes seem so incredibly far away from my hands. Over the summer, in the mornings a slow, creeping stiffness would start to take root in my lower spine first thing, and although I found that getting out of bed and getting dressed were starting to become irritating, I ignored it. Soon, the initial mild tightness began to develop into tearing sensations – the sort of feelings you get when a wound heals over with a scab and you have to move it. The cats had breakfast tipped into their bowls from a height, which sometimes worked and sometimes didn't – occasionally they ended up wearing their food as a hat, the chunks dripping down over their ears.

I carried my running shoes around like a child, wondering when I could get them on again, my mind ruminating on what ifs – I'm sure you know what I mean. Stupid, unhelpful, worrying ideas about potential future events that may or may not happen. It's interesting that humans do this, while animals don't; can you imagine a tiger thinking, 'I'm not sure if I can be bothered to go hunting today… I might not find any prey, I could break a leg, and I might get thirsty…'?

Then, one morning last summer, I really could not straighten up for ten long minutes. I immediately started to panic, my monkey brain winning and completely terrifying the life out of me. It chattered away frantically in my ear: 'that's done it now – you're finished. You can't work on patients anymore!' Of course, the logical part of my mind said: 'everyone injures their back at some point in their lives. Come on, Snaz, you know what to do and what to think – you know how to treat your back and how to fix it.' I just had to ignore my monkey brain.

FOUR RED KEYS

So, ignoring the monkey brain, my super logical neocortex said: 'let's revisit *The 4 Keys* – colours please for mind, lifestyle, food and drink, and fitness.' Now let's look at the scores on the doors... Guess who had been burning it at both ends (and in the middle)? And, due to unforeseen complications with business and work commitments, my lifestyle balance was – as usual – arse about face, and tipped on its head. Here's how my scores looked:

FITNESS KEY: Well, my mix of running, cycling, swimming and pilates had been mostly replaced with a summer of twice daily 2 to 3 mile sprints a day, on hard-surfaced roads.

FOOD AND DRINK: Yes to both. Due to working between clinics over a hundred miles apart, meals were disrupted, containing more sugar and less water. The body – and especially the spine – hates dehydration.

MINDSET: I drove my body like the car – it was thrust into gear and raced up and down motorways in bad weather, being forced to cope with too many long journeys between clinics. My body was showing signs of wear and tear, and the mind was ignoring it completely in order to achieve my urgent short-term goals. Exhaustion was ignored and the body hit back. Literally, BACK.

LIFESTYLE: Working in different parts of the country was stealing my friends and family time, as well as my beloved writing time. On top of all this, sitting in cars instead of sleeping or exercising in a healthy way was irritating the hell out of my joints.

WHAT DID THE KEYS MEAN TO ME?

I meditated on my body's wisdom, pondering what was it telling me about my red keys. It was like Groundhog Day – every morning I would reach for my trainers to go running, and every day I was met with a searing tightness in my back, restricting any chance I had of getting anywhere near my feet and making my head spin. My running was my stress-buster; every time exhaustion bit, I would run and come back refreshed and energised. The addictive high it gave me was a small price to pay for a small nagging doubt in the back of my mind that running such a lot on hard surfaces was bound to catch up with me at some point. This new experience of having a stiff back gave me a sickening feeling of vulnerability, and echoing in my head were my patients' voices saying, "You call yourself a back expert, and yet you have a bad back first thing in the morning? What have you got to say for yourself?"

My knowledge of spines and the 4 keys meant that I was able to prevent it from getting any worse, and I also managed to do this without missing even one day of clinics. I decided to use the incident as a blessing, and write about my own experience and treatments in a very open, honest way. It felt as if the universe had sent me the experience of being both a healer and patient just at the time I was writing the body volume, my hope being to connect with a larger audience in order to share my experience from both perspectives.

SNAZZY'S SPINAL HEALING JOURNEY STARTED WITH MRI

I went to diagnostics, lying down in a brand new MRI (Magnetic Resonance Imaging) machine to get my back scanned, so I could see which components were wearing out. As I lay there, I felt the fear of 'what ifs' again. What if the scans showed an imminent disaster that's about to stop me from creating clinics and treating patients and doing all the activities I love? What if I can't fix myself? What if something's really wrong? Such a cascade of vulnerable thoughts! Where was my faith? Part of the ritual of being scanned is to wear a white gown – one that exposes nearly everything – and in this instance, I frightened a little old man who had just arrived for a brain scan.

A week later, my MRI disc and letter arrived, and it felt more than a little strange looking at pictures deep inside my own body. There was good news on the whole: no cancer, no badly protruding disc, nothing serious at all. It seemed, however, that my cushioning disc at the base of my spine had left its cushioning days behind it, and was now a toughened old biscuit, slightly bulging towards my nerves while the disc above headed this way with a slightly bigger bulge. The facet joints were starting to show some rot, and the bone at the base of my spine showed endplate changes to the repeated shockwaves of running and walking and lifting patients, not to mention being bent over a treatment couch for a quarter of a century.

Looking at the images, I knew I was not to do so much road running in my future years – it was cushioning soled trainers I needed, and more old lady swimming, though I actually swim very fast and may return to sub-aqua, so there's at least some saving grace to growing old disgracefully and unconventionally.

Being out of the NHS and its slow cogwheels of change, I was now in a position to be able to experience first-hand my armoury of preventative health treatments. Being involved in bringing magnetic resonance (MRT/MBST) to the UK, my preventative, anti-aging MRT clinics help to regenerate grades one, two, and three (though not four) osteoarthritis, as well as torn or degenerate discs, plus helping thinning bones and worn tendons and muscles. Naturally, this was my first pit stop for Snazzy's spinal repair, to firstly repair the discs in order to avoid nerve irritation, and then to slow down the aging process of the old, already worn back. Thirty years of a flexed posture over patients is not a good thing for a spine.

Then followed nine hour-long sessions of disc MRT, squashed into my previous running times, whilst I constantly wrestled with finding the time to do it. I lay in the silent MRT machine whilst I proofread my Mind book, telling myself that being a patient was just temporary. I found that the soft, silent energy waves made me feel tired and emotional, but I told myself off for being maudlin, and instead instructed my conscious brain to get excited at the fact I could experiment on myself yet again in order to help others.

This clever MRT lessened the intensity of the pain and stiffness straight away, but the symptoms still persisted, though in a much less intense way than before. Of course, I expected a slow response, as I knew it would take many weeks for the tissue to heal. My first priority – the disc damage – was being addressed, plus the numbness and ache from the nerves. I still needed to feel my left foot for safety when going up or down stairs, and the rumbling discomfort was due to irritated facet joints and vertebrae, which I would later follow up with bone treatment.

MY GERMAN TIME MACHINE

I knew from my biology days that regenerating cartilage cells needed a good three months, especially when combined with the degenerative aging beneath the injury, and my mind flew back to Germany, when on one wet autumn day, the MRT scientists were explaining how it all worked. My husband and I were there, plus our surgeon and friend, Mr. Kathuria. To help explain this, you can imagine that every time a cell divides, it would ideally like an identical version of itself, and if we are in optimum health – well-hydrated, nutrient rich, with fewer toxins, viruses, and stress hormones within our bodies – this is much more likely to happen.

However, the reality is that cellular aging and natural rot is due to a poor photocopy of the original, with it becoming a little more faded as the years and replications go on. The healthier our lifestyle and the environment our cells are bathed in, the healthier and more youthful our experience. The science evolving from MRI (Magnetic Resonance Imaging) looks at how cells respond to electromagnetic fields, as well as measuring cell membrane potentials as a guide to physical changes happening from energy medicine, as opposed to biochemical triggers. This research fascinates me, hence my involvement.

SNAZZY SOFT SHOES

Anyway, back to Snazzy's next step of the recovery program. In the short-term, I swapped running so much for intensive, fast swimming and cycling like an old lady… though just for now, you understand. I swapped my trainers for softer soled ones – MBT (masai barefoot technology) – that my back loves and my biomechanical expert friends cringe at. I did make a note that I needed an update on my running style, and once my back was healing, I went and played on the Gaitscan analysis toys – more about this when I get to it. Then, to help with the discomfort and joint flexibility, over the next week or two I booked some physio and needling treatments with my friends.

HOMEWORK:
What plan do you have to prevent a painful back?

NEEDLES AND PINS IN MY BACK

I booked in the first couple of sessions with my experienced colleague to apply my clinics' combined approach of physio, acupuncture, and IMS dry needling – the latter taught by Snaz. As the needles plunged into my tight muscles, I experienced a cascade of different emotions in both body and mind; I felt deep vulnerability and fear at my own mortality. I also felt scared about how much I'd relied on a healthy physical body to be the vehicle in which to carry out my life's purpose. On top of all this, however, I felt proud that I had played a key part in honing the precision needed to locate and release the suffocating muscle contractures trapping the discs, joints, and nerves within their webbed, leathery strands.

As the fine needle tips teased away the tethered bands with surgical precision, the nerves sang messages to each other, calling to networks further away, and I felt warmth and feeling slowly returning to my feet. I was the observer within, witnessing my conscious and subconscious dance together as one, as both the physical flesh and energy matrix were manipulated by the healer within the mechanic. It was as if several switches were being flicked off and on in my autonomic nervous system, jump starting the relay circuits and relaying information back and forth between my mind and my body.

My monkey brain decided there was no danger in the treatment, my reptilian brain modulated the physiological responses, and my human mind decided on suffering and healing strategies. Like an orchestra of responses, the conductor within my brain controlled my breathing, heart rate, blood pressure, and flow, as well as my inflammatory and cellular repair process-es, rhythmically creating a crescendo of response – the snazzy treatment response overture. The watcher within is my conductor, and I felt a very strong sense of knowing that the treatment was being expertly adminis-tered, an innate body wisdom of felt sense.

I have often said to my patients that they should know if the treatment was right for them or not, and I was reminded of this as I went through mine. I always tell them to feel the way the treatment resonated with them, and to go within and feel the body's wisdom. After all my years of teaching, of being a guinea pig so practitioners could practice the art of needling on my body, now *I* was the patient. I could gauge the skills of doctors and physios, articulating pretend injuries in my body – this was a whole new arena. Hav-ing a real injury is a very powerful insight into a therapist's skill.

HOMEWORK:
What is it that you feel emotionally when you have treatment?

VANCOUVER GUNN CLINIC

The needling aroused a flashback to my very first visit to Professor Gunn's teaching clinic in Vancouver. A long flight on my own with an eight-hour time difference was a good excuse for me upsetting the passport security of-ficer when I got there. "Reason for visit?" muttered the officious officer, and guess what I said? That's right: "To study at the Gunn clinic." There followed a very unnerving few minutes of explaining that there were no rifles in-volved in the treatment, just painful needles inside plungers. No guns at all.

Vancouver was exciting and mostly safe, friendly, and full of health-conscious fit people keen on skiing in the mountains and exercising in Stanley Park by the waterfront. Half of the city's population was Chinese, which reminded me of my visit to the east, although my visits were more to further my instructor training than to do any sightseeing. The teaching clinic was located in a base-ment in central Vancouver, and it was here that I watched the masters' hands weave and pluck, teasing out painful muscle contractures in patients. There followed four more trips to empower my teaching skills, and to share this art in the UK – which I will no doubt ruminate on later in the book.

Let's get back in my time machine now to 2015, to address my diet key. Raised acidity would not help the inflammation in my back, so it was off to the farm shop to fill the kitchen with all the food I wrote about in *The Four Keys* (and that I discuss later in this book). I did this so I would be able to eat healthily at home, as it is so difficult travelling between clinics and eat-ing out all the time; it's not easy or practical to transport fresh food up and down the motorways without going limp – the food, that is.

Tonight, as I write this, it is the day after my birthday. The actual day was spent with patients, cards, flowers, and hugs, and was very special, although sadly all of the birthday weekend celebrations were postponed due to Alan getting a head cold. Illness needs warm, partly digested food (by cooking according to the Tao way of healthy eating), so, as I write this I am dashing back and forth to nurture a huge pot of homemade veggie soup, fresh bread and butter, plus jugs of veggie and berry juices. The fluids and nutrients will help with Grumpy's healing process (as well as my irritated back) and increasing his supplement levels of minerals and vitamins, omega oils, and hormone D3 with Vitamin C and Zinc will bolster his immune system.

LIFESTYLE KEY

I am spoilt with a lovely local spa to ease these dark UK skies that some-times make outside activities so uninspiring. 'If only time allowed' is my theme tune. When I am home and working from my Wolseley Clinic, there is a local health spa, set in what was once an old stately home. Over this last summer, however – with the project going ahead in Yorkshire – I told myself that I had no time to visit, no time to spend at the lovely big pool and pretty grounds, no time to give my body the correct mix of exercise relaxation. So in part, I am reaping what I sowed, with lots of impact-laden frantic running in cold, wet, and icy conditions. Feeling guilty about that, there will be no impact for my irritated bones today; I am off shortly to swim and cycle through red and yellow leafed woods, on a wonderful October morning. Delightful.

I *was* writing this paragraph with good posture on my fit ball – and I'm using the past tense here as Lara my cat just burst it. I knew the postures I had standing and sitting would affect my back recovery, so I prescribed myself my back exercises (again described later in this book), avoiding overstretching as I focused on gentle core and lateral stability workouts using a mixture of pilates and yoga moves that keep the lumbar spine rigid – much more about this later in the book. The daily breathing and stomach workout is essential to do with the lumbar spine static, and no inappropriate sit-ups that can stress discs.

The cats will no doubt claw the next ball too, which is still in its cardboard box and currently being sat on by them. Hence I am not sure of its shelf time, though it is probably a lot less than mine – or maybe not should it be clawed and explode, causing me to hit my head. Should this happen I apologise now for any deterioration in the quality of future writing.

As you can see, I am taking lots of little steps in different key areas in my lifestyle in order to heal the injury. Get my drift? I am not simply relying on a practitioner or machine to cure me, and you shouldn't either.

So what else am I doing?

THE HUMAN TOUCH

I met with my dear old friend Ken, June's buddy and a fascinating psychic. (As a side note, I just want to thank him for writing the foreword to my Mind book). When I spoke to him he asked, "What's the problem? You've been a secret healer since you were born; believe you can heal yourself and you will." He was very matter of fact about it, a case of 'that's sorted, now move on'. Unfortunately, I can't say it's ever been that easy to heal yourself.

So, in an attempt to tune into my self-healing reiki skills, I booked a relaxing massage and reiki session with my friend and practice manager. It's a big frustrating weakness of mine that I do not carry out enough meditation and self-healing sessions, especially as it's been seven months now since my friend June died. It was during my reiki session that it came to me: sharing my deeply personal experiences and vulnerability may actually help my patients and therapists find their voice, and I had a strong sense that my current back issue would wrap itself up with the final chapter to this book. I will be writing in-depth about my healing/shamanic and reiki training in my Soul book.

It's during healing sessions that you become aware of your fears, and how you talk to yourself about them. Being qualified in NLP (neurolinguistics programming) I knew the importance of the language I used when describing my back problem, and it's so stupid that I didn't apply it deeply enough. Instead, I let my fearful thoughts open the door to doubt, with hope being the main course on the menu. That's right, monkey brain, chomp chomp chomp – eat away at hope.

HEALING JOURNEY MAP

Now, how did I map out my healing journey? First of all I pulled out a notebook and scribbled some thoughts down. I had to reduce my stress hormones – which means looking at my lifestyle – and I knew I could still eat and drink better. Then I needed to get my mind-set into a state of, 'my back problem will resolve itself and I must see this experience as a gift'. Finally – and most importantly – I had to decide which treatments I still needed, and when and in what order I needed to have them.

This complex dilemma always smacks me in the face with each and every patient. The NHS is not geared up to fund these treatment pathways, and my clinics do not receive government funding as yet, so patients need to pay something towards the team's wages and the equipment they have to use. Of course, each and every one of us would like a quick, inexpensive, painless fix, and if this is not possible, there is a feeling of helplessness in the air – and at times, panic. It is only sensible to seek out long-term painkillers and surgery when good treatment and time cannot heal you.

Now, let me share with you my thoughts and experience regarding my back, and please remember that everyone's back is different. My vertebra and tiny facet joints were showing signs of wear and irritation, and the discs small bulges. That tells me that any manipulation needed to be gentle, not vigorous, for there was nothing out of alignment; it was just sore, with the inflammation causing stiffness.

With that, I wrote down some more notes for my preventative treatment plan.

WHAT KIND OF SOFT TISSUE MANIPULATION DO I NEED, AND WHO IS BEST TO DO IT?

So, did I seek out osteopaths, chiropractors, and/or manipulative spinal physiotherapists? This is such a vast subject that I cannot do it justice within this book. However, I will share my experiences with you.

When a joint is said to be out of line – which may be a birth defect or may be due to a biomechanical reason, such as years spent walking on a longer leg or a foot turned in or out (Goften & Trueman, 1971) – it could be down to trauma or a sudden lift or turn. It could also be due to repetitive actions, where a joint is always turned and loaded in a certain way (Schamberger, 2002). It could be poor posture (Key, 2007; Vleming et al., 2007) or it could be tight muscle contractures (Gunn, Simons & Travell, 1999). You have to play detective a bit here – go back in your time machine and work out why the joint is deemed to be out of alignment and in need of adjustment.

Personally, I have flat feet and one leg a little longer than the other, so I'm far from a perfect example of biomechanics! The way I walk and run on hard surfaces impacts my spine, and I discuss my biomechanics assessment later in the book.

In 1962, Carl McConnell – an influential osteopath of his time – wrote the following in his book, *Osteopathic Institute of Applied Technique Yearbook 1962*. I really liked what Carl said, and so did a man called Leon, who quoted it in his book on modern neuromuscular techniques (Chaitow, 2011):

"Osseous (bony) malalignment is sustained by ligamentous rigidity. This rigidity is incepted by muscular fascial and tendinous tensions and stresses. Every case portrays a uniqueness in accordance with location, architectural plan and laws, tissue texture, regional and strength ratios, resident properties, environmental settings, resolution of forces etc. Remember I am speaking of the solid biological background of individual pathogenesis, the veritable soil of prediseased conditions. The lack of either sufficient, or efficient, soft tissue work, is one reason for the mediocre technique and recurrence of lesions. The same is evident in the correction of postural defects."
- Carl McConnell

Loosely translated, in essence this means that there are many reasons why a joint might need help, and that there are many ways to achieve this through experience. Many physical therapists blend their manipulative skills with soft tissue work, and a current trend in soft tissue work is the neuromuscular technique (NMT) from America, which is now being taught in Europe. Its roots are shared within different disciplines, with the main pioneers being Lief and Chaitow in Osteopathy, Nimmo in Chiropractic therapy, and myofascial pain experts Travell and Simons – all of whom are referred to by physios.

NMT does not use technology; rather, it uses human touch – the fingers – to rub the body in specific places, using a certain degree of pressure and repetition. It is useful prior to manipulation, though it may relax a trigger point if not deep seated (though personally, I still believe needling is needed as well). It helps with circulation and drainage as well as elasticity, and it works towards restoring a more normal fibrotic, tight, muscular tissue. Additional manual methods to NMT include massage, muscle energy technique (MET), positional release technique (PRT), myofascial technique (MRT) and many variations of these soft tissue manipulations. There isn't enough space in this book to go into all of these in too much detail, but these techniques are superb in the hands of my gifted sports therapist and physios.

Clinical work in India – carried out by orthopaedic surgeons themselves working in rehabilitation with recent post-op hip or knee replacements – demonstrated the value of slowly applied isotonic-eccentric stretching in such cases, thus reducing fibrosis and speeding up the recovery, when compared with traditional passive stretching methods (Parmer, 2011). I remember working flat out for weeks on a delightful patient in a local hospital. The patient had had two false knees, and sadly, his body had formed a bucketload of scar tissue post-op. He had come to see me some weeks later, and we battled against it together, but to no avail. The problem was that the tissue was no longer elastic, and there was no way I could have called in one of the surgeons that works for me and asked if he could massage my patient – it just doesn't happen in England.

Anyway, let's get *back* to me – pardon the pun. I had several treatments that embraced a combination of approaches: muscle energy releases to relax the muscles around my sacroiliac joints, gentle cyriax mobilisation techniques – which helped with flexibility – and one manual traction that my back didn't like at all. I also practised postural low-grade McKenzie movements when standing, as prone lying was embarrassing when I had to crawl to my next patient (as I couldn't stand up quickly afterwards).

I LIKE MASSAGE – WHEN SHOULD I SCHEDULE IT IN?

I like massage. However, after hurting my back, relaxing on my front made me very uncomfortable, so being aware of the best posture to massage in is very important when it comes to backs.

I want to just pause here to discuss soft tissue, and what fascia actually is – this wonderful bubble wrap of energy lines where acupuncture does its miracles. This elegantly phrased quote, from a research article by Weppler & Magnusson, summarises this point brilliantly: "Skeletal muscles comprise contractile tissue intricately woven together by fibrous connective tissue that gradually blends into tendons... made of fibrous connective tissue that attach the muscle to bone. Although contractile tissue and tendons are sometimes evaluated separately for research purposes, they cannot be separated during routine clinical testing and stretching procedures, nor during functional activity" (Weppler & Magnusson, 2010). Nor, of course, during manual treatment.

Now, here's a rather nice excuse for regular massages after you've strained yourself. Mechanotransduction research describes the many ways in which cell behaviour changes as they respond to different degrees of load, such as pressure, tension, stretch, friction, etc. Research looked at fascial cells (fibroblasts) that are responsible for the early stages of healing traumatised tissues, as well as reducing inflammation. Research has shown that when these cells have been distressed by many hours of rapid movement, they start producing inflammatory chemicals. A brief period (for instance, a minute to 90 seconds) during which the cells are "treated" with the equivalent of myofascial release (MFR) or positional release (strain/counterstrain, or SCS) normalises them (Standley & Meltzer, 2008). This would also explain why folks say that massage is nice but that it's only a temporary pleasure, because if they continue with the activities that traumatise their cells, they will start to ache again.

A few years ago, just after the 9/11 disaster when problems hit aerospace, my husband left behind his career of running aerospace companies to help with the business side of my life-long dream: to have homely, comfortable clinics where folks could come to be healed. He decided to qualify in massage and Chinese medicine, briefly teaching patients before returning to a non-healing role of accounting, as well as managing all those tedious tasks that are vital in enabling clinics to function. Anyway, for a couple of weeks he decided to break all communications with the world so he could spend the time immersed in giving and receiving massage from a renowned expert, Mr Raynor, and buying entirely into the whole alternative health world – quite a change for a scientific doctor. Sadly, I only received one of these massages from him. This could be because I ended up swearing at him – the massage was much stronger than I expected, and that was that!

Brandon Raynor is a tall, strong man who teaches deep tissue massage. I went to visit him on their exam day, and his hands felt like they could crush my body in an instant. I understand that Raynor Naturopathic Massage is a holistic system of bodywork developed by Naturopath, Brandon Raynor. Its origins are in Ayurvedic massage, Chinese medicine, Lomi Lomi, reflexology, shiatsu, and yoga breathing work. I had some experience in massage within my physiotherapy and shiatsu training, so I felt I could easily grasp his approach. Brandon embraced the eastern theory that the physical body is a gross manifestation of a subtle body, composed of a life force (chi or prana), emotions, and other subtle energies, and that each are related and have an effect on each other. He discussed that physical or emotional stressors can lead to a blockage or disruption in the flow of chi or prana, and that this can cause bones to shift out of place or create tension in the body.

Bands in the body that are composed of muscles, tendons, ligaments, and other body tissues can also increase in tension with emotion, and underlying all of these physical manifestations of the bands are subtle energy systems similar to meridians in Chinese medicine, sen lines in Thai massage, or nadis in Ayurvedic massage. The knowledge and techniques gleaned from these ancient modalities were then integrated and evolved to form the Raynor Band Theory, which – along with its unique set of techniques, adjustments, stretches, and rhythm – suggest that its physical manifestation can be traced. The goal of this is to relieve a person of residual tension/ muscle tightness in a particular area of the body when it is at rest, before returning the body to its natural state of relaxation. I remember that whatever Alan learnt on that course, it took him a long time to wipe the smile off his face!

There are so many types of massage: aromatherapy, Swedish, sport and deep tissue… the list goes on. I remember experiencing aromatherapy and stone massages thanks to a delightful lady called Genevieve – sadly no longer living – who used to be my receptionist at my home practice before going on to learn all about the wonderfully relaxing and smelly massage. Aromatherapy has all sorts of soothing oils to help with ailments and is a really great way to relax. I describe the uses for some of these oils in my *4 Keys* book, though it is a vast subject that could fill several volumes. While it is a nice stress-buster, it will not alter fascial problems.

WHY AM I LESS BENDY?

The fascia's *sliding and gliding fascial functions* between muscles – or the separating of dense fascial structures from muscle or from other fascial layers – contain viscous loose connective tissues that allow a gliding, sliding function, protecting sensitive neural structures as well as facilitating pain-free, efficient movement and force transmission. This gliding function may be lost because of trauma, inflammation, or the natural process of aging, resulting in fibrosis and thickening (Pavan et al., 2014).

Talking to my in-house soft tissue experts, they tell me that massage is a good preventative treatment to have regularly, especially if you're constantly physically stressing your body. Andy, my experienced sports therapist, explained to me how there were train tracks of fascial tissue all linking our body parts together, and it immediately reminded me of tights; pulling them up too tight can make your toes move. The body moves in such complex ways.

He did some gentle release work on my thoracolumbar fascia (the spine between the neck and the bottom), and gave me some references for me to read up on. For example, Carvalhais and colleagues (2013) demonstrated how the contraction of latissimus dorsi – when you pull your shoulder blades together – turns the opposite hip outwards via the superficial layer of the thoracolumbar (spinal) fascia. Also, Stecco et al. (2013) showed how gluteus maximus (bottom) contractions directly influence the knee via a tight band on the outside of the thigh called the iliotibial band. Potentially, therefore, left-knee dysfunction could involve right latissimus dorsi behaviour. Awareness of such links come to light in the hands of experts.

Bearing all this in mind, I then went to see David in my clinic, which is good as it meant I didn't have to go far. He is a very experienced physiotherapist who uses a lot of soft tissue techniques, and he also worked on my iliosacral (pelvic) joints with muscle energy techniques (MET). He would ask me to push hard against myself, then in that reflex moment of relaxation, trick the muscles into stretching further than they normally would do in order to stretch out stiffened joints. It certainly helped, though I might add – it's not the most graceful of positions!

David had me reaching down in my Bridget Jones knickers to see how my pelvis moved with my spine – this would tell him which manipulations to use in order to correct malalignments. The pelvis comprises of two iliac bones linked at the back by a triangular sacrum that once had a tail growing from the coccyx. The 'reaching forward towards my toes' test is indicative of the *il-io-sacral* (pelvic bone moving on sacral bone) motion, while the 'seated bending forward' test is indicative of the *sacro-iliac* (sacral bone moving on iliac bone) motion. A positive test –meaning a movement dysfunction – is determined by the asymmetrical excursion of one posterior superior iliac spine (PSIS –a bony landmark on the iliac pelvic bone) whilst bending forward, the positive side travelling further and more superior (higher) than the other side. The explanation for this behaviour is that as the sacrum nutates (flexes, turns forwards) with lumbar spine forward bending (flexion), the fixed iliac crest of your pelvis is carried with it and draws the PSIS more cephalad (towards your head) than the uninvolved side. This means a certain type of manipulation is used. These tests are not this simple, and are in fact very controversial, with lots of research arguing that black is white and vice versa.

David looked serious, and after getting me to bend up and down in my Bridget Jones knickers, he assured me I was moving much better after having had the MET. I knew one sacroiliac joint used to be stiffer than the other from going on courses, as well as the fact that I had small scoliotic curves in my spine and a slight leg length discrepancy. Asymmetries in lumbo-pelvic rhythm, leg length, scoliosis, hip flexion, sacroiliac joint anatomy, hamstring, piriformis, and quadratus lumborum muscle length must also have a profound effect on pelvic symmetry during forward bending. Our bodies become walking books of clinical adjustments – it's all part of the job!

The growth in popularity of osteopathic muscle energy technique (MET) over the last two decades – with everyone from osteopaths and medical practitioners to physiotherapists, chiropractors, and remedial therapists – is likely a testament to its clinical efficacy. These techniques were originally devised and described by Fred Mitchell Sr. in the 1940s and 1950s, with the first technique being manually published in 1979 (Fryer, 2000). The explanation for the therapeutic action of MET in spinal dysfunction that has gained the widest currency is that of the shortened monoarticular muscles – which restrict joint motion – being stretched. I still find that Gunn IMS does this better, just perhaps a bit more painfully.

Myofascial unwinding is the movement-facilitation aspect of the myofascial-release techniques (MRT) and it is a more holistic approach that embraces the subconscious influence. In fact, Barnes – a myofascial release expert – believes that the mind-body's ability to self-correct via myofascial unwinding has been around since the beginning of mankind (Barnes, 2007). Arthur Koestler's book *The Ghost in the Machine* discusses how science considers terms like 'consciousness' and 'mind' to be unscientific, even stating that they are treated as dirty words. Furthermore, Albert Einstein speculated that rational science reveals only the external appearances of some deeper reality.

Barnes believed that "myofascial release allows us, now, to deal with that deeper reality. Traditional therapy missed a key component for lasting effectiveness, the treatment of the myofascial system – the conduit of consciousness" (Barnes, 2007).

The subconscious tightens against the unresolved trauma like a broken record that plays all day and all night. It doesn't matter how intelligent you are, how strong you are, or how hard you're trying to get better – it is not on the conscious level. This is extremely evident with my car crash victims. It is so very difficult as a therapist to find objective markers to account for so much anger and pain, and ignoring the subconscious' 'bracing patterns' has thwarted health care's ability to help people truly heal. It is very difficult writing up medicolegal reports with these subconscious issues swirling through fascial tissue. Medicolegal reports are to help determine the compensation that should be paid out for injury claims. The report asks questions about range of motion, nerve involvement, perceived pain, and function, as well as any obvious psychological problems. As pain is felt and not seen, the latter is so hard to measure.

The mind-body brake on healing will stop when all of the information from the past trauma – which has been buried in the subconscious, as well as in tissue memory – billows forth in the form of sensations, pictures, emotions, and memories. As this sensory information enters the conscious mind, the tightness from the bracing patterns softens and the healing can commence. Now that these repressed tissue memories have been retrieved, the subconscious releases its iron grip on the structures so that structural work will now be successful and lasting. The subconscious rules!

I remember very vividly one chap who had smashed his pelvis up in a car crash. Months later, after the bones had healed, his pain was worse than ever, and it took several sessions to get to that healing point. He had received MRT to accelerate and strengthen the bone healing, physiotherapy, and then Gunn IMS. His physical signs were good –walking well without crutches, having a full range of movement, and his strength returning – so I decided to use reiki on him. Low and behold, that morning he said to me, "I feel a grid of light, a criss-cross grid spreading throughout my body. I'm changing back to me, to the person I was before the accident." And that he did; the pain eased to a small niggle, and he got a new job as well. I ponder on what my body is hiding from me with my recent back problem; if June was still alive she would know.

I play special, relaxing music to get both patient and therapist into the alpha state of healing – the 'hypnagogic' state of consciousness just before you go to sleep or wake up, when you are daydreaming. I like my therapists and clients to achieve this healing zone so that they can both heal and enhance the quality of their lives. During this state, patients may experience the flashback phenomena, or they may experience therapeutic pain or fear. This is a memory, and I need them to be in a safe place in order to feel this. It is the lack of expression of tissue memory that perpetuates the holding patterns that inhibit our ability to heal.

Tentatively, science agrees that there is the possibility of a memory trace on the molecular cellular synaptic level. We know that we have the involvement of the amygdala (our chattering monkey brain) and the hippocampus (the library) of the limbic-hypothalamic system in processing. In my Mind book I talked about memory a lot, discussing encoding, and explaining that the recall of the specific memory trace may be located in many different places in the brain.

Now, this really interested me: when reading up on John Barnes' massage techniques, I found that he talked about the physical position the patient was in when they experienced the trauma. I had seen a lot of muscle tensions related to feet being slammed down on brakes on impact, hands gripping the steering wheel, necks rotated on impact and so on. However, thinking about this in more depth, if – as Barnes suggested – the position the person is in at the moment of trauma is encoded into their body, then of course it will adapt and develop strategies to protect itself from further trauma. The fearful memories make the body avoid those specific three-dimensional positions – for instance, my patients who fear bending over. They avoid it as much as possible, due to the fact that their back 'went' when they happened to be bent over. The emotions communicate this mind-body information through its network by way of juices called neuropeptides. Then, we get the crazy dance: the vicious interplay among the endocrine (hormone), neuro-peptides, immune, and autonomic neuromyofascial systems.

If this hormone dance continues too long, during therapy sessions the person can get stuck at the traffic lights – with their foot on the brake – and healing ends up not taking place, unless they have a very skilled practitioner. This unloading of the structure into therapists' hands allows the body's righting reflexes and protective responses to suspend their in-fluences. I can't tell you the number of times I've had patients say, "I can't get off the couch," before – to their absolute amazement – doing that exact thing. A delightful Russian doctor – who used to be my patient, along with her mother – recently came to see me. Her mother had been dancing in the square in Moscow, despite the fact that she previously said she couldn't walk or dance. Once the body and mind feel safe enough, the body can then move into positions that allow these position-dependent physiologic flashback phenomena to reoccur, fading and freeing up the body's tensions. Pain no longer haunts these positions.

WHAT ABOUT GETTING MY SPINE MANIPULATED?

Spinal manipulation often frightens people, as they imagine bones cracking and splintering. It is a therapeutic intervention performed on spinal articulations which are synovial joints. There are many little spinal joints, z-joints, the atlanto-occipital, atlanto-axial, lumbosacral, sacroiliac, costotransverse, and costovertebral joints. National guidelines (NICE) come to different conclusions about spinal manipulation over the years – not recommending it, saying it is optional, or recommending a short course for those who do not improve with other treatments first. NICE 2016 have put it back into physiotherapy guidelines for spines.

It is now seven months since my first episode of a persistent stiff back, and it doesn't really trouble me unless I've been laid out on the sofa or sleeping in bed – then it can take half an hour or more for me to get to the point where I can bend over again. It's very frustrating. I asked Dave – a member of my team and a senior physiotherapist – to manipulate my back, as it had been some time since he'd treated me. He IMS'd (dry needled) the right side of my spine, like I had taught him – the symptom-free side that was locked up – and I felt a twinge as he manipulated the needle into tight muscles and fascia at the lumbar 4/5 level (which is the disc second up from the base on the right). It was a brief, deep ache. Then David used a Cyriax (this is described later on) manipulation, where I lay on my spine and he rotated me to realign the lumbar facet joints. There was a satisfying click, click, clunk, then for the first time in a while, my more flexible joints could flex and extend further. It is important to retest movement after treatment, and chronic inflammation always causes the joints to stiffen. I will discuss what manipulative training physiotherapists learn later on in this chapter.

ELECTROTHERAPY

Just as a quick aside, I had some laser and ultrasound with my physiotherapy sessions, and both of these treatments are described in detail in the appendix.

CLUNK CLICK EVERY TRIP

I remember interviewing a chiropractor for my clinic, and part of that interview included a manipulation. It was very clever, accurate, and frightening all at once, like a rocket going off in my upper back. At that time, a dull ache in my upper back lingered for about three weeks before it was calling for another adjustment.

I liked her and was impressed by the knowledge she had, but she wanted four patients in the same room, with just 15 minutes per session, and a crèche in the same room – this didn't exactly fit in with my healing and counselling philosophy for the practice, not to mention the car parking issues! So, how does a chiropractic manipulation vary from anyone else's? This is a pretty complex answer, as other professionals manipulate as well; it's just the philosophy around joint cracking that stands them apart. The textbook explanation is that the original chiropractic adjustment approach is generally referred to as spinal manipulation, and may also be called the diversified technique or the high velocity low amplitude technique.

New chiropractic adjustment approaches typically evolve as a variation from an existing technique, and are often named after the chiropractor who developed it. Chiropractors are not the only health care providers who utilise spinal manipulation for back pain treatment, however; many physiotherapists and osteopaths will provide a variety of different types of spinal adjustments, such as spinal manipulation and mobilisation. For instance, McTimoney chiropractors are trained in Oxford in the UK, completing a gentler, shorter manipulative course.

Throughout its history, chiropractors have been the subject of criticism. The founder of chiropractic, Daniel D. Palmer – known as a 'magnetic healer'

– stated that vertebral subluxation was the sole cause of all diseases, and that manipulation was the cure for all diseases of the human race, along the same lines of insane rationales for cures. This, of course, did nothing for the future of bone clickers. A 2003 profession-wide survey found that most chiropractors still hold views of the cause and cure of disease consistent with those of the Palmers. Chiropractic had a bumpy start, rooted as it was in mystical concepts and salesmanship, and this led to an internal conflict within the chiropractic profession, which still continues today. Many chiropractors – including D. D. Palmer –were jailed for practicing medicine without a license, and in order to try and resolve this problem, D.D. Palmer considered establishing chiropractic as a religion. I can't say that was a very wise decision!

For most of its existence, chiropractic has battled with medics, sustained by the early unscientific ideas about the significance on general health with subluxation (the alignment of spinal joints). I think there is clearly a place for adjusting spinal joints, to help the health of the joints and the nervous system as well, and integrated within all the other modalities, it really is excellent. In my opinion, however, the point at which it loses its efficacy a little is when manipulation alone is used to constantly crack open joints, time and again for just quick 10 to 15 minute appointments. A holistic chiropractor that embraces a multi-disciplinary approach makes for excellent treatment, though sadly not all do this.

Medical chiropractic researchers have documented – whether rightly or wrongly – that both fraud and abuse are more prevalent in chiropractic medicine than in any other health care profession. It's certainly true that chiros have had a rough ride. These committees say that unsubstantiated claims about the efficacy of chiropractic have continued to be made by chiropractic associations. Orthodox medicine finds that the core concept of traditional chiropractic, vertebral subluxation treating every medical condition to be unacceptable, with the exception of treatment for back pain. Although rare, spinal manipulation, particularly of the upper spine, can also result in complications that can lead to permanent disability or death; these can occur in adults and children."

Spinal manipulation alone still gets very slamming and damning reports, with research often stating that it is unlikely to result in relevant early pain reduction in patients with acute low back pain. Personally, I have felt the sudden change in my own back with a chronic stiffening condition administered by a manipulative physio within my own clinic, even though it in no way solved the problem. I have also felt an instant change administered by a chiropractor that lasted a full three weeks before aching again. However, with acute disc damage and inflammation, caution definitely needs to be taken.

In my opinion, chiropractors have exceptional skills at manipulating spines, and can go beyond where most of us fear to tread. Sadly, I know one or two who are not holistic and are more like car mechanics in their approach – they do just a quick manipulation, spending only a short time with their patient and carrying out many, many treatments, and you know who you are. They may benefit from getting to know their patients a little better.

Joints need adjusting at times, and with the right posture, biomechanics, and tight muscle contractures being released, they do behave. If a joint needs to be repeatedly manipulated, however, the root cause has been missed. I just think that if physical therapists would only work together and not compete against each other, everyone would gain a much better ethical and scientific understanding of the importance of physical medicine.

SNAZZY'S MANIPULATIVE JOURNEY TO TOAD OF TOAD HALL

My physios are trained in several different schools of manipulation, and going back in my time machine to my early postgrad days, I also studied manipulation, taught in several different ways. There were the odd combined seminars for all physical therapists too, where it was lots of fun to share our views. Then I studied physiotherapy – specifically Cyriax Orthopaedic Medicine, Maitland, and McKenzie – all of which had different ideas about where to position the patient and when to treat them with different amounts of twists, turns, and force. Each had its own language to scribble into your notes so that your joint wiggle could be repeated by a colleague.

I remember on my Cyriax courses being told that the late Dr. Cyriax always wore green and painted a lot of his rooms green, so of course I kept imagining a large TOAD! He also carried a frog clicker in his pocket, and he used to say that beyond the physical effect of manipulating the joints, hearing the click was the most powerful healer. The course went into various detailed orthopaedic assessments, with mild moderate and bad arse strong manips. My Orthopaedic Medicine qualification improved my diagnosis and non-operative treatment of soft tissue lesions around the body, as the scope of the treatment included lesions of ligaments, tendons, bursa, and muscles, along with lesions of the cervical, thoracic, and lumbar spines.

Cyriax employed an orthodox western medical approach, teaching when to manipulate, and when to inject or use physiotherapy modalities. The late Dr. James Cyriax was an internist and orthopaedic surgeon in England, and he developed his system of Orthopaedic Medicine over an extended period, starting in the early 1920's. The diagnostic and manipulation exams were followed by his orthopaedic injection course and exams, a distinctive feature and one of the most useful of the Cyriax methods being the capsular pattern.

This *capsular pattern* denotes inflammation of the capsule, such as in an inflammatory or traumatic arthritis, a fracture, or a cancer, which extends close to or into that joint. It is associated with a specific pattern of limitation, with the various passive movements at the joint, and each joint having its own distinctive capsular pattern. A *non-capsular pattern* implies that the capsule is not involved and that intra- or extra-articular tissue is inflamed or injured, and is therefore the source of the pain. Either pattern will be consistent on repeated exams from one day to the next. The London courses always included a wonderful eclectic group of enthusiastic teachers with whom I would visit delicious restaurants, and after just a year of postgrad, I'd made up my mind that if I could have fun like this, I would teach as well.

GENTLE JOINT JIGGLING DOWN SOUTH

The Maitlands course was a year of weekends spent in various hospitals in Bath, Yeovil, and Chichester – not to mention a hell of a lot of driving

– and the techniques ranged from tiny delicate mobilisations to strong manipulations.

"The Maitland Concept of Manipulative Physiotherapy (as it became to be known), emphasizes a specific way of thinking, continuous evaluation and assessment and the art of manipulative physiotherapy ("knowing when, how and which techniques to perform, and adapt these to the individual Patient") and a total commitment to the patient."
- Geoffrey D. Maitland, 1924–2010

Maitland was an Australian physical therapy visionary and innovator with a career spanning more than four decades. A pioneer in the use of mobilisation for pain modulation, his models for practice and his descriptions of examination and treatment techniques are still used as methodological standards by manual therapy researchers today. In particular, Maitland has been heralded for fostering patient-centred care, awareness of "the nature of the person", and its impact on treatment. Maitland's treatment can be so very gentle and soothing, and the belief was that it sang a lullaby to the nerves. Now, I'm going to go into a brief summary of nerve physiology here, so get your seat belts on!

Nerves transmit information to and from our joints. The size of the nerve fibres is an important consideration, as the bigger the nerve, the quicker the conduction, and additionally, conduction speed is also increased by the presence of a myelin sheath (insulating coating) – subsequently, large myelinated nerves are very efficient at conduction. This means that α-Beta fibres are the quickest of the three types, followed by α-Delta fibres, and finally, slow old C fibres. Gentle, rhythmical, sexy manipulating oscillations block the pain signals travelling through these guys.

PAIN PHYSIOLOGY IN SWITZERLAND

Now, back in the time machine we go to 2011, and my light-hearted lectures on pain in an amazing hotel in Montreau – the scenery was lovely, with the mountains and the beautiful lake. Anyway, back to the interplay between these nerves, which is very important. As you can see, only two of these nerves are pain receptors; **α-Delta** fibres are purely sensory and sexy in terms of touch. All of these nerves synapse onto projection cells, which travel up the freeway called the spinothalamic tract of the CNS (Central Nervous System) to the brain, where they continue via the thalamus (router) to the somatosensory cortex (the part of the brain where you feel sensation), the limbic system (the monkey brain), and other areas.

In the spinal cord there are also inhibitory interneurons which act as the 'gate keeper' (though not like in Ghostbusters), and when there is no sensation from the nerves, the inhibitory interneurons (the gate keepers) stop signals from travelling up the spinal cord – as there is no important information needing to reach the brain, the gate is 'closed'. When the smaller fibres are stimulated, the inhibitory interneurons (the gate keepers) do not act, and therefore the gate is 'open' when pain is sensed. When the larger α-Delta fibres are stimulated, they reach the inhibitory interneurons faster and, as larger fibres inhibit the interneuron (the gate keeper) from working, the gate is 'closed'. This is why after you have a lot of Maitland's mobilisations, you are stimulating the α-Delta fibres which close the gate. If you imagine you are pain, driving an a beta or C car, and you're sitting and waiting to get out of a junction on a busy road full of a delta drivers, but you can't pull out. So, in this case, pain can't travel to the brain.

NECK MANIPS CAN KILL

I remember it being drilled into us to be very cautious when manipulating the neck, and to always ask about the patient's blood pressure before doing anything to do with the neck. Personally, without X-rays to show the extent of osteoarthritis and osteophytes, I always err on the side of caution. I mean, I have a body bag ready just in case, but really I go very carefully.

"Because of the proximity of the vertebral artery to the lateral cervical articulations, caution must be used during manipulation of the cervical spine (MCS). It is thought that stroke can be induced as a result of MCS

by mechanical compression or excessive stretching of arterial walls but the pathogenesis of ischemia is unknown."
- ***Di Fabio, 1979.***

MR PUSHUP ALIAS MR MCKENZIE

Robin McKenzie, a New Zealand physical therapist, taught a combination of exercises and specific stretches with postural advice for discs, moving into manipulations where appropriate. The McKenzie disc centralisation phenomenon was developed by McKenzie in the 1960s, and in his practice, he noted that extending the spine could provide significant pain relief to certain patients, and allow them to return to their normal daily activities. This discovery happened by accident one day in 1956 when a patient got stuck in what looked like a very uncomfortable extended position for five minutes, causing his pain to completely vanish from his leg. With the McKenzie approach, physical therapy and exercise are used to extend the spine, which can help 'centralise' the patient's pain by moving it away from the extremities (the legs or arms) and to the back. Back pain is usually better tolerated than leg pain or arm pain, and the main theory of the approach is that centralising the pain allows the *source* of the pain to be treated, rather than the symptoms. Also, for some patients – such as those with large disc bulges or those with lumbar spinal stenosis or facet joint osteoarthritis – extending the spine can increase their pain. Therefore, the physio needs to be experienced in order to gauge the appropriate amount of extension.

The long-term goal of the McKenzie Method is to teach patients who are suffering from neck pain and/or back pain how to treat themselves and manage their own pain for life, through using exercise and other strategies. While it may seem counterintuitive, McKenzie pushes the notion that exercise is usually better for relieving sciatic pain than bed rest. Of course, patients may rest for a day or two after their sciatic pain flares up, but after that time period, inactivity will usually make the pain worse. I agree in principle with some of the gentler extension exercises, but I do think that missing out all the other modalities of treatment –

including dry needling – is detrimental to a fast recovery. At the time of writing this, my back did not like the McKenzie treatment, but I remain hopeful – as it repairs, I can get up off the floor more easily and I have been doing some McKenzie stretches.

NAGS AND SNAGS

Now, Mr McKenzie had a buddy, Mr Mulligan. Brian Mulligan was trained as a physiotherapist at the New Zealand School of Physiotherapy, qualifying in 1954. He and his colleague, Robin McKenzie, were the principle teachers on the newly-formed postgraduate program for the Diploma of Manipulative Therapy in 1968 – when I was still in nursery school. The concepts of mobilisations with movement (MWMS) in the extremities, and sustained natural apophyseal glides (SNAGS) in the spine, are logical continuations of this evolution, with the concurrent application of both therapist-applied accessory and patient-generated active physiological movements.

During assessment, the therapist will identify one or more comparable signs as described by Maitland. These signs may be due to a loss of joint movement, pain associated with movement, or pain associated with specific functional activities, and the therapist will investigate various combinations of parallel or perpendicular glides in order to find the correct treatment plane and grade of movement. While sustaining the accessory glide, the patient is requested to perform the comparable sign, which should now be significantly improved (i.e. increased range of motion, and a significant decrease in – or better yet, absence of – the original pain). There is an art to this so you don't feel you're wrestling with the patient. The goal is to achieve a movement to full range without pain, and this may need many glides – even up to 30 in a session.

NAGS and SNAGS is a handy tool to enhance some of the Maitland work. I remember watching his skilful hands and gentle sense of humour at a course in Eastbourne of all places; the local inhabitants – all of whom are mostly retired – would have snapped like twigs having this treatment. Let's just say the location was far from glamorous, but it did save a long flight to NZ.

I have to say that the major thing missing for me with all these schools of manipulation is that if the patient has peripheral nerve pain and you don't manipulate or extend... you pray, or suggest alcohol or strong meds. That's where GUNN IMS dry needling is so powerful, yet sadly the UK physios were not and still are not interested, even though gentle Chinese acupuncture does not do enough for tight muscle bands and nerve pain. I've had this same conversation in London, Korea, China, and Canada, and the neurosurgeons, orthopods, and medics abroad were much more open-minded. Certainly, the late AcuMedic Professor Mei's Chinese Medicine courses agreed that IMS stands alone and above when it comes to pain relief.

However, the combination of the postgrad training in orthopaedic medicine and Gunn IMS is excellent, and Professor Gunn was very strict in insisting that you had to have completed these postgrad courses before commencing his training. Unfortunately, the British Orthopaedic Society refused to let me write a research project on it – I remember a very tearful Snaz walking across London after a very derogatory response to my request.

SNAZZY'S EXERCISE DRILL

This basically involves brisk walks interspersed with short, fast jogs, then the McGills drill – as described in detail in the anti-aging fitness chapter – and swimming.

MY SUBCONSCIOUS FEAR

I was in my teens when my mother's back 'went'. Now, this was a long time ago so back in my time machine we'll go, this time to the early 80's. I'm afraid my memories are far from clear, however, I still remember the emotions that came to the surface during the countless visits to so-called physical therapy experts, all of whom failed to tame this elusive creature, pain. I do remember very well the short-lived excitement of, "this is the one, the cure, the gift!" quickly followed constantly by tears of frustration.

Many of my teenage years spent being the one in the waiting room, and all of those unsatisfying visits, are etched deep into my subconscious. On top of this were the daily changes I had to make while my mother was in pain. I helped to wash and dress her, took my little brother to school, cooked, and kept the house tidy, as well as attending school and studying. My father helped when he could – he had a busy job that often required him to be abroad – and my eldest brother had left home several years before to study chemistry at university, and in his spare time DJ at live gigs and on the radio. We cruised the many, many streets of therapy for the latest cure, pill, manipulation, exercise, and machine, without relief. We were going nowhere fast.

Years passed of living in a house full of repressed, angry, despairing energy, battling Mr. Pain who had by now completely moved in – pain enveloping and circling every daily activity, every attempted social engagement. Pain sucking the life blood out of youth, wrecking the simplest of pleasures such as the taste of food, putting pretty clothes on, dancing to music, and all the innate creative expressions of the physical body. The futile attempts of the laying on of hands, which while they soothed the soul, left pain curled up in the spine. If I look deep into my psychology, I realise that this haunted me until I could play a key role in fighting the dark side of pain myself, as pain is a lifesaver only in acute episodes.

These teenage years confused my psyche when it came to career pathways, my desire to use my healing gifts on patients becoming almost extinguished at times with the sheer exhaustion of living with someone in constant pain, not to mention the frustrations of modern physical medicine being absolutely powerless to help.

Every trip home from physical therapists meant that Mr. Pain got into the car with us, putting on his seat belt and getting ready for the ride. He was here for good, or so it seemed.

My recent experience of a troublesome back sent me right back down memory lane, making me think about how I ended up being the Sherlock Holmes of back pain.

WHY DID I STUDY THE PHYSICAL BODY?

Back in 1988, I went away to universities for six long years, going down the route of being a student of biological sciences so I could go back to the roots of our own existence. I learnt that we are a colony of a trillion cells, and that our existence depends on the health and communication of these cells. At the time, my thoughts were that if I could research how cells functioned, and how signals were received across the cell membrane, maybe I could find the hidden secrets of pain. Afterwards, I went on to study the evolution of single cells into multi cellular organisms and then into humans. I looked at the possibilities of the mind's impact on cells, something not found within my psychology modules.

Armed with this knowledge, I studied physiotherapy to give me access to hospitals where I could end patients' needless suffering, but my training left me needy, as I was really not equipped to tackle the complex issues of pain. My diagnostic skills gave me a safety net in which to explore the need for less well-known or accepted treatments and technology, and they also gave me the opportunity to at least communicate with physios and medics in their own language. While frustrating, the lack of time and the lack of belief in non-drug based treatments gave me the opportunity to grow my own health business from the ground up – in essence, to marry together orthodox treatments with less well-known 'unorthodox' advances in medicine, technology, and healing skills.

Medical doctors specialising in musculoskeletal problems, and chartered physiotherapists, are both seen as practicing an orthodox medical approach in the UK. I chose the latter to enable me to spend the time I need with patients and to weave together a healing, hands on, patient-centred approach. Time is needed for counselling. In the 1950's, a GP practice was about looking after the community in a preventative way, and managing chronic illness with a personal service at home. Working within my own company, in an orthodox way and with a holistic approach – with the local GP's full blessing – has improved to date (just in the last decade) 10,000 patients' lifestyles. Now, get your seat belts back on: we use an approach that is not drug based, but lifestyle based, with a centre to call on should hands on treatment be needed.

I taught surgeons, doctors, and physios internationally, and I enjoyed presenting to the public alongside talented speakers on health. As my body is now showing its very first signs of structural aging, and as my patient list has grown far beyond my ability to personally touch every one of them, I'm very glad to have a talented team to treat many of my patients. This has allowed me to find a little time for me to glean great comfort in sharing my thoughts through books and radio.

As I write this, I still treat four, and at times five to six days a week, even though I am supposed to be backing off. I write very, very late at night whilst everyone sleeps, and these times are so special to me. Through my life and eyes and body, I can share what I have learnt. This is my life's purpose and it is a true blessing.

So, within the covers of this book I can re-evaluate my human garage from within my own body. I'm just glad I'm not teaching surgery!

Physical medicine is about accessing the body's self-healing abilities through the body's own wisdom. It is also about understanding and accessing the mind's healing power through touching the body, and flicking switches on and off in order to create preventative self-healing programs. To fire fight at times when illness and injury have taken over.

To end this chapter I'm going to turn to my analogy of a jellyfish, the brain reaching every part of your body through several long tentacles. As a therapist, I can tickle its tentacles and avoid the sting.

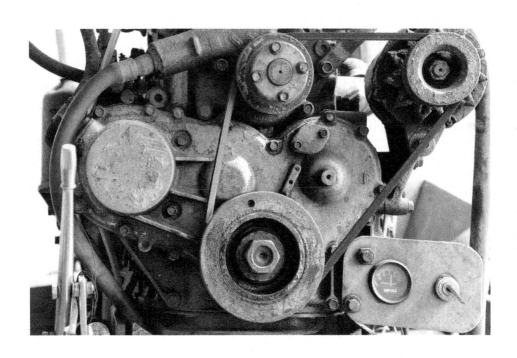

Chapter Two

"There is a fountain of youth: it is your mind, your talents, the creativity you bring to your life and the lives of people you love. When you learn to tap this source, you will truly have defeated age."

– Sophia Loren

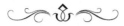

We are a colony of billions of cells

"The greatest revolution in our generation is the discovery that human beings, by changing the inner attitudes of their minds, can change the outer aspects of their lives."
- **William James**

ARE YOU A RESPONSIBLE OWNER OF YOUR BODY?

"Take your life in your hands, and what happens? A terrible thing; no one to blame."
- **Erica Jong**

When you get a problem with your car you take it to a garage, where a car mechanic looks under the bonnet, runs some diagnostic tests, then goes to the store and orders replacements for the faulty parts. You let them go about their business, with your only responsibility being to pay the bill. Or is it really just that? Do you actually have more responsibility than this?

Now, let's look at the parallel of this scenario in the medical industry, where you buy drugs to keep your vehicle/body going, in order to make it run properly and smoothly. Too often you view your body like a machine; if it's faulty, we see the body as something that is letting us down, like an unreliable car. We blame our body or our doctor for whatever's gone wrong, never ourselves; when we are ill, we look to our genes, to our blood biochemistry and viruses, just like a car mechanic does.

We would be shocked if the car mechanic interviewed us, and said, "Would you like to tell me how you drive this car? How often do you polish it? And do you make sure you keep its oil and fluid levels topped up?" In response, we would no doubt get rather indignant: "Are you saying that just because I'm the driver, I am responsible for this mechanical breakdown? How ridiculous!"

If you had two identical cars for sale – one owned by a mature, lady owner and one owned by a nineteen-year-old lad – which driver is likely to have a healthier car that would last longer than the other? This simple analogy of a driver seeing no relevance to responsible driving can be related to our conscious awareness about health; poor driver education means a lack of responsibility for car defects, and reckless driving is more likely making scrap merchants richer.

In a scrap yard, we find all kinds of things: smashed-up cars due to driver failure in accidents, beaten down cars that were driven too hard, were poorly looked after, and were poorly serviced, and then the really unlucky cars that are written off and sent to the scrapyard, aged far before their time. Get my drift?

CELL CITY

Cells are tiny humans. They have a membrane, like our skin, and they also have a kind of brain in the membrane and in the nucleus, its DNA carrying our blueprint. Mitochondria (see the glossary for all of these terms) are like lungs, the endoplasmic reticulum is like the liver, with vacuoles being the stomachs.

Moreover, we build our cities just like our bodies and like our cells. If we consider the city as a reflection of the cell, we can see that the cell membrane is represented by government buildings, passport offices and tollgates. Protein chains are echoed in the infrastructure of roads to carry materials in and out of cities, and agricultural fields for creating food and supplying supermarkets equate to the stomach. Hospitals and police stations represent the immune system, whereas the toilets and sewers are the bladder and colon. The library, schools, and lawyers would be the cell nucleus, and power stations would be the mitochondria. Phone systems would be the innate intelligence and Qi (this is chi or prana, the life force energy). Go on, look closely at a cell, then think about the town or city you live in. It's all the same design.

DOES YOUR CELL GET THE RIGHT VIBES?

As a biologist back in the late 80's (so it's back in my time machine again, folks), I had the opportunity to look at cells through powerful scanning electron microscopes. I was researching what effect environmental triggers, such as chemicals – in my case, ionophores – had on cells, as it seemed that the cell membrane had, simply put, a key and lock mechanism in order to allow specific electrochemical or electromagnetic signals to create reactions that happened deep within the cell itself. I could take images of what happened within the cells after these keys were inserted at the cell membrane, and the key caused staggering changes within the cell.

At the turn of the century, the double helix of Watson and Crick was born, and scientists finally thought they had it all figured out. Genetic engineering and designer humans were all the rage, and the central dogmas of biology were born. This went against the work of scientists such as Bruce Lipton who said things like, "Human beings are a consequence of collective amoebic consciousness," as well as, "We need to put the spirit back into the equation when we want to improve our physical and mental health" (Lipton, 2005).

These controversial ideas fascinated me, as I had grown up with the scientific dogma (belief) that the nucleus holding the DNA was the control centre – a bit like the old belief that the earth was in the centre of the universe, and we all know how that turned out. The basic sciences that I studied at university – such as cell biology and biochemistry – were said to define the mechanisms of life on which modern allopathic medicine is built. The central dogma here was that the 'flow of information in biological systems' shaped the biological characteristics of an organism, and this flow of information was carried as if in a car travelling down a motorway from city to city.

The information was presumed to express itself in a linear, unidirectional path that originated with genetic DNA (see glossary), which was translated into RNA (again, please see the glossary for these terms) and then proteins. These were the physical and behavioural building blocks, the dogma literally being that the DNA blueprint of proteins determined the quality of your life; that what you ate and thought, and how much you played, had no effect on your appearance, happiness, or health. That's it, that's your lot. Well, bollocks to that disempowering theory!

Now, for the scientists among you, hands over ears and seat belts on, please! Healers add into this that an innate intelligence – a vital energy – flows from the universe, possibly via the pineal gland into the brain, through the nervous system or meridian network in the fascia, and into all tissues and cells. This innate intelligence has a role to play when it comes to genes switching on and off, as well as cell behaviour. Eastern medicine (including Ayurvedic) leans more to this theory than the former, though having studied both, I can see a combination of the two ideas being much closer to the truth.

GENES CONTROL OUR BIOLOGY? I DON'T THINK SO

The old western model of genes alone controlling our biology – as well as the biological process employing Newtonian mechanics – is at last outdated. The Earth is not at the centre of the universe anymore, or hadn't anyone told you yet?

The results from the Human Genome Project made it clear that it was even more unlikely that genes alone controlled our lives. In summary, David Baltimore (a Nobel Prize winner) stated, "What does give us our complexity, remains a challenge for the future" (Nature, 2001).

Now, to make up a human you need 150,000 proteins – not many in the grand scheme of things. Like a little spine of joints, each protein comprises of its own specific combination of amino acids, and just like how muscles pull a spine into position, electrical charges push and pull at the protein shapes, making them dance. These sexy dancing proteins produce specific functions for contracting muscles, digesting, breathing, circulation, and so on.

I am excited by the theory that vibrational energy configurations (NOT physical chemicals) can make proteins dance, that they can alter the electromagnetic charge around a protein and actually cause its configuration to change. My allopathic, biological, and physiotherapy background was all about Newtonian mechanics, as well as chemical signals such as hormones and drugs affecting our health, rather than focusing on something we couldn't see. This slowly evolving new age of epigenetics – including biophysics and its quantum principles – suggests that vibrational waves move proteins more effectively than physical chemicals.

So, if we fall ill, is this because we have a dysfunctional protein? It is very unlikely, as less than 5% of the causes of illness are down to genetic defects. This suggests that it's our communication system – the way we signal the cell to make changes – that determines our health, and this empowers us to 'drive' a healthier lifestyle, and therefore be more accountable for our health.

Basically, with falling ill, this could be one of three faults: damage to the signal pathway, not having enough chemistry to make a signal, or the nervous system giving faulty messages due to problems such as trauma, toxins, viruses, and thoughts. Hence an environmental trigger affects the brain, then the spinal cord, then the organs, tissues, and cells – and ultimately, our health.

We know that cells move towards more energy and away from less; simply speaking, they carry a negative charge inside, and the greater the difference across the cell membrane (positive to negative), the more energy the cell has and the healthier it is. The cell senses its environment by reading the energy field around it; if it is losing energy it moves away, and if it is gaining energy it moves towards. It is constructive and destructive interference, like the song says: good vibes... good vibrations... This actually puts me in mind of a cocktail party: some people really drain your energy and you have to move away, whereas others make you feel alive and you just want to be near them.

THE COMBUSTION ENGINE

An immigrant bacteria (called mitochondria) fused with the human cell billions of years ago, though they still have separate cell walls and DNA. Mitochondria take in sugar and oxygen and push out the explosive dynamite ATP (adenosine triphosphate – please see the glossary). They are the essential powerhouses of the cell, and they have a big role to play in cancer because they need to kill faulty cells by flooding them with calcium. If faulty cells live, the human can die.

Normally, the mitochondria picks up signals from the body that the cell is in the wrong place or doing the wrong thing, and consequently it flicks the kill switch. Cancer is powerful, because somehow it gives the body permission to let it live through wrong signalling: a failure of micro-architecture, a failure of Qi. Pre-cancerous changes mean that cells are losing their lines of communication, and that some stressful influence is allowing the programming to fail. It's amazing that an immigrant all those years ago is critical to our existence today! Mitochondria also need good nutrition in order to heal us.

As an aside, I came across a novel way of looking at cancer thanks to the biophoton emission experiments conducted by Takeda et al. in 2004, which I have included as a reference in this book if you're interested in reading further on this subject. Some much less known research involves the emission of biophotons from living creatures, believed to originate from mitochondrial DNA, which can be found in the near ultraviolet spectrum. Now, here's a spooky fact for you: a paper written by Cohen et al. in 2003 discovered that biophotons are emitted most readily from fingers and toes, and that they are released quicker with illness and when close to death.

CELL MEMBRANES UNDER MY MICROSCOPE

Now, let's look more closely at how YOUR human cell experiences the environment. The old dogma of the nucleus being the most important part of the cell was not the case in my experiments – what unfolded in front of my eyes told a very different story. The cell membrane – or rather, the mem'BRAIN' – was a critical decision-maker in what could lock in and initiate a protein building blocks sequence of events. In my imagination I saw the protein shapes as boulders of chiselled stone, moving and locking into position, and if this is a true model of what happens at the cell's surface, what we eat and think does ultimately have a huge impact on our body.

More recent scientific theories suggest that the cell membrane adapts the cell to whatever environment it is in. Signals that are recognised by receptor proteins on the outside of the membrane bind to effector proteins, making them dance, changing their configuration, and switching on internal cell behaviour. This receptor-effector sense, if you like a lock and key action, is the cell tasting its environment.

The membrane is made up of phospholipid molecules. It has liquid crystal properties much like a semiconductor, and the receptors taste the inside and outside of the cell via channels. Back in 1986 in a newsletter for the Planetary Association, Bruce Lipton discussed that the membrane can be likened to an information-processing transistor, or an organic computer chip. Lipton describes his delightful theories in his *Biology of Belief* book (2005), in which he sees the receptors being like keys on a keyboard, while the membrane is like a computer chip, receiving signals to modify all its functions – including the possibilities of turning off and on genes and re-writing DNA code sequence, the nucleus' role being like a read-write hard disc with genetic programs.

BINDING IS MOLECULAR SEX IN THE CITY

That's right – if you think about it, our very existence requires the consented union of two molecular beings on the surface of the cell membrane. Sound familiar to how babies are born? Right, get your seat belts on, as I'm about to talk down and dirty to you. Right now, millions of molecules are having sex all over your cells' membranes. That's trillions of cells – with millions of receptors per cell – all bonking. How disgusting, you might say. Well, it's how life is created and maintained.

Cell membrane receptors (and there are literally millions of these per cell) sit there waiting to connect with their very specific partners. They are all very fussy, sitting on the edge of the dance floor and waiting to see who is going to ask them to dance. These vibrating amino acid receptors flex and wriggle, snaking between the outer and inner part of the membrane, looking very much like little beaded sexy snakes. Once they sense a buddy – as these guys are our cell's eyes, ears, and nose – they sing and wriggle and vibrate and change shape, usually to one of three forms. Their buddy (called a ligand) fits into them like the male anatomy into a lady's 'front bottom', as my friend June called it. This 'key in lock' procedure changes the receptor's shape, and then bam! The message – or rather, the command – is delivered into the cell. There is a bumping and grinding and slipping off – just like sex – until the receptor and ligand really make that gear change (or orgasm) and the cell hears the scream and obeys.

At this moment, the cell roars into life, and at this point the internal factors may start doing many things: producing a replica cell or specific proteins, closing or opening more ion channels, or adding or throwing out more calcium or potassium or various energetic chemical groups. This makes the cell more or less energetic and vital by altering the electrical potential magnitude. The cell is negative to the outside fluids, and a greater gradient is indicative of health, which is good news for anti-aging. I must point out here that receptors of 'locks' are very specific – ladies, we don't want any old key in there, do we?

Just a little more science here, so make sure you have a stretch and a few deep breaths as you'll need some oxygen for this bit (and perhaps a quick flip to the glossary at the back of the book). There are basically three physical keys, and who knows how many electromagnetic ones. The three physical keys are the following: the first set are neurotransmitters – tiny, simple brain juices that (mind the gap) carry messages across synapses. These amino acids are made in the brain. The second set of keys are made from cholesterol, and give us our sexy hormones and our fight or flight juices. These are steroid keys. The third set – which forms 95% of the keys (ligands) – are peptides, which are necklaces of amino acids.

Right, now back to my lab. Looking into these cells, I could see massive reactions when the receptors in the membrane received the signalling ligands/keys; the cell would start making structures and churning out molecules. In the case of my mast cell experiments, large vacuoles filled with histamine poured out. I still have some of the pictures. I learnt that if you take out the nucleus, the cell can live for some time, however, if I ruptured the membrane, this would result in instant death. I also learnt that if there was even the slightest dilute toxic cleaning chemical in the petri dishes or glassware, the cells were affected or even killed, hence the environment was critical to survival.

Since these early experiments, researchers have looked at how lifestyle can alter gene expression through the lock and key receptors, as well as looking at how signals can dictate genes being activated or shut down.

THE TELEVISION ANALOGY IN YOUR CELL

In my presentations – especially when I'm faced with a sensitive or elderly audience – I use an analogy of TV aerials on a rooftop, with the rooftop being the cell membrane, and the aerial being a receptor, receiving a signal for the BBC or ITV. The TV set in the lounge selects and runs the channel, and in a similar way, once the signal arrives and locks into the cell membrane, the cell's internal workings create what is asked of them. Cytoarchitecture – that is, the inside structures of the cell – remind me of a little city of buildings, and if I knew my audience well, I could mention the fact that signalling proteins are f***ing all over your cells in order to create and maintain your health.

Could scrutinising the cell's ultrastructure really give me clues regarding healing and pain relief, or was I barking up the wrong tree? In the future, how could I measure the impact of electromagnetic signals? The cell membrane electrical potential seems to be just one basic scientific explanation, and my Quadscan equipment has a basic interpretation of that. I hope that after reading this chapter, you wake up, have a coffee/tea break, and understand why the 4 keys approach to health is so important. Our cells are our senses, and everything we say, think, and eat – and every energetic, electro-magnetic field – affects our health and our happiness.

JANE'S SPINE

One day, a woman called Jane came into my office and pushed a large enve-lope into my hand, adding, "Professor X says my spine is f***ed, and doesn't want to do any more surgery. He says you may be able to help with my quality of life. I've heard of your reputation, and now you have to prove it to me." Prove it – how often had I heard that? She carried on: "I need to be pain free; I need to get on with my busy social life and walking the dogs. I lost my husband due to ill health and I am healthy and far too busy to have a bad back, so just fix it and I can be on my way."

My eyes flickered towards the magic wand I'd bought for my nephews, with its flashing lights and tingly music; I kept it there to keep my sense of hu-mour from letting my mind become too overwhelmed. I had already helped so many people beyond what even I felt was possible, but when you start the journey to recovery, there will be sticking points along the way where you either can or can't push through. Like footprints in snowfall, it's not clear where they came from or where they want to go, and it will only ever be transient; you just do your best to walk alongside and guide them, for their footsteps will vanish and new ones will come. It's inevitable, but every walk is different every time; the important thing is for the footsteps to be leading somewhere, wherever that might be.

I wrote *The 4 Keys* and now *The Human Garage* to enable me to empower people, getting them to the best optimum health that their age and disease allows. Those are my footsteps, wherever they should lead to.

Anyway, back to my patient, Jane. I loaded the MRI scans onto my computer, cleaned my glasses, and peered at the pictures of the spine. The discs looked like narrow pieces of burnt charcoal, and the vertebra had what looked like chewed holes in them, evidence of Scheuermann's disease (please see the glossary for more information). On top of this, the little sculptured facet joints had ragged edges, and had lost the smooth, pearl-like edges you find on hinged shells. The muscles had fatty deposits and looked tired.

"So," said Jane, "you've seen the scans, what do you think? Do I need to come back or can you fix it today? Professor X at Oswestry said you were a miracle worker." When she'd finished talking, I sat very still, only too aware of my body language. I chose my words carefully, and in a slow, measured answer I said, "Your body has done a lot of living, so let's take it in small steps. Shall we make our first goal to walk a little further without any pain? OK, let's go through your 4 keys to see where you can give your body the best chance to suffer less."

Pain and damage is not directly related to suffering; the brain decides (in an emotional way) how to translate tissue damage into pain. I want to tell you a true story now of an elderly nun who was sent to me by my in-house orthopaedic surgeon. She had discomfort in her shoulder, and whilst she was in the hospital, we X-rayed her spine. It was crumbled to dust, and yet she had felt no pain. Now, it was not for us to alert her mind to this. Somehow, her faith and lifestyle had allowed her mind to discount this problem – she was simply not suffering.

When I see evidence of worrying scans and X-rays, and I need to avoid disheartening the patient, I share true stories of destroyed joints that caused no suffering. Recently I saw some research on the lack of correlation between osteoarthritic damage and pain. What we believe about a problem plays a key role in our recovery – if we perceive that we cannot improve, then we will struggle to do so.

This patient had an amber key for mind-set, as she had a mixture of grief and a lack of meaningful purpose in her life, but she was still very grounded and secure. Her diet was good, but chronic painkiller usage would have affected her gut and nutrient absorption, so it was amber here too. Her fitness key was green, as she did lots of exercise and activity despite her problems. Lastly, her lifestyle was amber, as she was financially secure, retired, and had lots of hobbies and friends – however, she had no family or close friends.

There were some issues she could have worked on in order to get her four green keys, but as she wasn't uncomfortable enough to change anything major, it was unlikely that I'd be able to achieve this for her.

Now, back to her scan. I examined it over and over again, looking for clues where she could be getting the symptoms. There was scar tissue from surgery she'd had to remove parts of discs that were trapping nerves. Compressed nerves invariably become neuropathic, and this could be helped with Gunn IMS treatment. They can also be wrapped up in scar tissue like ivy, therefore making it very difficult for me to help. The facets looked arthritic and the bones were thinned, both of which could cause juicy inflammatory pain dependent partly on the immune system, as well as bone pain from the osteopenic bones.

Her core stability could be improved with specific prescribed exercise such as McGill, both to stabilise the spine and to ease tension in the smaller muscles. Stiffness and general pain could be helped with gentle physiotherapy spinal mobilisations, as well as acupuncture and electrotherapy. Magnetic resonance treatments for the disc pathology and degenerative bones would help as an anti-aging (grade 1 to 3 osteoarthritis only) preventative treatment to slow down the deterioration, and improve cartilage and bone cell repair processes within the cells. Adding in juices and smoothies and supplements – with her GP's consent, of course – would help with bone repair processes.

Jane had a map to recovery in her hand, as well as her scans. However, being a healer as well as a mechanic means dissecting cells down to nuts and bolts, but this only presents part of the picture to me. What of energetic matrixes and meridian lines?

WHY GET ARTHRITIC JOINTS?

The doctors tell us that it's just unavoidable wear and tear, that we should simply learn to live with it as nothing can be done. If our body has been evolving over millions of years, why do we get so much body rot? As Einstein said, "The problems we have created cannot be solved at the same level of thinking we were at when we created them."

There are basically two types of arthritis: the wear and tear osteoarthritic type, and the more serious rheumatoid type, where the immune system goes into overdrive and actually attacks its own joints. This form of arthritis is thought to be triggered by a virus, and is in part genetic. Jane had the former and the start of osteoporosis. This is getting very common now, with one in three patients breaking bones over the age of 70 due to osteoporosis alone. This is made worse by several factors: a lack of oestrogen, progesterone and Vitamin D, weight bearing exercise, a lack of magnesium, parathyroid or thyroid problems, diabetes, alcohol, and a poor diet.

At my age – which is 50, if you were going to ask – 80% of people have osteoarthritis, and a quarter of us experience pain from it. We get stiffer, less flexible joints, and our smooth cartilage dries out and dies, leading to further bone damage. The joint juice gets sticky and inflamed, and lifestyle factors further affect arthritis, especially diet and posture. Good nutrition, walking, and a good sitting posture are all key.

FASCIA, WELL WE COME HYGIENICALLY BUBBLE WRAPPED

Now, this isn't something we paid a lot of attention to in anatomy classes, but fascia can get inflamed and can sometimes get too tight (compartment syndrome, see glossary). Fascia is a kind of biological ordering; surgeons use it to go between planes, avoiding the need to cut too much and minimising scarring.

In Chinese medicine, fascia is a big deal – in fact, they dedicate two organs/meridians to it: the pericardium and the triple burner meridians. These meridian lines carry Qi, the life force. The pericardium is said to protect the heart from physical damage and emotions, whereas the triple burner is a concept unique to Chinese medicine and controls the entire circulation of body fluid. The Yellow Emperor's classic of internal medicine (HuangDi NeiJing) – the most important ancient text in Chinese medicine – is still open to a lot of interpretation. A more modern, well-known Chinese medical classic about health and wellness – the Nanjing, which is 2000 years old – describes the triple warmer meridian as having no form.

The three layers – or burners – of the triple warmer are loosely described as being within the pelvis elimination of energy, abdomen transformation of energy, and the intake at the thorax. This meridian moves solids and fluids, and produces and circulates nourishing protective energy, as well as regulating the activities of other organs. Of course, there is little space to even touch on Chinese medicine in just one book.

The body vacuum packs everything with fascia, and a tear can mean death. Fascia is connective tissue, rich in collagen cells, and is also impenetrable to biological substances; water, blood, pus, electricity… everything just slides off it. Fascia creates compartments for the heart, lungs, kidneys, pelvis, and abdomen, much like you do in your socks and pants drawers.

Interestingly, fascia is also piezoelectric, which is the effect certain materials have to generate an electric charge in response to mechanical stress (Minary-Jolandan, 2009). Some would say that fascia holds the secrets to the acupuncture channels/meridians, plus the transport of Qi (life energy) through the body.

YOU ARE MADE OF STEEL

The steel in the fascia is actually collagen, which is very strong, like super glue – its name is actually Greek for 'glue creator'. It is the steel within so many structures, including vessels, nerves, bones, cartilage, tendons, and ligaments. Far more exciting than being the support, however, this special protein is a double helix with a twist – yes, a triple helix – and it owes its semi-crystalline electrical properties (piezoelectric properties) to this structure (Tomaselli and Shamos, 1974).

COLLAGEN IS A WEB OF ELECTRICAL CHANNELS

Collagen holds, generates, and directs our body electricity, and is also thought to have a role in directing stem cells. It is believed to guide the position of cells in embryos in order to determine what they grow into, as shown by Feng et al. (2012). It is far more than fabric bubble wrapping; it is a life-giving, gentle – though controlling – electric force field. To me, it makes sense that acupuncture relates to fascia, and my IMS dry needling to muscles. Both do different jobs and both merit importance.

SUPER GLUE TO BONES

Bone has a mixture of collagen and hydroxyapatite crystals of calcium and phosphate, making it feel metallic – I think about it as being similar to stirring crystals into cement, until it gets thicker and solid. Electric fields in the fascia are said to determine the density (Hartig et al., 2000), so guys, for a healthy bone smoothie, get enough vitamins – especially C for collagen, and also D, as well as minerals for bone cells. Recently, we used MRT (magnetic resonance) to treat a lady who point blank refused to eat veggies and fruit, and/or supplements. Her results were poor, and still we could not convince her to give her body the nutrients it needed, so we declined further MRT until she would reconsider, for her own good. In the meantime, we gave her gentle massage treatment instead.

ROLFING

There are so many different names for soft tissue work, and 'Rolfing' is one of them. Ida Rolf began working on clients in New York in the 1930's, with the theory that the human structure could be organised 'in relation to gravity'. Rolf was teaching her work across the United States, and in the mid-1960's, she began teaching at the Esalen Institute in California. Rolf theorised that 'bound up' fasciae (connective tissues) can restrict muscles from functioning correctly. She aimed to separate the fibres of bound up fasciae manually in order to loosen them and allow for effective movement. She also claimed to have found an association between emotions and the soft tissue. In addition to the physical manipulation of tissue, Rolfing uses a combination of active and passive movement retraining; moving is so important in getting the collagen to stay elastic and to help in tissue regeneration.

Movement makes the collagen fire these little currents and also allows the bone-making cells to create bone. "Piezoelectricity could predict sites of formation/resorption in bone remodelling" (Fernandez, 2012). This way, we strengthen where needed, and gravity plays a key role in this electrical happening. Without electricity, we die – it's as simple as that. If I revisit my A level biology notes about cells, I know that the cell is negatively charged. It has pumps that throw out three positively charged sodium ions in exchange for two positive potassium ions coming in. As soon as the pumps stop, the cell dies in minutes.

We are silent electrical webs of energy. Our eyes see with photons, our heart is paced with its pacemaker, nerves transmit electricity, our brain thinks with it… get my drift? Without electricity, life simply stops.

ANATOMY TRAINS

Anatomy Trains is a unique map of the 'anatomy of connection' – whole-body fascial and myofascial linkages. The Anatomy Trains concept joins individual muscles into functional complexes within the fascial planes – each with a defined anatomy and 'meaning' in human movement. Mr. Thomas Meyers – a genius 'body worker' – started to be heard in the 1990's, when he got a team of soft tissue experts together in order to help promote these enlightening ideas about human architecture. Historically, we were so hung up about bones and muscles that connective tissue was a bit of an after-thought.

Anatomy Trains knowledge is said to improve stability and coordination, as well as resolving long-standing dysfunctional postural and movement patterns. It involves looking at body connective tissue in 3D, and thinking about why we are built and how we can maintain the architecture, from the individual cell to the social sporting activities, such as how we get stuck in poor postures and how we mature and grow out of such restrictions. Mr. Meyers calls this 'Spatial Medicine', and he talks about body intelligence and a kinesthetic quotient – I guess a kind of 3D body awareness in space.

BREATHING INTO YOUR SHOULDERS

Taught in Anatomy Trains, this is an easy but telling assessment for the way your shoulders move by watching their response to the breath. Watch first with a normal tidal breath (this is how you breathe naturally), but if that is too small to produce any shoulder movement, gradually increase the depth of the breath until you see some movement response in the shoulder girdle (this is the scapula humeral rhythm. The scapula is the triangular-shaped bone on your back).

Generally, you will see one of the three following patterns. ONLY THE THIRD IS CORRECT.

HOMEWORK:
Look in the mirror at how your shoulders move.

• The shoulder girdle moves straight up with the in-breath and back down on the exhale. In this case, look to the muscles that hold the shoulder to the ribs (the serratus anterior and pectoralis minor). **This is WRONG.**

• The shoulder girdle hardly moves, even with a deeper breath. In this case, the shoulder is hanging off the neck and head, and you should look to the stressed muscles (trapezius and levator scapulae) that hold the shoulder girdle from above. Also, the neck muscles (the scalenes), which are not normally listed as shoulder muscles but do attach fascially to the arms, can often bring good results for this pattern. **This is WRONG.**

• The shoulder girdle moves up and out on the inhale; down and in on the exhale. The shoulder is loose enough to ride and glide on the ribcage in response to the breath. **This is CORRECT.**

HOMEWORK:
Feel how you breathe, then find a friend to work on the tight muscles.

IS HAVING BUBBLE WRAP A BIG DEAL?

Fascia is, in fact, our system of biomechanical regulation – just as our circulatory system is a chemical regulator, and the nervous system is a timing regulator – and it therefore needs to be treated as a system, rather than as just a series of parts. Anatomy textbooks tend to reduce us to Newtonian biomechanics of forces, vectors, and levers, as if we are manufactured from parts – just like a car. Of course, this is a very simplistic and limited viewpoint and is rapidly falling before Einstein's theory of relativity, fractal mathematics, synergetic systems theory, and tensegrity geometry as applied to biological systems – all of which are far too deep for this book.

My embryology lecture notes suggest that the fascial system starts about two weeks into development as a fibrous gel that pervades and surrounds all the cells in the developing embryo. It is then progressively folded by the motions of development into the complex layers of fascia we see in adults. ECM (the extracellular matrix) is a collagenous network of products and connective tissue cells (bone cells, cartilage cells, mast cells...) and these equal fascia. This dense leathery mesh found in bones, cartilage, tendons, and ligaments forms different layers of wrapping paper or cling film, and the muscles are surrounded by and invested with a loose but strong network (though looser mesh is found in structures like the breast). Every bone has a tough plastic wrap layer around the outside, while every organ is bagged in a fascial sac.

Unlike buildings – where bricks are placed one on top of the other with straight, compressive lines – fascial continuity suggests that the myofascia acts like an 'adjustable tensegrity' around the skeleton; a continuous inward pulling tensional network like the elastics, with the bones acting like the struts in the tensegrity model. This is a floating compression; isolated components in compression inside a net of continuous tension, in such a way that the compressed bars/struts don't touch each other or the pre-stressed tensioned members.

Courses for massage therapists demonstrate how these fascial trains/meridians transmit forces and strains. There simply isn't enough time to go into details within the covers of this book, but I'd just like to say that for those of you keen on massage, take a look at Thomas Myers' brilliant book, *Anatomy Train* (2010).

SQUID

No, I am not back in the ocean, so what am I talking about here? Well, I mentioned earlier that fascia is good at conducting electricity. "Have we any science to back this up?" I hear you say, and the answer is: yes. A Superconducting Quantum Interference Device (SQUID) magnetometer can detect the tiny biomagnetic fields that are projected out from your head or heart to quite some distance outside the body. We know that all cells produce tiny electrical currents, and these currents generate tiny magnetic fields in the surrounding space. Our nerves are actually coated in perineural sheaths that pulse with biomagnetism.

There will be much more about this in the Soul book, but briefly, Qi emissions are the eastern interpretation of this. Healers emit detectable frequencies between 0.3 and 30 Hz, and in fact, all of our tissue produces specific magnetic pulsations that are collectively called a biomagnetic field, which is projected several feet beyond our bodies.

As an aside – and to wind up my editor – the importance in measuring tiny electrical changes was mentioned at a meeting last week (October 2015), with one of the magnetic resonance bosses. In a pretty chapel room in Hoar Cross, he relayed information from their German scientists, stating that they had measured the difference in cell membrane potential as a scientific indicator of the status of the cell. They saw the detection of differences in the degree of positive and negative electrical energy across the cell membrane as critical to cellular health research, when comparing the effectiveness of treatment.

SAT NAV FOR CELLS

In the body, there are believed to be nodes that are embryological points that control growth with an organising centre (OC), and in 1935, Spelman was awarded the Nobel Prize for this discovery. This OC uses juices called morphogens, which are growth factors, and in 1995 Nüsslein-Volhard named an OC she'd discovered 'Sonic the Hedgehog'. She showed that relative concentrations of these juices – the gradient – was the key to what these cells made themselves into, and this tiny essence of growth juice diffuses through spaces between cells. She got a Nobel Prize for this. It reminds me of a business plan, the body being an ever-changing conglomerate of OCs controlling their zone of cells.

There is a school of thought that meridian points/caves are also sites of stem cells. The CEO of this operation is a mystery, as the ultimate control did not appear to herald from the brain or via nerves. It remains a mystery, though perhaps it is to do with innate intelligence, meridian lines, and Qi – no one knows as yet.

THE THIRD EYE – IS IT THE PINEAL GLAND?

Now, it's that time again: hands over ears, scientists, and get your seat belts on. Is this the missing link between the source of communication and infinite intelligence? Could this be the seat of the soul? I pondered in my Mind book about where the soul resided in the brain. The Ayurvedic medics – along with many different shamans – talked about the pineal gland being the 3rd eye; it sits above the third ventricle of cerebral fluid in the brain, and beneath it is the pituitary. Could it receive a subtle transmission like the old-fashioned radios?

Also, the pineal gland contains crystals. I remember listening to a discussion with Bruce Lipton when he talked about nerve dendrites touching the crystals like the wire whiskers of old radios. As everyone has a unique collection of dendrites, they would therefore receive a personal transmission.

So, we have a possible theory of a mass consciousness, of universal energy and infinite wisdom, giving our soul an input of information to the pineal (the 'radio station'), before the signals travel from the pituitary, through the brain to the spinal cord, and down nerves and meridians to the cells. Is this the missing link? Is this the source of Chi? What really controls life? We just don't know.

I remember in the 80's – back in my biologist days, if we can briefly take my time machine to those years – there were several weird cloning experiments going wrong. Cloning seems to have gone out of vogue a bit now and instead it's all about artificial intelligence. Anyway, back then they would take an egg with half the DNA needed, then they would inject mature DNA in from the mother's cell. And it was the 'mature' part that was the problem – they created monsters. The one thing that made a difference was a tiny electrical current that kicked the cell into life. What are we playing with? The word 'Frankenstein' certainly comes to mind.

CAN WE PERCEIVE DIVINITY?

In 1973, Edgar Mitchell – an Apollo 14 astronaut, who two years earlier had become the sixth man to walk on the moon – founded the Institute of Noetic Sciences (IONS), also coining the term *noetic sciences*. Mitchell described his trip back home from space as a *samadhi* (or 'blissful divine') experience: "The presence of divinity became almost palpable, and I knew that life in the universe was not just an accident based on random processes... the knowledge came to me directly" (IONS website).

From this experience, Mitchell came to the conclusion that reality consists of a lot more than he'd previously been led to believe from his scientific training, and he thought that a deeper understanding of consciousness could perhaps lead to a new understanding of our reality. It is good to have an open mind as to how cells know how to function, and where their direction and intelligence comes from, asking questions such as, 'who designed us?' There will be more of this in my Soul book.

A WALKING, TALKING COMPASS

Scientists know that a variety of animals are able to sense and react to electric fields, including humans – they can sense electric fields and move along them. This is evident, for example, in wound healing. In this case, the actual sensor mechanism has been found. In the late 80's I was looking at sensors in the whiskers of little fish, producing large pictures of these guys by scanning electron microscopy.

"Like tiny crawling compass needles, whole living cells and cell fragments orient and move in response to electric fields – but in opposite directions, scientists have found. Their results could ultimately lead to new ways to heal wounds and deliver stem cell therapies" (Davis, 2013).

Stem cells are undifferentiated cells, which means they are undecided as to what they want to be when they grow up. When an embryonic stem cell is at the first stage of its development, it has the potential to grow into any type of cell, and some unknown intelligence tells them who they will become. "Using an electric field to pull stem cells through a fluid, a team of researchers from Scotland has now demonstrated a way to easily distinguish undifferentiated embryonic stem cells from later-stage stem cells whose fate is sealed" (Velugotla et al., 2012).

Back in May 2013, a team of scientists at Oregon Health and Science University were able to reprogram human skin cells back into embryonic stem cells at the stage where they didn't know who they wanted to become when they were older." It is believed that stem cell therapies may hold the promise of replacing cells damaged through injury or illness; diseases or conditions that might be treated through stem cell therapy include Parkinson's disease, multiple sclerosis, cardiac disease, and spinal cord injuries."

DOLLY

As the first mammal to be cloned from an adult cell, Dolly the sheep (from The Roslin Institute) is by far the world's most famous clone. However, cloning has existed in nature since the dawn of life – i.e. from asexual bacteria. In basic terms, clones are all around us and are fundamentally no different to other organisms; a clone has the same DNA sequence as its parent, making them genetically identical. To achieve this in a lab, somatic cell nuclear transfer (SCNT) is used in embryonic stem cell research, or in regenerative medicine where it is sometimes referred to as 'therapeutic cloning'. It can also be used as the first step in the process of reproductive cloning.

In SCNT, the nucleus – which contains the organism's DNA – of a somatic cell (a body cell other than a sperm or egg cell) is removed and the rest of the cell discarded. The nucleus of an egg cell is removed at the same time to allow the nucleus of the somatic cell to go in its place. Interestingly, the somatic cell nucleus is reprogrammed by the host cell. The egg – now containing the nucleus of a somatic cell – is then stimulated with an electric shock, and will therefore begin to divide. This reminds me of shocking a heart in order to restart it.

After many mitotic divisions in culture, this single cell forms a blastocyst (an early stage embryo consisting of approximately 100 cells) that features almost identical DNA to the original organism. Long before the infamous Dolly, several clones had been produced in the lab, including mice, frogs, and cows, all of which had been cloned from embryo DNA.

In being the first mammal to be cloned from an adult cell, Dolly really was remarkable; it was a major scientific achievement as it demonstrated that the DNA from adult cells – despite having specialised as one particular type of cell – can be used to create an entire organism. "From 277 cell fusions, 29 early embryos developed and were implanted into 13 surrogate mothers. But only one pregnancy went to full term, and the 6.6kg Finn Dorset lamb 6LLS (alias Dolly) was born after 148 days" (AnimalResearch.info).

I remember seeing a picture of Dolly and her baby lamb, Bonnie. She mated, having lambs in a normal way and leading a pleasant life until she was euthanised in 2003, 6.5 years after her creation. Sheep can live to age 11 or 12, but Dolly suffered from arthritis in a hind leg joint and from a virus-induced lung tumour that is common among sheep which are raised indoors.

So why did she age so fast? The DNA is held in chromosomes, and in the tips of these chromosomes are telomeres, little clocks that count down.

Dolly was created with the nucleus of a six-year-old sheep. Also, the mitochondrial DNA had been inherited from the donor mother. This was an eye opener into how it might be possible to avoid diseases caused by the mother's mitochondria, such as muscular dystrophy. The anti-aging problem still hasn't been cracked – as far as I know, anyway. There's always time.

IF YOUR HEART'S SPARK PLUGS AND VALVES FAIL, YOU GET AN ENGINE BLOW OUT

In my last book I talked about the heart-mind link and the brain cells within the heart. In my Body volume I will just briefly mention that this organ is a pump. The pacemaker sparks the beat, and this electricity is then conducted through the heart and cells within the atrioventricular node, which slows down the contraction in order to allow an emptying of the atria to happen before the ventricle. The heart strings pull the valves shut to allow the heart to fill, and open to allow blood through. When the aortic valve opens, the blood rushes out. The electric resonance allows our hearts to beat with a rhythm necessary for oxygenating our body at different levels of activity, and it can be measured by ECG electrocardiogram, a first-line diagnostic test used by paramedics.

GOOD RHYTHM, GOOD HEALTH

Heart rate variability – the change in the time intervals between adjacent heartbeats – is directly related to the body's regulatory systems, their efficiency, and their health. "An optimal level of HRV within an organism reflects healthy function and an inherent self-regulatory capacity, adaptability, or resilience," McCraty and Shaffer write (2016). Although generally, the greater the HRV the better, they note that too much variability, or instability, "such as arrhythmias or nervous system chaos is detrimental to efficient physiological functioning and energy utilization… Too little variation indicates age-related system depletion, chronic stress, pathology, or inadequate functioning in various levels of self-regulatory control systems." The authors here are HeartMath Institute (HMI) Director of Research, Rollin McCraty, Ph.D. and Fred Shaffer, and in conclusion, they write: "Numerous studies have provided evidence that coherence training consisting of intentional activation of positive emotions paired with HRV coherence feedback facilitates significant improvements in wellness and well-being indicators in a variety of populations." I had the privilege of trying this out onstage with Patrick Holford, and I presented this technology at a Swizz Z Factor event as well. Also, my dear friend Joseph McClendon – and his co-presenter, Tony Robbins – fully engage with this stress-buster.

HOW HARD SHOULD I BE REVVING MY ENGINE?

Your heart rate – the number of times your heart beats within one minute – is a good measure of both cardiovascular fitness and how hard you are working out. Most athletes know that measuring your resting heart rate, then comparing it to their rate whilst during a workout, will tell you about your current fitness, as well as your potential fat burning and cardiovascular fitness. The time taken to recover back to your resting rate after stopping exercise is an indication of fitness too.

Many things will affect your heart rate, including emotions, fitness level, medications, and how fat you are. Keeping fit strengthens your heart, making your muscles more efficient at using oxygen. The amount of blood pumping through your body at each heartbeat is then increased, resulting in a lower resting heart rate. A resting heart rate is generally between 60 and 100 beats per minute, unless you're super fit in which case it will be lower. Your target heart rate is the number of beats per minute you should be aiming for when working out, and you can monitor your heart rate periodically during your workout to ensure you're on track. Simply put, it is 50% to 85% of your maximum heart rate, and general guidelines state that your maximum heart rate is roughly 220 minus your age. From that, you can determine your target heart rate by calculating both 50% and 85% of your maximum.

NOT ENOUGH NORFOLK SAND TO RUN ON

I had such fun in a running shop in Norwich, choosing an orange tracksuit and a trendy pair of running shoes; I had a quick check on the treadmill in the shop and ended up with two lovely pairs of trainers. Although I could run faster in them, they lacked the shock absorbency my old pair had, and consequently my back reacted to it. I thought about the Dolly story and genetics, pondering that it is important to consider our genetic predisposition to sport. A sheep has little hooves to cope with wet terrain and grass lands, whereas a greyhound has incredibly spritely legs – and then there's me. Road running is not kind to aging joints no matter how strong and flexible we are, and the invention of tarmac did nothing for arthritic joints.

I went back to my practice biomechanics lab to see how much greyhound and how much dachshund were in my feet, as well as looking at the points at which the pressures transmitted up through my feet as I ran. I was called Flipper at the hospital because I have size 7 feet that are a bit flat. When I was very young I was a ballerina, and I was given exercises to help the flatness in the arches of my feet – insoles for young children is a controversial subject. As I walk across the GaitScan plate, 4096 sensors are set to scan the plantar surface of my foot in motion. The GaitScan system records timing sequences during walking and captures the relative pressure for each of ten distinct anatomical landmarks.

The result is the detection of imbalances and other indicators of common lower limb pathologies. It can also be a predictor of lower limb osteoarthritis. The data from Gaitscan –together with a thorough history and biomechanical assessment done by one of my experts – helps to determine if my foot function is related to my back problem. 25% of my bones are in my foot; I have one in my skeleton box in my office – so many little nuts and bolts of bone.

Each day we are told that we take (or should take) around 10,000 steps, and it is the complex interaction of my foot on the ground and the correct alignment of knee, hip, and pelvis over my foot, that will affect my spine, especially with the shock-absorbing powers of my lumbar discs now leaving me. The best biomechanical fit in the way my foot hits the floor will enable more efficient, pain free walking and running. Abnormal foot function can result in common conditions such as localised foot pain (metatarsalgia, bunions, neuroma), heel and ankle pain (plantar fasciitis/achilles tendinosis), and other lower limb problems such as shin splints and patellofemoral pain.

PRESSURE MAPPING

GaitScan gives you the ability to view a patient's plantar pressure distribution in both 2D and 3D. The synchronised mode allows for a direct right and left foot comparison and displays the centre of pressure or "gait line" of the foot throughout the gait cycle, while detailed images allow for the easy identification of high-pressure areas and existing biomechanical inefficiencies. My feet lack a certain springiness, and my right toe joint takes a hammering. I may well need to wear some insoles; I'll let you know…

YOUR THIGH BONE'S CONNECTED TO YOUR KNEE BONE

I need my muscles to move in the correct sequence in order to walk. Attached to my bones are about 700 named muscles that make up roughly half my weight, with each muscle being an organ of skeletal muscle tissue, blood vessels, tendons, and nerves. Muscle is also found inside the heart, digestive organs, and blood vessels. Skeletal muscle is the only voluntary muscle tissue – it is controlled consciously – and every physical action I consciously perform (e.g. speaking, walking, or writing) requires skeletal muscle.

The function of this skeletal muscle is to consciously contract in order to move parts of the body closer to the bone that the muscle is attached to. Most skeletal muscles are attached to two bones across a joint, so the muscle serves to move parts of those bones closer to each other. Type I fibres are very slow and deliberate in their contractions, and are found throughout our body for both posture and stamina. They are very resistant to fatigue because they use aerobic respiration (oxygen) to produce energy from sugar. We find Type I fibres near the spine; very high concentrations of Type I fibres hold the body up throughout the day. Without these muscles we could go limp, which could be very embarassing indeed.

Just a quick aside, we also have Type II A and Type II B fibres. Type II A fibres are faster and stronger than Type Is, but they do not have as much endurance. They are especially prevalent in the legs, where they work to support your body throughout a long day of walking, standing about working on patients, or shopping.

Type II B fibres are even faster, stronger, and paler, have even less endurance, and lack myoglobin, an oxygen-storing pigment. We find Type II B particularly in the upper body, where they give speed and strength to the arms and chest at the expense of stamina. Do you ever notice how arm swinging doesn't last quite as long as the walking does, and how carrying shopping makes your arms ache quite fast? Skeletal muscle cells form when many smaller progenitor cells lump themselves together to create long, straight, strong, multinucleated fibres. These are called myofibrils, which are like a train, while the carriages/units are called sarcomeres.

The sarcolemma is the cell membrane of muscle fibres, and it acts as a conductor for electrochemical signals that stimulate muscle cells. Connected to the cell wall are transverse tubules (T-tubules) that help carry these electrochemical signals into the middle of the muscle fibre. The sarcoplasmic reticulum (the storage facility) for calcium ions ($Ca2+$) are vital to muscle contraction. Mitochondria (the power houses of the cell) are abundant in muscle cells in order to break down sugars and provide energy in the form of ATP (adenosine triphosphate) to active muscles.

When the immune system is attacked, muscles can suffer problems in a similar way to joints. For instance, polymyalgia is a rheumatoid-like condition triggered by stress or a virus. This is a rather debilitating condition but it does improve and resolve over time.

Muscles respond to our lifestyle and what we feed them with. How I walk with good posture and eat healthily for my muscles is all visible to an expert eye watching the way I walk, so there's no hiding – be fit and walk the walk.

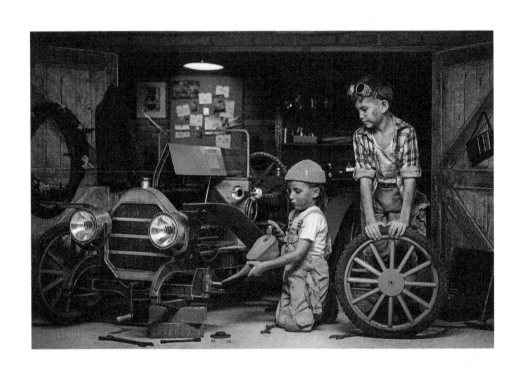

Chapter Three

"The key to successful aging is to pay as little attention to it as possible."

– Judith Regan

Treating and healing through the body's wisdom

HEALER, HEAL THYSELF

"The modern world has sought to deny the sacredness of human life. But it has not denied it absolutely. Rather, it has distorted it. It has done away with the notion of sacredness altogether. It has merely replaced it with relatively superficial notions such as the equality of life."
- Donald DeMarco

"If you talk to a man in a language he understands, that goes to his head. If you talk to him in his language, that goes to his heart."
 - Nelson Mandela

I grew up attending a darling little village school across the road from a church, and as a young child the Bible readings were taught to me so well that I could actually recite them. It was about a healer called Jesus, who came to this planet – sent by his father, God – to remind us of the soul within humanity. By placing healing hands on people, he eased their suffering. Then he got crucified for it. Not a very positive message for a little child, I thought – heal the sick, but make sure you look out for pieces of wood with nails in them.

This concept of the laying on of hands transcends cultures and time; I have sat with shamans and priests and vicars, all of them having their own specific ritual and their own Gods. Despite their different beliefs and backgrounds, it struck me that there was a large similarity in all of their rituals, in that they all lay their hands on the suffering and then open their heart and empathy to their 'victim' – with one eye open for a wooden cross!

I grew up in a Christian community – Church of England – and when I was a teenager, a delightful Catholic priest holidayed with my family in Tenerife. I have sat down with wiccans and spiritualists and buddhists and all kind of shamans. I've studied with Chinese, Korean, Malaysian, Canadian, Mexican, American, and European doctors, and my respect for so many different points of view just keeps on growing. Constantly learning about different beliefs and different ways of approaching health can be incredibly eye-opening.

TO TREAT OR NOT TO TREAT HOLISTICALLY

There seems to be a natural progression of physical intervention between patient and practitioner, and this has been echoed over many centuries and throughout the entire world. The ritual starts with building a trusting connection, in order to converse and communicate in the language of the patient. This then proceeds onto communicating with a light exploratory touch using various methods. Some shamans start working in auric fields, praying to Gods or touching lightly, followed by a heavier touch – with hands, stones, bamboo canes, or needles – into learned points.

In many cultures these learned points are often acupressure points, whereas in the western hemisphere it is more likely to be the perceived area of injury or tension. Then, if deemed necessary, surgery is prescribed to cut it out, using either psychic surgery or actual surgery. In later years we started to benefit from pain relief during surgery, whether it be hypnotism, acupuncture, or anaesthesia. Physical therapy is in part intellectual, but it is mostly intuitive, experimental, and is improved with experience. It is an art, with a blend of many techniques, giving a unique fingerprint to the practitioner's touch. Just like language, it is a colourful combination of learnt words.

The stark difference I experienced when studying the western approach in England, Europe, Canada, and America, compared with the more eastern/ holistic approach, was in the prescription. The western orthodox treatment dosage is prescribed by the practitioner to the patient, with little intuitive feedback. In the role of an instructor to peers, I am asked to prescribe exactly the position, depth, frequency, time duration of the said treatment, and the prognosis. Now, and here's the worrying bit – so get your seat belts on again – it is expected to happen with no mention by the practitioner of the patient's interaction with the treatment. I will say that again: with no mention of the patient's interaction with and participation in the treatment.

This is the sticking point: in my early days of teaching – which made me look further afield, taking myself abroad and away from universities to understand the dance between patient and therapist – nearly every course I attended always talked about how to deal with the patient's problems. Nothing was ever said about the importance of the therapist's wellbeing in this interaction.

I am writing this at the stage in my life when my colleagues are retiring from physical treatments. My friend Andy has done soft tissue work for many years in my clinic, and at 55, his body's wisdom is talking to him – he's looking to teach more and is leaving the clinic next month. Another friend of mine, Pam (who is between mine and Andy's age), has just qualified in nutrition to cut back on the demands of long sessions of physical exertion and posture in healing. Another friend (who has also worked at my clinic in the past) is thinking of leaving surgery as weariness is biting hard. This made me feel old today, and I had to give myself a strong talking to.

I have been physically working on patients for nearly 30 years – with very little time off or time away – and now, for the first time in my life, my body is weary and my hands and back have started complaining in the mornings, not to mention after a long day in the cold. Also, the brief times I've spent away from working on patients were mostly so I could learn or teach treatment techniques, so it wasn't time 'off' exactly. The nature of the posture we maintain whilst working is not conducive to a healthy body, and therefore these books are aimed at both the patient and the therapist, so you can gain an understanding about the need to keep as healthy as you can, in everything you do. All of our bodies have a sell-by date, and suffering the pains of early aging must be tackled rather than endured.

I am now witnessing and experiencing the damage that we as practitioners do to our bodies whilst rescuing others with bad posture, not to mention lifting, and the repetitive use of our own limbs to impart physical changes in the patient receiving the treatment. Furthermore, the unrelenting stress of listening to people's suffering, and feeling the exhausting responsibility that the healer must cure the patient, and (incorrectly) have the sole responsibility of achieving this, takes its toll. We are called Human Beings, not Human Doings. No, that sounds wrong – haha.

As practitioners, if we don't listen to our body's wisdom, how can we expect our patients to? If we're not setting the correct example, we will destroy our own bodies well before time.

SHOULDER ON ICE

I'd just like to give one example here about coming at something from a different angle, and that is my investment in studying how to treat frozen shoulders – a very prolonged, painful pathology. There is no known reason for it, but speculation suggests a combination of wear and tear, stress, hormones, the immune system, and changes in the cervical disc heights – hence nerve conduction, or the ongoing irritation of rotator cuff tendons, and so on and so on. No matter how it starts, it leads to a leathery thickened bursa and lots and lots of pain.

I am spoilt in that I have two friends who are shoulder surgeons – Mr Vinod Kathuria and Roger Hackney – both of whom kindly allowed me to study their assessments and surgical approaches. Both are rather handsome too, so it's very easy on the eye to observe their surgery, if you know what I mean, ladies.

I spent many weekends in my early twenties on orthopaedic courses with names like Maitland and Cyriax and McKenzie, the idea being to make sure we could be accountable, and to replicate a precise treatment modality and record it in our notes for our colleagues to follow. We needed strong hands, shiny badges on pressed white tunics, and a disciplined mind with attention to detail – not to mention a sound understanding of the need for painkilling meds.

In my opinion, accountability stifles creativity, but we live in the world we live in, and sadly pain is often wrapped up in fear and anger, leading to some people accusing others of malpractice, even if it is totally unjustified. So, it's in order to safeguard our friends and fellow practitioners that we batter them with rules about note-taking and exams. Also, to a certain extent, I do understand that as a patient, trust is earned by knowing that the treatments are regulated and honed, with the practitioner being up to date with their education. As I've said before, the training in the NHS is an excellent grounding.

Therefore, in the early years I worked on shoulders in my very strictly trained way, with everything having to be recognised and approved. For one of the many recognised treatments for a frozen shoulder (adhesive capsulitis), the patient would have to lie on their back. Armed with extensive training on the anatomy of the shoulder – plus the treatment modality training book of how to stretch the shoulder in a precise way – you would then carry out the said treatment on the patient. You would continue to do said treatment unless the distressed patient was screaming loudly (rather than quietly; it's OK to scream quietly). You could alter the angle if it was allowed and if it was accepted practice, and you noted the exact pressure and frequency of manipulations. You kept the hand positions in the correct place as recognised by the society of chartered physiotherapists, and you noted down the taught symbols so a colleague could replicate the treatment in the future.

You were allowed to make appropriate polite conversation, whilst also listening to the conversations in the cubicles either side of yours, which were divided by thin white curtains. You then gave an outcome code for the patient, and agreed the next treatment goal – say, 10 degrees more elevation of the arm, and a 2-point change on the VAS (visual analogue scale) on pain. You were convinced you had given a good treatment to the anxious, sore, and bewildered patient, who went away with home exercises that they feared due to the pain they would go through doing them. Good job done! You noted the number of repeat visits before discharge – whether they got better, or whether they needed an injection and then surgery. There was an outcome code for everything. Then, if the patient did not return, it would help the waiting list and department funding. I was amused to read the wide range of outcome codes, from '5/5 excellent shoulder recovery' to 'R1', meaning death. Apologies for being a little, shall we say, tongue-in-cheek, but I'm just being honest.

It was taking courses in alternative approaches and fusing the best of both orthodox and alternative medicine that was the catalyst to igniting a strong healing response. Not only did my patients blossom, but they also actually enjoyed their treatments. The writing up of notes wasn't really feasible here; if I wrote up my notes with the details of what I really did, it would take up an hour or two per thirty minute or hour appointment, restricting my treating time to the bare minimum. Also, unless my colleagues had trained for nearly 30 years – with ongoing studying and having taken various courses in alternative medicine – they would not be able to replicate the results from my notes anyway. So, instead, I chose to write the briefest of notes on the techniques covered within the remit of my colleagues' chartered training and postgrad courses I knew them to have taken. Then I made a promise to myself I would write books that would include all of my knowledge (or at least some of it).

When Prof Gunn trained me to be one of the leading lights in pain relief with IMS dry needling, the teaching had to be extremely exact and precise, and I thoroughly endorse the need for seriousness and precision in training; after all, you have someone's life in the palm of your hand, for living with pain is a nightmare. Poor skills can leave the patient in more pain than they were before, or at worst, even kill. So, you can take your seat belts off now; it's not that I'm anti-good, traditional, clinical practice, I just believe that teaching must create a sound platform for the inexperienced. Overall, I believe in learning the other arts that complement medicine and allow preventative health to blossom.

JULIE'S SHOULDER FROZE

Right, now it's back in my time machine to the 90's, and another manic day in outpatients. I was in my twenties, still fit and enthusiastic and armed with a wall of certificates to prove I could sort out stiff shoulder joints. I could surely force a misbehaving shoulder to start behaving again – you just had to move in it certain ways with a certain force, and it would give. Anyway, that day my shiny pager went off: it was a post-op MUA (manipulation under anaesthetic), last week's failed shoulder case from my physio department.

I had spent countless weekends manipulating healthy physios' shoulders on orthopaedic courses to prove I could cure just this kind of case, so why had we failed again?

It was another late Thursday evening and another patient, this one sent down for injections then surgery in order to stretch the shoulder out under anaesthetic. Only this time, something clicked into place. As usual, I was paged to go onto the ward and see a patient post-op, and I found the patient with her arm tied to the bed, sobbing with fear that the physio would come and hurt her. It was imperative that the shoulder be stretched out to make sure the torn adhesions did not glue together again, and as I looked at the patient, my soul was screaming, 'there has to be another way!'

Her notes suggested red keys: traumatic home life, overweight, unfit, and stressed up to the hilt. My eastern courses had taught me that her path to recovery was more of a well-choreographed dance of energy and movement between this lady and her therapist, something alien to my orthodox training. Now, let me share my thought processes regarding blending her treatment modalities to allow a comfortable approach to promote healing – I'll just pause the story here a moment to explain about the eastern treatments I used.

Japanese shiatsu is very much about the ease of joint movement, positioning, and feeling the nine levels of energy on meridian points. Hands are placed on specific acupressure points whilst moving the joints, whereas with western physiotherapy you just place your hands on the body without sensing energy or tapping into meridian points.

Reiki – and a less well-known technique called ohashi – is all about the therapist working in a state of meditation. It is about using both hands to constantly gain receiver/patient feedback, and adjusting the position and strength according to that feedback. It is not giving what you think is needed from theory, but giving them what their body actually asks for. This is the bit that excites me, as it is a healthy way of physically treating; it heals and exercises the practitioner's body at the same time as the patient's, rather than destroying it like many other treatments can do.

One of the practitioner's hands is called the mother, sensing patient feedback, while the other is the messenger, giving treatment. The practitioner needs to learn 'oneness' with the receiver and leave preconceived ideas about what treatment they think the patient should have behind. It is the art of being and not doing; you are there to help the receiving patient facilitate their healing through a state of being in the zone, and awakening their body's wisdom as to what needs to be done by themselves. Also, you need to work towards a quiet acceptance, if healing is not possible or even if death is imminent – and in this instance, I mean the patient's!

Therapists should be aware of their way of life and lead by example. For instance, physical fitness, plus good balance and a state of focus meditation make it possible to physically treat people. Did you know that Pilates is a western child of Qi Kong and Tai Chi with a mind/soul disconnect?

HOMEWORK:
Go and ask a friend to massage your back, then ask why they chose a certain strength of touch. Also ask them what they are reading from your body in order to do it that way.

When working in a close, energetic way, your personality and vitality will have an impact on the experience of the patient, and in order to attune your treatments to a synergistic approach, you need maturity, a lot of experience, and a good scientific or medical training background to keep your feet on the ground. I do not recommend this work for the uninitiated youthful enthusiast. Communication on this level with allow both the giver and the receiver to take part in self development – spiritually, physically, and psychologically. Carried out correctly and in moderation, this will enable treating to continue beyond the years that physical therapists retire from treating; energy medicine is a wonderful addition to sound medical or physiotherapy knowledge.

I miss my weekly healing tutorials with my friends June, Ken, and Lesley; I didn't appreciate just how much they kept my physical body healthy until those sessions ended this year. That total honesty of mind, body, spirit, and trust in letting go is just not appreciated in our culture. I will share with you some of our incredible experiences, for the first time, in the next volume: The Soul.

Anyway, back to Julie now, the lady with the frozen shoulder. I'd decided that there had to be another way, and after a decision comes the action, otherwise a decision on its own is powerless. Armed with the skills of Reiki and Shiatsu – as well as the information I'd gleaned from various soft tissue courses – I decided to brave it out and integrate it into my orthodox traditional training.

I discreetly placed my hands on the patient's skin, and while she thought I was simply helping her to move her arm, I was actually putting my hands on the chakra points, listening to what her body told me. The tears soon stopped and I promised to get her up to my department the next day to start work. I was on call, and it was just another Sunday morning on duty.

The next day I laid her on the couch, on the side, with her sore arm upper most, just like I was taught in shiatsu – except that it was deliciously comfortable for me compared to the floor boards of the draughty old hall I was taught in. As with Reiki, I asked permission to work, and with Acupressure I held those points; with my physiotherapy knowledge, I knew how far to push the hot, sore joint. I took a deep breath and steadied myself. Then I started to pace my breath with hers, moving her arm as I felt she was telling me to do through my listening hands.

Briefly, I gave her a soft tissue massage that also massaged her meridians, which are called the large and small intestine, the triple warmer, lung, heart and gallbladder, and the pericardium, gently pausing over the acupressure points that called to me. I stimulated the elbow chakra PC3 and post throat chakra Gov14. Then I used a laser at these points, as well as at any tight tender places, which are called ashi points. I cradled the scapula (the shoulder blade) and gently circled the arm. The arm moved easily and painlessly – so different to the doing method.

Had the shoulder not just been manipulated under anaesthetic, I would have added in mobilisations to the lower aspect of the neck, as well as IMS dry needling to the tight fascia around the shoulder. Then, if the pain was under control, I would finish with shockwave treatment to help any calcified tendons or tethered fascia, which may have avoided the need for an anaesthetic. I had no idea how to write my notes up (well, not the alternative part of my notes, anyway); although trained and certified in these techniques, if the patient complained and the shoulder stiffened, it would be clear that I was off protocol.

I continued to piece together treatment protocols that were on a good foundation and grounded with recognised treatment modalities, then I weaved in the aspects of healing that allowed me to achieve the results both the surgeon and the patient wanted. I chose home exercises that embraced more of a linked mind-body approach, and that still had the same goals of strength, flexibility, and pain relief applied.

I made sure this combined approach was sound and not deemed out in 'woo-woo' land. However, the downside was that I could not teach these ways outside my clinics, as they were deemed by many medical and physiotherapy professions as being 'unorthodox' approaches. This fascinating knowledge, steeped in the history of thousands of years of experience, was just thrown out, using instead a relatively short-lived evolution of orthodox remedial massage/physiotherapeutic treatments. Sadly, even that approach is now becoming extinct at the hands of a rapidly evolving, hands off, exercise prescribing, and over-intellectualised group of practitioners.

This patient did regain shoulder movement and keep it moving, with no need for ongoing painkillers, and she even went on to join pilates and yoga classes before starting to teach her own. Yes, her preventative program kept her shoulder healthy. She exercised with care, and consistently ate healthily and shared her knowledge with others.

HIS CALF ACHE WAS JUST AN EXTENSION OF HIS SPINE

When I have a new patient, I usually ask why they have come to see me, whether or not they believe they can get better, and what kind of therapy they feel comfortable with. Some patients request physical treatment only, as they do not wish for any deeper healing, and this must be accepted and honoured.

THE STORY OF EDWIN

One autumn morning last year, a rather handsome, quiet, middle-aged clinical professor came to see me because he found his gym workout was irritating the hell out of his elbow and ankle. He was only too happy to show off his slim, toned body, and it made a pleasant change from far too many patients who eat far too much and exercise far too little.

First, I watched the way he walked and sat down so I could choose movement patterns that could be altered for him. Then I went over the 4 keys, to which he scored green in food, water, supplements, and fitness. He scored amber in lifestyle – he was working a little too much. Family life had been fraught with problems until recently, and on the whole he loved his work. He just couldn't quite get his life/work balance right. His mind was amber and at times red, as he found teaching at university stressful, and he also found it difficult to switch off. I intuitively sensed some deeper issues, and it made sense that keeping fit calmed his mind. Although he held both scientific and holistic beliefs, he was very guarded and not comfortable with the spiritual aspect affecting him.

114

"I haven't injured myself or upped my workouts or done anything to cause these pains; they've just crept up on me," he stated. This clearly irritated the hell out of him, and when he dug his thumb into the offending areas – grimacing to show me his pain – his face said it all. "My pain is deep and aching, not sharp, and I haven't done anything to cause it," he repeated, at a loss as to why this was happening to him.

This made me decide to explore his physical body for neuropathic pain, and to reach into the deeper spinal muscles and relevant joints and ligaments. It seemed wise to be wary of energetic healing and to leave out the fascial energetic matrix – the home of acupuncture – till later. This aspect of healing needs a deeper level of understanding and trust between practitioner and patient – the symbiotic dance needs a trusting relationship built slowly over time.

I attended to the symptoms in his physical body – palpating along the muscle bands of his lower back – and it was clear that he was tighter on one side. This could have been disc irritation, or it could have been his biomechanics; the way he sits and walks, and either a fixed or habitual posture. Telltale signs of collagen lines on his lower lumbar/back and lower cervical/neck suggested a thinning of the underlying discs, especially over lumbar 5, the base of his spine. His buttock was acutely tender over the gluteus medius (see the glossary for these terms) and deep into the piriformis. His hamstring was slightly more tense, with sensitivity being increased again over the division of the sciatic nerve at the back of the knee, tight bands in his calf muscles, and a moving tenderness where his ankle flexors wove around his ankle.

This was all pointing to neuropathic changes to his L5 nerve root, as well as mild peripheral nerve changes, causing small contractures down the limb and the ache. This type of problem is insidious, and is often a normal part of aging related to postural issues, causing disc narrowing spondylosis and changes in nerves, from very mild to severe neuropathy.

Now, let me share with you the postural exercises I taught him.

HOMEWORK:

Let's look at head posture. Use your phone to take a picture side-ways on, then get a friend so you can look at their alignment of ear over shoulder – with a pointed chin held just an inch forward, the leverage meaning twice the pressure goes through unsuspecting neck discs. Poor head posture is rotting your discs. Do you sit as if your legs are the front legs of a chair, taking your body weight both through your legs and your bottom through the real chair? Or do you slouch? Could you sit on a fit ball at times? Think about your posture and how it could be improved.

During a follow-up appointment, the shaman in me would have looked to help him heal issues in his auric body, balance his chakras, and use key acupuncture points in his fascial plane. However, the orthodox physio in me believed that just for now, the approach should be gentle; single acupuncture needles, laser and physiotherapy mobilisations seemed appropriate for his mind to accept and his body to facilitate a healing response.

VANCOUVER, AND SHERLOCK HOMES IS HUNTING DOWN MR. NEUROPATHIC PAIN

Now, I'm going to allow my time machine to drift back to a cold, wet, January morning in the Vancouver clinic in 1999. Professor Gunn was half dressed in a suit he was getting adjusted for a presentation later that week. The jet lag was biting, and it wasn't really helped by the healthy glass of water I was drinking.

I was attending another training session on lecturing on Gunn IMS, and it was a day we were reviewing diagnostic physical signs. We went into one of the teaching cubicles where a shy doctor – a student of IMS – was needling a patient. Prof turned to me and asked me to quiz the attending doctor about the patient's x-rays, scans, bloods, and routine orthopaedic assessment, which invariably misses the culprit, Mr Pain (you can read more about this in an article I wrote for a magazine entitled 'The Pain Jungle').

The prof said, "although most musculoskeletal conditions appear as separate entities – i.e. tendinitis, plantar fasciitis, and tenosynovitis – this is often not the case." He turned to me. "What do we look for, Ms Snazell?"

I knew he needed me to go over the physical signs that we need to hunt out in order to find the elusive Mr Pain, but as I was daydreaming and jetlagged to hell and back, I jumped when he mentioned my name, stuttering a parrot-like response: "Sensation can be enhanced, and be more painful over the affected skin/dermatome. Muscles will be tender over their shortened contracted muscle bands and above motor endplates, the effect called allodynia."(I explain all of these terms in the glossary).

"Go on," said the prof. "Describe what our autonomic nervous system is showing us."

Feeling like I was back in school, I went over in my mind the names of what sounded to me like Japanese motorbikes. "We have to find vasomotor, pilomotor, and sudomotor changes, Prof." Lots of funny words, I said to myself; the medical language sure does like Greek and Latin mixes. I went on: "It means that if the nerve is faulty, the part of the body it looks after shows subtle changes. The area feels colder, features vasoconstriction, and after activity, more sweating is seen (sudomotor) in the affected dermatome. Goosebumps can be seen, and if you press on a tender point, it can jump (pilomotor). You get hair loss in the area – which are called trophic changes – and if you push a matchstick gently into the skin, it leaves a dent called trophedema. Muscle contractures are palpable and tender and often have 'trigger points'; they can restrict joint range and accelerate osteoarthritic changes. The tendinous attachments to the bone are thickened and tender."

"All this should be documented as evidence that this type of painful problem is not just some syndrome given yet another name," said the prof in response, though he should have added: 'and needs a poke with my needle'.

Just then, my time machine threw me back into my clinic room into October 2015, where the patient was thrashing around and saying his arm had gone dead while hanging it off the couch in a weird position.

CASE STUDY PART 2
HIS ELBOW WAS AN EXTENSION OF HIS NECK

On his second visit, Edwin asked me to also look at his arm pain. I wondered how much I should explain about his problem regarding my physical and psychic sightings, then decided that body rot is not a cheerful conversation, and clearly his mind was closed to discuss deeper issues. So instead, I gently eased some of his muscle tension with soft tissue work, and used unwinding release techniques and Maitlands mobilisations over his lower back. I used a small number of acupuncture needles placed in Chinese bladder meridian points that are good for back issues, later using an IMS dry needle technique to alleviate his symptoms by releasing deep, silent muscle contractures to fire up reflexes to his nerves and talk to his brain.

I made a mental note that if the disc was inflamed and degenerate, then technologies such as pulsed shortwave – or better still, (nuclear) magnetic resonance – would help with the repair process and the inflamed degenerate cells. He would also need to look to his posture and spinal flexibility.

Next, I turned my attention to his elbow issue. The skin on the back of his neck showed a clear crease line at C5/6 (cervical disc five and six). Testing his neck movements by sideflexing (doing a head tilt) and rotating to the right showed that he stopped at two thirds of his full movement, closing down soft tissue around his C6 nerve root. This was giving him his pain. The muscles around his shoulder blade had palpable tight bands. The levator scapulae (which lifts the shoulder blade) and traps were tight on the right. Then, as I felt his right arm tissue, his muscles that enable him to bend his elbow, his biceps, and the supinator were tender, and the extensor digitorum brevis (the muscle that helps in extending the elbow and carrying shopping with the first two fingers, or writing) was very leathery and sore. He was showing signs of tennis elbow. Again, it all related to posture and use. As I had learnt from my trips to Canada, all of the physical signs were there in his neck and arm: the coldness, goosebumps, hair loss, and tight bands.

Tight bands or muscle contractures are often painless, so why can they become so painful? The answer involves many different reasons: neuropathic nerve, chronic overload of a muscle, repetitive actions, poor posture, leaving a muscle in a shortened position for some time, virus, emotional stress, strains due to arthritic joint instability, and so on. When I asked him, it turned out that Edwin had been driving and typing for long periods of time without stretching. Muscles must be able to receive and respond to nerve impulses, as well as being able to shorten, be stretched, and be elastic enough not to look like Bridget Jones's knickers after use, instead being able to return to their original shape.

It wasn't until the end of his visit that he told me he'd sustained a neck injury some time ago, something that could account for these changes. I knew then that he would benefit from shockwave and IMS into the thickened part of the extensor tendon, then progressive stretches to the tendon with laser and MRT, plus any healing modality to help tendinopathy – the thickened tendon – which attaches to the bone at the elbow and tends to be angry and degenerative.

Just a quick time travel trip back to operating theatres in Leeds now, at around the year 2010. I can remember a friend and surgeon, Mr Roger Hackney, correcting me during one of my theatre observations, saying that tennis elbow is a degenerative condition, not an inflammatory one.

Back in the time machine again now to a course in Chichester in the 90's, where I remember looking after a fascinating Professor Janda, who had polio, the poor thing. He came from a teaching hospital in Prague where spinal pain came under the faculty of all neurological problems, not in orthopaedics – hence his ward of patients could be victims of stroke, Parkinson's, motor neuron, or back pain.

He spoke of the evolution of muscles, evident throughout the animal kingdom. He said that muscles were either one thing or the other (which as a biologist, fascinated me), being more postural in function and always partially contracted, or more able to move specific joints with rapid contractions, some muscles always heading towards tightness while others moved towards the look of a baggy cardigan.

Unhealthy muscles do not return to their nice, elastic, full length after contracting, hence joints get tighter, lymph more sluggish, blood flow less, and with it, less oxygen. The taut bands cannot enjoy being flexible and pain free like their buddies. The faulty nerve input to these muscle bands hinders the overall performance of the muscle in response to nerve stimuli about contraction, the intensity, the proprioception (sense) of position, balance, and strength. After treatment the muscle functions well again, which is essential in sport.

This was all going through my head as I looked at Edwin's body. His tight muscles needed some deep muscle release with Gunn IMS needling, as well as laser to make him more comfortable. However, his mind was not ready for the shock of such an invasive treatment, so instead I used a gentle needling technique around the nerve root in his spine, his neck muscles, shoulder blade, and around the elbow. The reason for this was to improve the range of movement, reduce the sensitivity, and promote healing through the release of local healing factors.

This treatment approach was aimed at the effects of the neuropathic nerves on his muscles, built up over years of postural issues. It couldn't make any structural bony changes; it would just give the discs more breathing space, and the nerves, the muscles, and the joints a little more play. The release of muscle contractures should take most of the neuropathic pain away, and I like to review this on a follow-up visit, where the patients' 4 keys are green.

Massage, acupressure, acupuncture, reiki, laser, and ultrasound all gently ease distress and pain from inflammation and hypoxic muscles. In terms of

Edwin's treatment, at this stage it would not be appropriate to work in a shamanic way to make a big impact on his subtle body, something I will explain in the next section. After all, Edwin had booked a physiotherapy session, not one aimed at energy medicine. The more orthodox approach needed to follow a gentle physiotherapy approach, hence my plan was to include Gunn IMS to take away pain from muscle contractures. Both strengthening and stretching was needed in order to improve muscle tone, bone density, and disc compression, and cell repair can be helped with treatments such as magnetic resonance (MRT). This could help the spinal disc and irritated tendons around his shoulder and elbow, but the appropriateness for this advanced therapy partly depended on the scan results for his spine.

Edwin took away notes on maintenance sessions regarding soft tissue mobilisations, and massage and posture advice. These sessions – which would take place every few weeks or months – would keep an eye on his mind state and the condition of his body, and then (if appropriate, and if Edwin was ready), reiki could be used to tease out some deeper issues. Core stability in the form of home Pilates exercises would also help with his posture and premature disc rot.

Edwin continued to be too busy to carry on with his treatments, so I followed his session up with an email on home exercises and postural advice. I then wrote a letter to his GP with these facts enclosed: 'the patient had no evidence of muscle tears, ligament tears above grade 1. Mild facet joint subluxation likely in neck at C5/6 on the right, also mild inflammation/ arthritis. Very minor and not acute disc bulge likely at C5/6 and L5/S1 and no frank disc protrusion, no fractured vertebra, only mild nerve root irritation, mild chronic neuritis of the nerve. Mild tennis elbow and calf strain. These mild strains made worse by postural issues, causing spinal mechanical dysfunction.'

This was a difficult case of juggling what treatments I felt he needed, with what he felt he had time for.

"The fruit of silence is prayer.
The fruit of prayer is faith.
The fruit of faith is love.
The fruit of love is service.
The fruit of service is peace."
- **Mother Teresa**

PAUSE, LISTEN TO THE BODY'S WISDOM, AND PUT DOWN YOUR BAG OF TOOLS

Those of us who are practitioners and healers see our patients in a – now how shall I say this? – more multi-dimensional way. That said, it is still important to have undergone orthodox training in order to take a case history, make a provisional diagnosis, and make notes. Then you are safe to step aside from your logical brain and let their body's wisdom talk to you.

In order to read a body in this way, you have to stop and just be present in the moment, to step outside your cluttered analytic brain and listen to what their body needs from you. I find that if I can be in this state of mind – helped by a little soft music – I can literally climb inside the problem to both see and feel where the source is. This approach is more holistic, but no less safe or intelligent. In fact, it simply puts aside the mechanics toolbox and opens up several different channels to healing.

My training in physiotherapy was just that: treating the *physical* body – with a splash of psychology thrown in – and no mention at all of the body's energetic system until postgraduate teaching; I was trained to simply diagnose and treat through the physical body. Forgetting at times (in the early days) the connections to the mind, organs, and hormones, I puzzled over what appeared to be random reactions to treatment. We were trained to treat the injury, then – time permitting – the physical postural compensations that were created secondary to the injury, in the bones and muscles only, leaving everything else that needed to heal to chance.

In my early years in the hospitals, nearly all physios specialised in acute sports injuries. There would be a nice, straightforward, easy diagnosis, the injured area invariably smashed up with bruising. The body could usually heal itself given time, even without our help, and the psychology is straightforward, especially for sportsmen: the patient is injured, and it needs to heal in x weeks in order for them to be match fit. Prescribed rehabilitation and assisted treatment is useful to speed up the healing process, and that's it – job done.

I remember Prof Gunn giving a pep talk out in Vancouver in 2000, during a meeting with us instructors. The aim was to set up international guidelines for teaching his work, and to persist after his retirement. I remember this mostly due to a rather embarrassing moment when a phone was placed in front of me and the committee – it was my father ringing from England, with some apparently very important request. He told me that my cat, Pooh Bear, was missing me and that he'd stopped eating. With a red face, I whispered down the phone: "Dad, I'm in the meeting room in Vancouver, teaching with an international team and creating the future of IMS. *And* we're on a deadline," to which my father replied, "I don't give a damn! Sing to your cat; I don't want to be burying him." So I did, and to this day they thought it was my son! I didn't bother correcting them. And yes, I got the first fellowship award – despite these kinds of traumas – which just shows that anything is possible.

Chan Gunn went on to prepare us for the bumpy journey ahead, saying something along the lines of, "For those of you wanting to heal those folk that nobody else can, it's a lonely journey. Your peers will be irritated at you if you succeed where they couldn't, and by the time the patients find you, they will have run out of time, money, and politeness, and will be angry, depressed, demanding, and at times downright rude. You will struggle to make ends meet, and you will always be looking and studying for answers, rarely getting thanked for your hard work and commitment. Those of you who would rather do acute sports injuries, go now with my blessing."

So yes, you guessed it – numpty here stopped her masters in sports medicine and enrolled in a lifetime of learning how to treat H.C.'s – that is medical shorthand for Hopeless Cases.

Then, due to my past life of watching my mother's life-changing case history of chronic back pain, and because very few physios liked treating spines – guess who became a renowned expert in spinal hopeless cases? Yep, I'm a real glutton for punishment.

However, how bloody fantastic it is when you crack it! It's the Rubik's cube of a bad back. Every problem is unique, with a combination of every system in the body sticking its oar in, and the traditional way of getting a distilled down, bottomed out, specific diagnosis stifles the creative genius lurking within practitioners.

Now, medical jargon – or 'it's gobbledygook to me' as my patients call it – can be a little difficult to understand, so I've included a large section in the back of the book explaining the pathologies of everything I treat. In my opinion, it would have led to a very dull book if it had filled the chapters, and to show you what I mean, here is an example of my clinic notes:

'Provisional diagnosis: postural dysfunction, no evidence of anything other than mild osteoarthritis, no evidence of osteoporosis, only possible mild disc degenerative disease, mild chronic neuropathic nerve conditions likely.'

Get my drift? The above is medical jargon for symptoms in the physical body. Now, before we return to the physical realms of treating, I want to share a very brief introduction to the Harry Potter world of physiotherapy.

THE TABLE EDGE IMPALED MY BACK

Some injuries are etched into our bodies with indelible ink. Last month, an elderly gentleman walked into my office with an aura of quiet distrust; the atmosphere became heavy, and standing in his auric field, I started to feel weary and edgy – I sensed this would be a difficult consultation for both of us. He needed to feel in control and respected, and no kind of healing could happen without first building a good patient-practitioner bridge for him to hobble over. His knowledge of his physical problems was at most poor.

"Tell me your story," I said, and settled down to listen to his perception of the problem he'd brought to me. I wanted to know if he felt that he could heal, and what his prior knowledge of me was. His 4 keys assessment was at best poor, with his mind-set red, lifestyle red due to his stressed view of it, food knowledge red, and fitness red. I knew any kind of treatment would be slow – like trying to light my hearth at home with damp matches – and I explained that we would try three sessions, then review if I could help him.

I managed to glean his bitterness at his failed knee replacements, leaving him with more pain, not less. His right leg felt dead to him – he relied on a stick, though he had no idea why – and he had no trust whatsoever in the medical establishment. I scanned his physical movements to see which one to change first; the way he stood and sat, or perhaps his limp. I then intuitively tuned in (this part is a gift and hard to teach), sensing – on an energetic level – a small hole in his lumbar spine, before starting to piece together his physical state with a thorough orthopaedic assessment.

His physical examination clearly offered clues to a spinal stenotic problem (see appendix), with a clear lack of sensation down his right leg. He had poor light touch, and vibrational sense and joint awareness in his knee, which had been replaced twice. His quads were poor at best. His hips showed wear but in keeping with his age, and were not responsible for his symptoms. His Doppler tests (regarding circulation) told me that he showed no 'plumbing' problems with his blood pipes.

His spine on the right at lumbar 3/4 gave pain on palpation of the facet joint, and his leg symptoms classically belonged to his spine. As Prof Gunn would say, "The legs are merely an extension of the spine, Nicky." A dry needle articulating in deep muscles around L3/4 gave a massive positive grab, and I could also feel an indent in his soft tissue. The grab is indicative of a neuropathic nerve (see glossary). The muscle memory then jolted to life, the muscle releasing some of its tension around the nerve root and facet joint.

"Ah," said my patient, "I did impale a cupboard corner in my back, just before my leg felt dead… I just made the link," he muttered as if an after-thought.

I felt it best to take a very orthodox, orthopaedic approach to his treatment, and I did not want to mention the less orthodox approach of combining healing. It is important to match patients' beliefs and understanding to the treatment approach. Also, you should never be negative about any other practitioners' approach; not only does it break creeds of practice, but it also destroys faith.

Follow up treatment was a blend of acupressure and soft tissue meridian massage, laser, Gunn IMS, laser with electroacupuncture, then ultrasound (see the appendix for more details). Then, whilst discussing exercises, I gently placed my hands over acupressure points to assess his energy levels – as I had been taught in both shiatsu and reiki – while at the same time (in my head) asking permission for chakra balancing, which was not granted and blocked. It felt like a door slamming in my face and I stepped back.

After one of his treatment sessions, a frustrated Mr X phoned up, saying he wasn't cured yet and asking how long it would take before he was better. Again I went through an orthopaedic assessment to settle his concerns, though there was a degree of memory loss as most of what I did was lost to him. He could not lie on his front, so I changed the Maitland and Cyriax manipulative approach to gentle shiatsu side mobilisations. Then I used a combination of dry needling, laser, and acupuncture to ease his nerve pain. Again he rang up even more fed up: not cured yet, how long will this take?

On the third visit I was ready to explain that I could not help him. His body was not able to take the next step and make the change with so little treatment, and he did not wish to spend more time on something he had little faith in. It was like pouring water through a sieve. He went home, sat in a chair, did not exercise, told his body there was no cure, and started eating food with little nourishment in it. So, I decided to be a bit stronger with him – it was his last visit, after all, so there was nothing left to lose.

This time he let me treat him, and as soon as I started balancing his base and sacral chakras with reiki, he explained how he fell. He then went on to tell me more about his recent near death experience and how much it had frightened him. I gently mobilised his spine, and this time once the electroacupuncture kit was set up, he said he could feel warmth and light touch down his leg, causing his pain to melt away. This was the first sign his body had given that it could make a step change towards being more comfortable.

"All healing is essentially the release from fear."
- **A Course In Miracles**

It was as if the fear of a near death experience had been trapped in that fall, and the brain had hardwired the spinal reflex coming back up from the injury site to fail, preventing the immune system from using the catalyst of the treatment modalities. As he now felt a knowing of his body's wisdom, orthodox physiotherapists and medics could help him again.

COMBINING ENERGY MEDICINE WITH PHYSIOTHERAPY

"When the soul collects all its interior powers within, and when the body collects all its external senses and unites them to the soul, the Holy spirit approaches and breathes into this union quietude and peace."
- **Father Andrew Leonard Winczewski, O.S.B.**

I have been intuitive/psychic since I was little, and this was safely ground-ed by a 'feet on the ground' upbringing, with lots of helpings of science to protect me from ridicule. When I was small, I always knew if someone was in pain, and I'd also know where it was in the body just by walking up to the person, even if they were a stranger. This was deemed as being 'weird behaviour', and the gift lessened with time. My parents told me I would say things like, "It's obvious they feel this," or, "This will be happening next." Due to other people's responses, I soon learnt to hide this gift.

June – my reiki teacher and dearest late friend – however, would find all this very normal. It was like enrolling at Harry Potter's School of Magic, studying with psychic healers over the last quarter of a century. They would talk about the BODY in a very different way to my anatomy lectures; they included the energy field around a physical body as an energetic body. The ancient eastern medical teachings suggest that seven chakras seed seven energetic layers around the physical body, and I remember June referring to them as etheric (1st layer), emotional, mental, astral, ethereal, celestial, and causal – which I will cover in my Soul book.

My friends would describe these energy fields in terms of patterns and colours, saying that if we are closer than five feet to a stranger, we are in their astral body, feeling their thoughts – a creepy feeling, eh! They would say that if they did not see auras around people about to get on a train or plane, there could be a major tragedy. I suppose it depends on who the people were – just kidding. In my shamanic, reiki, and wiccan teachings of ancient medicine, the physical body is just one aspect of our total body, part of it being energetic.

The practitioners amongst us who prefer to work as car mechanics will have wisely put the book down and gone off for a brew now.

ENERGY MEDICINE IN BRIEF

Right, get your seat belts on; there's more weird stuff heading your way! The healers amongst us believe that an injury or disease has far reaching implications with hormonal, visceral (concerning internal organs), energetic pathways, as well as emotional and spiritual repercussions. Simply treating a symptom – or worse still, cutting out the offending article – does not get to the root cause. If you think about it as a therapist or as a patient, to physically be treated you are standing in each others' auric fields, which is a pretty intimate thing to do.

June would teach me how to feel the etheric – both its physical and emotional aspects – the former just up to ¾ inch above, and the latter four inches. It is said to house the blueprint of both physical and emotional patterns, with the energetic matrix being seen as a web of energy threads called nadis. She described it as a thin, greyish-blue outline and would say that you can you feel the energy change. All creatures, including plants, are said to have this.

I guess it makes sense for reiki healers to hold their hands within four inches of the physical body to palpate the subtle body, and for physical therapists to touch the body with hands or needles, for this layer is believed to transmit, receive, and assimilate vital life force energy (or 'chi') in and out of the physical body via the chakras. This vital energy has many names: chi, prana, ki, huna, animal magnetism, universal energy, life force, and so on.

I have met medics brave enough to admit that they are also gifted healers, but it is very seldom they ever want anyone else to find out. And guess what? Their waiting lists are so much longer than anyone else's; it's as if their patients know of their unspoken gift. Even just this week I was at a conference with speakers who were surgeons and physiotherapists. They would read people and reach out intuitively to each other with healing hands, yet they would disclose nothing on stage.

I can remember when studying Japanese physio that every acupressure point was believed to have nine levels, and you had to balance the points with your energy in order to fill them up or empty them – this is called tsubo or kyo. Studying energy medicine taught me that the next level 'out' is called the ASTRAL body, and that this is all about emotions. It flows freely outwards to 10 to 12 inches, overflowing the first layer, and it is said to be harder to see, feel, or interpret, for obvious reasons. Negative emotions can badly affect healing times for treatments, and while I can find little scientific proof of this layer, I clearly remember how healing sessions using reiki, shiatsu, and spiritual approaches all had big impacts on my emotional state, and also how accurate my colleagues were about hidden emotions.

At my first meeting with June (my late reiki master), she told me there was a dark patch in my auric field over my heart. I thought, 'how strange', and a quick spell in hospital confirmed her opinion. She taught me that thought forms are said to be housed in a mental body up to 30 inches outside our actual body, so people's thoughts can be literally inside us and can affect our health, not to mention our own thoughts.

Spiritual healers who stand back whilst healing will only be in this field, and they may see this as a pale whitish light around them. Hence loving, compassionate, happy people bathe their bodies and others in their healing light – quite literally. I will touch more on this in the next book.

GOT A PASSPORT PICTURE OF YOUR AURA?

I can't see colours in auras; I'm afraid that at June's 'Harry Potter's School of Healing' I simply could not do this bit. It is said that Tesla photographed the aura, then in 1939, the Soviet scientist Semyon Kirlian used electrical currents to photograph the aura. In 1980, full spectrum cameras developed by Guy Coggins showed that the auric colours changed with mood and illness. The picture of mine was very red!

David Tansley – who wrote *Radionics & The Subtle Anatomy of Man* – believed that the energetic map held in the ethereal layer connected through to every cell in the body. Perhaps this is the missing link in the mysterious infinite intelligence that guides things, such as where and what stem cells should be.

CHAKRA THERAPY

Eastern medicine teaches us to embrace chakras, acupressure points, and meridian channels, and these teachings go back to ancient Sanskrit (an ancient Indo-Aryan language), and Tibetan. Each of the seven energy chakras or centres are thought to go through the physical body, the spine having the yang, masculine, musculoskeletal aspect, and the front the ying, organic, and emotional aspect.

In Sanskrit records, these chakras were each associated with acupuncture points, endocrine glands, organic association, spinal level, key points, specific meridians, spiritual phenomena, certain muscles, autonomic nervous system changes, colour and sound associations, and differing rotating vortices revolutions to mention just a few of some 22-odd connections. Therefore, the ancient shaman's ability to listen to the body's wisdom should not be sniffed at. I will cover this more in the Soul book, as well as the ancient use of herbs, oils, crystals, prayer, plants, and medicine.

In my healing tutorials I would be shown reiki, wicca, shiatsu, soul retrieval, past life regression, soul midwifery, chakra and acupuncture points, crystals, and pendulums, as well as being taught how to feel and diagnose subtle bodies – very different to the physiotherapy taught to me in UK universities, and absolutely mind blowing at times. Now, get your seat belts on for a brief summary of some ancient knowledge.

Energy coupling relationships are said to exist between the crown, bridge, and base chakra, the throat with the sacral, and the heart with the solar. Eastern healers may place a hand to each – as if weighing up the differences – or they may swing a pendulum over the patient, as I have seen a lot in my reiki training.

Furthermore, the chakras relate to their smaller chakra cousins, and this determines the placing of healers' hands: for instance, the crown with foot and hand, the brow with clavicle and groin, the throat with shoulder and navel, the heart with ear and intercostal, the solar plexus with spleen, the sacral with spleen, and the base with knee and elbow. My mother studied chakras and crystals in depth, and she helps me to fill in the gaps where my own knowledge is missing or confused.

Energy medicine touches on hormone changes, and is open to many contradicting interpretations. John Cross – a physiotherapist – concurred with other writers that the crown chakra was associated with the pineal gland, that magical and mysterious gland that contains crystals and is thought to be a transmitter of universal intelligence (Cross, 2006). He also states that the brow energetic system connects the pineal gland with the hypothalamus and pituitary, the throat chakra with thyroid, the heart with thymus, the solar plexus with pancreas, the sacral ovaries with balls, and the base adrenal medulla with the adrenal cortex. Physiotherapists trained in energy medicine work on all levels.

Now, if I wasn't already confused enough, each chakra is associated with bits of the body; the crown chakra with the right eye and brain cortex, the brow with the reptilian brain, the nervous system with the left eye, and so on... there will be more of this huge subject in my Soul book.

How about meridian channels? The crown chakra is associated with the triple energiser meridian, the brow chakra with the gallbladder, and so on... This ancient system of medicine interwove the endocrine and the nervous and central nervous system/brain by flipping energetic switches.

FREQUENCIES AND KEY ACUPUNCTURE POINTS FOR MUSICIANS

When combining healing chakra work with acupuncture or acupressure, there are certain keys that open up the energetic system. The crown chakra – with a resonance frequency of 0.25 Hz – has a key acupuncture point called Con4. The brow chakra –frequency 2.96 Hz – with acupuncture point Gov4. The throat chakra, 81.2 Hz, Con6. The heart chakra, 7.8 Hz, Gov7. The solar plexus, 23 Hz, Con17. The sacral chakra, 81.1Hz, Gov12. The base chakra, 81.1Hz, Con 22. June would use her fingers or a crystal on these points, though you can use laser, acupuncture, or a tuning fork (or whatever you are trained in) instead. Ancient caves are said to be chiselled out to resonate at specific healing frequencies when sung into.

Now, it's time to get your seat belts on again, as we look at something for the clever nerds. The autonomic nervous system connections with the chakras are as follows: the brow chakra is the superior cervical ganglion (sup. C.G for short), the throat is the inferior C.G, the heart chakra and solar plexus chakra are linked to the celiac plexus and ganglion, the sacral chakra to the inferior mesenteric ganglion, and the base chakra to the pelvis plexus (see glossary for all of these terms). As well as these, muscle innervations associated with the chakras are as follows: the crown chakra muscles are supplied by the nerves from the cervical (C is shorthand for cervical, the neck) C1, 2, 3, 4. The brow, C1, 2, 3, the throat chakra, C5, C6, C7, T1, T2 (T is shorthand for thoracic spine between the shoulder blades), heart chakra is innervated by many T2-L3, solar plexus, L1- L2 (L is lumbar/lower spine), and sacral plexus (S is the sacral nerves from the sacrum, the triangular bone in your seat), L2 to S3.

Emotions are associated with chakras and sensed by healers, as follows: the brow is anger, the throat is shyness, the heart is fear, depression, anxiety, and detachment, the solar plexus is anxiety and depression, the sacral chakra is lust and envy, and the base chakra is phobias, insecurity, and uncertainty.

Now, let's look at spiritual sense in physical therapy – does it have a place in our modern scientific society? This is a big subject in itself, and I will discuss this more in my Soul book, so for a brief summary about chakra energy, here goes.

The crown chakra is associated with the spirit and higher self, the brow with intuition, the throat with communication/expression, the heart with – an easy one here – love, the solar plexus with grounding, earthly connection, and stability, the sacral with joy, and the base chakra is all about the physical realm – wink wink.

June used to see the swirling chakras like dense or faint petals of energy; the more dense, the more physical the problem, whereas the more faint, the more emotional the issue. She would also talk of closing down and opening up the vortices following shamanic reiki treatments.

Just to mention this briefly, colours and sounds are also associated with chakras: the crown with violet and gold and tuning fork pitch B, the brow with indigo blue and pitch A, the throat with blue and pitch G, the heart with green and some pink and F, the solar plexus with orange and E, the sacral with orange and D, the base with red and pitch C. Crystals and aromatherapy are also associated with chakras, and I will go into all of this in more detail in my Soul book. I needed to mention this in my Body book as more intuitive therapists and doctors also interweave these alternative modalities into their treatments.

My belief is that combining the ancient healing arts with modern medicine is an intelligent, holistic – or wholistic as it used to be called – way to treat patients. Linking a healing touch – with such arts as reiki (with or without crystals), meditation, shamanism, shiatsu, aromatherapy, herbalism and nutrition, yoga, Qi Gong, Tai Chi, NLP and hypnosis, and acupuncture – with modern physical therapy modalities is an exquisite combination.

Where we place our hands with the focused intention to heal, and the words we use, alter the results. Every treatment is a unique combination impossible to replicate, a dance between therapist and patient at that moment in time. I see adding in modalities such as laser, shockwave, massage, manipulation, and acupuncture like keys on a piano; the tune we create is having more effect than we realise.

Modern day medicine, physiotherapy, osteopathy, and chiropractic all have their place in the hands of open-minded healers, but once we become segregated into all of our own specialised jobs and conferences and teachings, we lose the power of holistic healing and the possibilities of cure.

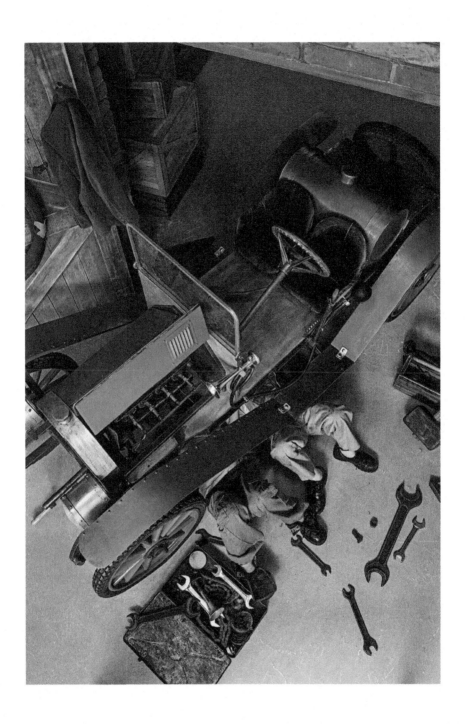

Chapter Four

"Beauty is not who you are on the outside, it is the wisdom and time you gave away to save another struggling soul, like you."

– Shannon L. Alder

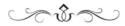

For treatment modalities, please see the appendix

IN THE WORKSHOP WITH NUTS AND BOLTS AND NEEDLES TOO

"If my body was a car, I would be trading it in for a newer model. I've got bumps, dents, and scratches, and my headlights are out of focus. My gearbox is seizing up, and it takes hours to reach maximum speed. I overheat for no reason, and every time I sneeze, cough, or laugh, either my radiator leaks or my exhaust backfires. This is from your friend and bestest old banger."
- Mrs Shelly, a wonderful patient of mine

Now, in this chapter we'll be looking at a continuation of the treatments mentioned in chapter three, looking not only at upper limb and spine problems, but also the lower limb.

HIS GOALSCORING LEG WAS JUST AN EXTENTION OF HIS SPINE

Right, we're going to jump in my time machine again now, heading back about nine years to a bitterly cold day in late November, when I received a phone call from a rather well-known football club. It seemed that their shooting star – who had previously played for his country – was no longer shooting, and I was asked if I could drive out to the hotel they were staying at and assess him, in order to advise the medic and physio if there was another approach that could be taken. I was asked to be discreet, as social media is hot on scandal/gossip, and a player who was due to play the next day being injured is not a very good advert.

I can remember getting into a lift with several beefy footballers, being surprised at how broad their shoulders were while I wrestled with my steamed-up glasses. Well, it was snowy outside – that's my excuse and I'm sticking to it. I could just about fit in the large hotel bedroom, where there were many guys fussing around a tall, slender chap. His aura was one of quiet desperation, however, with so many people in the room, it was difficult to tune into him intuitively.

"It's my hamstring; it just keeps feeling like it will snap," said the handsome, foreign-looking chap in his late thirties. He went on to tell me that he'd had dozens of ultrasound scans to look for tears, and lots of bum-numbing time out sessions on the bench.

I was hoping that the doc or physio would be one of my postgrad students, but they were not in this case, so I polished my glasses and began an examination of his spine and hamstrings – a thorough appraisal to see why it was happening. I cannot disclose who this chap was; I can only say that he was close to forty and his body had been hammered with an intense and successful career.

His biomechanics were spot on – I watched him walk, sit, and squat – and he'd previously had detailed biomechanical assessments and the correctly aligned trainers. His hamstrings were notchy in places, with evidence of scar tissue that shockwave and deep tissue massage had helped to heal. His core was strong for only short periods of time and his lateral spinal stabilisers struggled to fire consistently.

Now, let's get back in my time machine to travel back another six years to a course I taught at Shugborough Hall in 2000. Being the eccentric soul I am – and knowing that Prof Gunn liked culture – I thought why not teach in a National Trust building rather than a hospital? There is nothing I like more (when time allows) than visiting National Trust and English Heritage places, where all this great history dwells, so combining the two made sense. You may be thinking why has this meandering fool gone off track? Well, like Ronnie Corbett's stories, there *is* a point to it.

Whilst the late Lord Lichfield threw a party downstairs, we played a Downton Abbey version of an IMS teaching program and exams, with Prof Gunn assessing twin ex-professional footballers – you know who you are guys, as you still come to the clinic from time to time. He explained how repetitive hamstring injuries and sensations of tearing are so often due to the nerve roots being neuropathic and causing muscle contractures deep in the muscle of the lower lumbar spine and secondary contractures in the hamstrings, giving the feeling of strains. We taught the course participants how treating the lower lumbar spine will significantly reduce this type of chronic sports injury.

We had so much fun on the course, and many great memories were forever etched on my mind. There was Dr Cassons – having driven over from his French practice – with a four-wheel drive loaded with champagne for elevenses, not to mention the prof saying, "I am bored now, I want to speak now, Nicky," in a loud voice during one of my lectures. At times he would be asleep, sitting next to me and snoring in front of our post-grad docs and physios; he coped with the jet lag from Canada better than I did.

Armed with this poignant memory, let's jump forward in my time machine to December 2006 again and the footballer. I arranged several treatments back at my home practice, as we were at the point of moving the clinic to Cromwell House. The footballer was a charming, intelligent, family man, who knew his wine and his restaurants – hubby and I enjoyed his company a lot. The treatments were a combination of spinal robotic manipulation and a revisit to core, Gunn IMS dry needling, as well as NLP, as he carried so much fear that his hamstrings would go and he needed to score goals again. Luckily for me, the old magic still worked and he felt a lot better afterwards.

A. Hutton – a delightful Australian dry needling lecturer – quoted on his website: "In the hands of a skilled practitioner, dry needling can be used in most cases the majority of the time and with less energy expenditure on behalf of the practitioner and equal or better effect than other manual techniques currently being used. If practiced well there is also a remarkable absence of the 'post treatment tissue soreness' often experienced by the subject following other manual therapy interventions."

At 6 a.m. last weekend, I got a text asking if I wanted to go over needling techniques on a walkabout on a sunny May day in Coventry; Andrew had flown from Australia to Coventry for his workshop and was flying back to NZ that afternoon – amazing dedication.

> **HOMEWORK:**
> If you've suffered with sporting injuries, get your back checked out and make sure you keep your spine flexible and your core strong. This is even more important if you have dry needling treatment.

WHY DRY NEEDLING AND NOT WET ONES?

I am often asked, 'what is the difference between dry needling, injections, and acupuncture?' Well, dry needling is a broad term used to differentiate 'non-injection' needling from the practice of 'injection needling', which means a big mother f***ing hypodermic syringe and involves the injection of an agent such as local anaesthetic and/or corticosteroid into the tissue or joint, usually in aseptic (not dirty) conditions. In contrast to this, dry needling utilises a solid, filament needle – as is used in the practice of acupuncture – and also relies on the stimulation of specific reactions in the target tissue for its therapeutic effect.

I have completed extensive training in joint injection techniques, including a rather lengthy training period at Cannock Rheumatology department many years ago. My toes still curl when I remember failing miserably to get a large needle into a badly arthritic knee – during an exam.

Years later up in Sheffield, I took an orthodox orthopaedic revision course in order to hone my skills. Back home in my own clinic, my delightful friends, Mark and Vinod – foot and shoulder surgeons, and so clever at injecting – held my hand whilst I honed my harpooning injection skills. There is a place for injecting drugs, though personally I would rather leave that to the medics and instead concentrate on a more preventative approach.

The term 'dry needling' is also used to differentiate the use of needling in a western physiological paradigm from the use of needling in an oriental paradigm, which is referred to as acupuncture. The needling of points is done on meridians in the body, also referred to as energy lines, and which in the past were referred to as healing points, caves, or switches. Needles can boost, harmonise, and remove blockages in the flow of energy throughout the body, and this Chinese medicine has spread throughout Asia and the western world. Chinese medicine involves acupuncture, moxa (heat to needles), herbs and diet therapy, and exercise in the form of Chi Kong or Tai Chi, not forgetting several forms of massage or manipulative therapy (tuina, for instance).

Oriental medicine uses a system of physiology that describes channels/meridians through which vital energy (Qi) flows around the body. These have branches that go deep into the organs of the body and are the conduits through which the flow of energy in the meridians affects organ function and visa versa. Much like our planet has ley lines to guide animals in migration, and like early sailors used the galaxy of stars to navigate, the body's meridians were the early doctors' guide to navigating around the body.

In ancient times, bodies in the east were not dissected like they are in the west, so several beliefs were held without this knowledge being available. The internal organ system can be compared to a turbine and pump system: in a simplistic way, it extracts energy from the air and food, refining it and pushing it around the body. Wastes are also excreted by the organ system. When imbalance arises in the organ system, energy flow in the meridians can be disturbed, resulting in pain, tissue tightness, or other symptoms. Chinese medicine suggests that where there is insufficient energy, or where it becomes stuck in the meridians, symptoms of discomfort, pain, and tissue tightness arise. The oriental model – just like the holistic western approach – agrees that our health is a combination of the cumulative effects of our environment/lifestyle, our spiritual or psychoemotional state, our activity, and our diet, all of which impacts our genes/DNA. This is why I called my first book *The 4 Keys To Health*, as it looks at all four of these major areas.

Life places all sorts of stresses upon us, and our systems can only resist those stresses for so long. When this no longer becomes possible to do so, we experience disease. Acknowledging the influence of the 4 keys and seeking preventative treatment can allow us to exist for longer periods of time in a pain free and disease free state.

If there are temporary changes for the worse, or gradual deterioration in one or more of the above aspects of our being – our lifestyle, exercise levels, diet, or psychoemotional state – our ability to resist the stresses of life will be reduced, predisposing us to pain or disease. I see this time and time again with my patients when they come to me in pain, and seeking out answers to the 4 keys is extremely illuminating – rarely do we fall into disrepair when carrying 4 green keys with us. Of course, acupuncture treatment cannot make up for problems with the mindset or environment, or a lack of good food, love, or exercise, but it can, however, nudge the body back towards health by giving the patient the ability to cope again.

Western Acupuncture utilises meridian points, but applies it with 'western' reasoning, with particular consideration given to relevant neurophysiology and anatomy. It also does not utilise any traditional Chinese medicine assessment methods or paradigms. Points are stimulated to create local, spinal segmental, or supraspinal pain modulating effects – this can be called 'trigger point needling' if the focus is on tight muscle bands – and Gunn IMS is an advanced, specialised form of this. Employing a plunger device to enable microsurgical tiny incisions, it also incorporates the use of highly skilled and varied adaptations of traditional needling techniques, the effects of which are explained within an anatomical and neurophysiological paradigm famously described by Cannon and Rosenblueth's work in *The Gunn Approach To The Treatment Of Chronic Pain*. These techniques are then applied in order to stimulate changes in movement and tissue physiology based on neurodynamic and orthopaedic screening. I use a combination of many different types of needling, but IMS has and always will have my heart.

ACTING OUT DEATH, AND I HURT MY NECK

One spring morning I got a call from the ITV team saying that a delightful leading actress – who was filming a local TV series – had injured herself. Apparently, her mother enjoyed reading my monthly health pages in the county mag and had insisted they phone me. At the time I lived on my own, and I explained that I could help, but that I had to get home to feed the cat and hang up my smalls before I could come over.

I can still remember my amusement whilst hanging up said smalls – well, more like Bridget Jones knickers – when a smart black limousine showed up. It was back in the days when I had a home practice, as well as working long hours in hospitals – and was used to strange cars turning up with fascinating souls to treat.

Well, the chauffeur opened the door for me with a slightly irritated manner – as it turned out, his last job was Mel Gibson so I was one hell of a come-down. He could drive just as fast backwards as he could forwards, and as I got into the back seat, he shut me off from him with the glass window that went up and down between the front and back of the car.

They were filming from a big old Manor House, where there was a bus that had been converted into a dining room, and where caravans in a muddy field served as changing rooms. Once we were there, I was ushered into one of these caravans where I assessed the neck strain of a delightful and talent-ed actress. I will keep her name a secret – as it is not my story to tell – but I will say that her man is very handsome, and his drama series kept me on the edge of my seat. He, however, didn't have any injury, so I didn't need to worry about steamed-up glasses and shaky hands.

Anyway, back to my lady in question. I found Prof Gunn's teachings (that transcended physiotherapy and acupuncture for pain) so very helpful in fixing the problem, and my intuitive healing gifts also helped. This particu-lar treatment session was carried out in her caravan on the set, surround-ed by her stunt team, producer, and make-up artist – I was just glad they couldn't fit inside; I would have been rather squashed!

On one occasion, her team were waiting to put ropes on her for a flying scene, and another time she was preparing for a deathly boring scene in a coffin. I was able to reduce the neck pain with gentle physiotherapy mobilisations to the spine, as well as soft tissue work to tight muscles, with laser and IMS dry needling. Lunging about in a caravan rather than my treatment room is always a challenge on film sets, but it makes for an interesting time. When I was done, her stuntman was so pleased that she could take part in the 'flying' scene, and I have to say, so was I – I didn't fancy being a stand-in for anything even vaguely risky.

On several occasions since, I have had the excitement of going out to see members of film crews, directors, and cameramen, whose postures upset their backs, not to mention them having to deal with huge dollops of stress with regards to deadlines. Sadly, they usually come to me instead of the other way round, so I haven't had many exciting flights out to exotic locations.

I remember one patient who was a cameraman for a James Bond movie that was filming in Prague. He had a horrible backache from leaning over with cameras on all sorts of tracks, so next time you're enjoying a movie, give a prayer for all those hard-working cameramen's backs. I can't count the times I've been delivered to bedrooms armed with my laser and needles to help locked-up backs, and I have to say, it must look a bit weird for any onlookers: hearing screams and grunts and thumps, then seeing me come out to the waiting limousine with my hair on end, clutching my laser.

HOMEWORK:
Check your working posture; how do you stand and sit when you feel stressed out at work? Get a friend to take a picture of your stressed out posture. I've treated quite a few scriptwriters over the years, from films to weekly soaps of Coronation Street, Emmerdale, and so on, and these creative souls forget their posture when hunched over their laptops – it's as if the mind leaves the body, only to return later to an achy breaky spine.

HOMEWORK:
Put your feet flat on the floor, so the weight goes through the feet and bum. Breathe deeply into the tummy, then roll your shoulders back and place your head over them, not poked forward.

MY LEG HAUNTS ME

This is the story of an elderly lady named Mary. She was immaculately made up – her hair combed back, smartly dressed – and sadly she was profoundly deaf. She hobbled on sticks into my northern clinic, carrying with her a secret that was locked deep inside her body. Due to a past experience, she held an imprint of a trauma that occurred so long ago and was so deep that it had caused premature aging in her knee.

The deafness meant I could only listen to her telling me about her perceived problem, then I would have to try to act out the replies, as we both knew little sign language! Her aura was a mixture of quiet desperation and irritation of what the aging had done to her, though she was not about to give up, being both frustrated and stoical about her poor mobility.

I eased her quickly onto the couch, lifting her legs up where she couldn't fall. They say that the knees can reflect pent up emotion and grief, which is why we say that her knees 'went'. I remember seeing this when a colleague's knees literally did just that as her husband's coffin was being carried down the aisle. Reflecting on that memory, I wondered if there was a deep-seated emotional link to Mary's problem.

I carried out an orthopaedic assessment of her lower limbs. Unsurprising for her age, she had flat feet with the arches weakened, and her arthritic ankles were straining. The knees were clearly worn, grating as I moved them, and the kneecaps creaked like old rusty gates. The hips struggled to rotate and carry the pelvis, and there was a degree of pelvic torsion (twisting), plus stiffness of her left sacroiliac joint (the joint in her pelvis). Basically, everything had the signature tune of severe osteoarthritis, and even her back refused to move under my hands. The lumbar spine had a slight curvature (scoliosis), as well as locked facet joints with narrow discs, again in keeping with her age and adding to a leg length difference. However, with all of these problems, she interestingly only complained about her painful left knee and her lower leg, where there was a hidden large scar. "I feel old and ugly with these damn legs; they don't work," she kept telling me.

146

With her poor hearing and mild memory issues, I could not easily understand what her preferred treatment style was, so with her husband looking
on, I went for an orthodox approach to ease the knee pain, using laser and
electroacupuncture to tap into her pain receptors, working from the lumbar
spine to the knee. Aiming to settle some of the inflammatory pain caused
by the osteoarthritis, I carried out mobilisations for the kneecap and the
main knee joint (the tibiofemoral) with gentle stretches, manipulations, soft
tissue massage, and home exercises. Technology like MRT could only really
help her if she could understand me and commit to exercise, which was
very unlikely. My suggestion of gentle Tai Chi was not possible as yet, due
to such poor balance and her ears.

The next morning, my receptionist got the 'day after phone call' we all expect at times like this – "I'm not cured, what a waste of time!" – and of
course my darling patient could not hear the reply due to her hearing issues.

So, that was that, or so I thought until I saw her name on the list again. I
thought this could be because I'd used an orthodox approach with her husband's treatment (who had also come to see me with his own problem), and
had weaved in energy medicine in a discreet way. He evidently felt more at
ease with my approach and had encouraged his wife to return by instilling
trust within her regarding my treatment.

This time I asked for permission to treat her in a Shamanic way, as orthodox
physiotherapy simply would not crack this nut. I needed to see what catalyst
had caused this specific problem, and for this I needed to travel back in time
in my trusty machine.

I needed to see what had focused her pain into just one place in her body,
as I have learnt time and time again that damaged areas are painless, and
the pain actually lies hidden in seemingly healthy tissue (perhaps in brain
wiring, or if you believe in energy medicine, in your subtle body or soul).

I used some gentle laser, then turned her on her front before starting with some neuropathic work to ease the sensitivity from her spinal nerves to her knee. Then, with gentle chakra balancing and Reiki, I let her slip into a light trance – perhaps back to a time in her life when she could hear me. In my head, using Shamanic healing arts, I laid out a timeline to the first time her knee hurt:

I was back in an old hospital ward 66 years ago, in 1950.
The ward reminded me of the old ones I used to work in when I was on call.
I saw crisp white sheets lying under a rather swollen, infected, oozing wound over the knee. Her legs were sown together and fluid seeped into the sheets. I looked up at a young woman's face in her late teens: she had startled, fright-ened eyes.
I asked this version of her if I could be allowed to hear what was going on that day, and she explained that although the surgeon was delighted with the skin graft, her knee was so burnt he didn't know if he could save it.
I asked how long she had to have her legs stitched together – her inside calf to her knee – and she said six months.
"Is it sore?" I asked, and she heard me.
"Yes," she replied, "where he took the skin graft and where the burn was on my knee."
"How do you feel?"
"Old and ugly," she said.
"Where does it hurt?"
"In my knee," she replied.
Now that I understood where the pain had come from, I could work on easing the suffering it caused her.
The primitive surgical methods had upset her nerves in the skin, and the fas-cia in her leg, not to mention the meridians and chakras; her knee chakra felt dead. The osteoarthritis was just part of the pain.
Now I knew.

So, with that I came back in my time machine to 2016, before working on all levels of perception for a holistic treatment approach – one that left me feeling completely exhausted.

After I was finished, she sat up and said, "No one has ever done anything like this before; my leg is warm and not numb, and there's no pain in my knee." With her age and her memory, I didn't really expect a miracle, but even a small improvement that gives a better quality of life is a blessing and not one to be given up on at any time in your life.

She felt some ease in the symptoms that stayed with her, and she seemed to have more faith in life. She also understood that the surgeon had done the best he could to help her with the knowledge he had at the time. I am hopeful that she may come back, undertaking the discipline of gentle mindful exercise, and considering physiotherapy, acupuncture, and magnetic resonance for her arthritis. I won't hold my breath, however, as I feel it is a bridge too far for her to cross. So, for now I will just send her distant healing and hope she changes her mind.

'ANOTHER THERAPIST TO BREAK!' THINKS THE PATIENT

It was one of those tiresome, long, clinical days filled with successful retired businessmen with broken bodies and minds – a day that, if it doesn't kill you, makes you stronger, as the song goes.

During one particular session, a cross, tired-looking, disillusioned seventy-year-old man sat huddled in my waiting area, his eyes scanning the room with disdain. I knew he would have to find something to criticise as his energy field felt toxic – like diving into cold, stagnant water. I had already had a long day of discontent patients reaching out for help with one hand while punching with the other, which was actually pretty normal in my line of work: I represented the enemy, one in a whole band of warrior healers who had, in their eyes, failed them. This man was angry that money could not buy him a new body.

It's strange how five feet can make all the difference: whether I sit next to them as a fellow patient and sufferer, or cross over to sit on the other side. In such a case, chairs positioned to make an imaginary line easier between patient and therapist does little to change this kind of energy.

His piercing, hungry, distrustful eyes met mine, and I knew that his big, bullying, business world needed him to say how powerful and rich he was, how many surgeons he had bought to befriend him, and how he had family connections with drugs companies, and so on and so on. And yet under all this defensive bravado sat a little boy who just wanted a hug and desperately needed someone to take his pain away. Despite all the advice from his rich and powerful colleagues, somewhere deep inside his head he wanted to be here. He wanted to get better.

I took a deep breath and waited for the first insult. "Someone's pissed on your loo floor, you should know," was his opening greeting.

"Yes," I replied, smiling and keeping calm, "it's only water from the tap; it's a little strong and can wet the floor if turned on full."

"It's the tap in your toilet that wet my shirt! If it sprays when turned on full, can't you change it?"

"Perhaps after your treatment," I said, still smiling.

The man thought for a moment. "It is not obvious from the map on your website where this place is; I could have missed it."

I nodded, responding with, "Yes, you could, but luckily for me the map *did* get you here." A little tongue in cheek, I know.

He gruffly replied, "So, are you qualified in anything? You're in all the local papers with pictures of your hair down. Why is it tied up today?"

"I don't like to get spilt blood in my hair," I explained. I couldn't help it; he was winding me up.

However, he smiled at that point, realising that I wasn't going to give up on him without a fight. "You gonna look at my body or what? Do you need a chaperone?"

I didn't reply; the sadness in his eyes said it all. His frail, broken body struggled to stand up, while his arthritic hands struggled with his clothes. The compassion I felt for this broken man filled the room, and entangled in his aura of anger, the energy change was small but tangible. The dance had begun.

"My surgeon friends say that if they operate, I could have more pain; there are always risks, and no guarantees that it will improve my quality of life." Surgery after chronic pain issues is rarely successful, unless targeting a specific outcome such as cutting free a nerve exit or pressure on the spinal cord, or stabilising a crumbling spine.

I had a pile of the man's medical notes in front of me. He'd had at least some degree of pain since a car crash some 40-odd years ago, when his car spun out of control, causing spinal vertebrae damage. Countless MRI's showed degenerative changes beyond his years, and old fractures, not osteoporotic or malignant. There were no crushed nerves to warrant surgery, although they may have been neuropathic due to disc narrowing, and the spinal cord was free of any compressions. He had weak muscles due to apathy and pain associated with movement.

His bloods were normal for anaemia, inflammatory markers, bone profile, liver, and thyroid, and there was nothing to suggest anything sinister. The medics had been very thorough. None of the procedures he'd had alleviated the pain, and he'd had a lot of treatment before coming to see me: spinal injections into facets with corticosteroids, epidurals, rhysilopathy (nerve burning), opiates, muscle relaxants, anti-inflammatories, chiropractic (72 sessions), acupuncture, osteopathy, and physiotherapy with exercise.

Here were my clinical findings: his balance was poor, and without his stick he could not stand up. His deformed toes gripped the floor. He was very stooped and twisted like a willow tree, his spine weaving and rippling like a snake, and his muscles spasming as he tried to find a comfortable posture. He wheezed breathlessly and spoke in hoarse whispers.

His reflexes were weak, his muscles poor, though his hip movements were in keeping with his age. His replaced knees moved reluctantly with poor muscles, and the back... well, where do I start? His facet joints were stiffened, distorted, and sore, his disc spaces narrow, and his muscles also sore. With an assessment for neuropathic pain, there was some evidence of it being part of the picture, with some strong muscle grabs in the lumbar spine in response to dry needling.

His personality and the degree of damage his body showed would need a great deal of commitment for therapy to even take the edge off his problems, and I did not feel at this time that I was the right person to help. He needed to find a strong-minded male practitioner to see if a combination of physical therapy, dry needling, MRT and counselling could ease his suffering in the later part of his life. He also needed an involved neurological assessment to rule out motor neurone disease, amongst other pathologies. Here I paused his treatment and wrote to his doctor to run further tests – it is very important to know when to ask for help.

He did actually return to see if I could instantly weave some magic, and I tentatively released some tight muscle contractures within his spine using laser and IMS, with core muscle exercises to reinstate stability. I taught breathing exercises and safe balance work, and after a couple of attempts, I wrote back to the medics to explore further. When a body is this broken, it needs a commitment to proceed with a longer course of treatment than I could provide, but I could at least send my prescription on to his doctor.

HOCKEY WRECKED MY HIP

It was a sunny Saturday morning, and having a long clinic list left my heart heavy. I longed to be out in the sun, either walking or cycling. Still, I did some deep breathing, cleared my mind, and got into the correct state – I thought about those people's lives I would help today, and imagined myself relaxing on Sunday with a feeling or accomplishment. Or not...

Just then, a tall, confident, middle-aged lady swept into my room, wearing a smart tweed suit and a stern, wilting expression on her face. My heart sank; now, being inside on a lovely summer's morning was even harder. "I have parked my Porsche next to the Ferrari," she told me. "I assume it is safe here?"

She continued. "I've read up on you in the papers and the internet, as I don't like my time being wasted. I will read up on what you suggest today and make my own mind up about whether I value what you say. I will text my chiropractor and physio up in Harley Street as they will tell me if they think what you say holds water. You were ten minutes late, so I need a very big apology. I have a yoga class next, so don't overrun. Have you not got a helicopter, to avoid traffic issues?" She'd said all this without taking a breath.

I was suddenly glad I'd changed out of my running shorts and into a suit, as this lady was very typical of the arrogant rich. I guess that in life, you can be so busy acting a certain way that you are incapable of changing whilst in the company of someone so very unimpressed by this bullying behaviour. The Hippocratic Oath does not give one a let out when treating unpleasant individuals – unless you're being physically rather than emotionally beaten up by them.

"I have bought my scan from the family Harley Street consultant, and a diagnosis and prognosis. I have a labral tear and hip dysphagia. I don't suppose you know what that is, so I wrote it out for you. My husband has a good job in banking, and my late father left me a comfortable private income, so you see, they only want the best for me."

I nodded knowingly, while quickly googling 'labral tear' to double-check my facts. The hip labrum is a cartilage ring which deepens the hip socket by adding a rim, allowing flexibility and motion. A labral tear can be caused by degeneration due to overuse and can be seen in early osteoarthritis, congenital pathology (i.e. shape of the head of the femur in socket), or acute trauma with dislocation and sudden twisting. Labral tears are difficult to diagnose as they are so similar to hernias, snapping hip syndrome, and bursitis. Also, although a labrum may be torn, it doesn't mean that it is the cause of the symptoms. Typical signs are groin pain, clicking in the hip, and limited movement of the hip joint.

My heart lifted at the memory of treating a delightful tall lady with this problem earlier in the summer, with a very rewarding outcome. She was a darling and an inspiration to help. She was also rich, but she had not married to gain wealth and status; she was a self-made success story with a purposeful life. The love she felt for people shone out of her like a beacon. Even though she was a saint, however, she didn't suffer fools gladly, and she may well have been tempted to run over the other lady if they had met in the car park.

"I need it fixed quickly," my current patient stated, "my hip aches at night and when I go horse riding my groin and buttocks ache for hours. I have already had the best chiropractic treatment, so don't mess up and upset their great work."

I was amused at this, as here was a lady still evidently in pain, telling me how good her treatment was – it is strange how folks can be so defensive when requesting help. I asked what could still be aggravating her hip.

"Well," she started, and I mentally braced myself, "for starters, I don't work – I don't need to, unlike the likes of you. I did play hockey and ride, and I did like long walks, but all of those things make the pain unbearable now. I still enjoy very gentle yoga, that's about it! I don't suppose you know what hip dysplasia is?"

Luckily, I knew that hip dysplasia is a condition where the head of the femur is not the correct shape for the cup shape of the socket. My sister-in-law suffers with this. If we look at it from a human garage perspective, we can think of it like a car tyre: if the tyre shape or pressure is uneven, it affects the tracking. Certain changes can be made to help preserve the life of the hip joint, and current methods rely on lifestyle changes, MRT, or stem cell, and if severe enough, surgical treatments. Lifestyle changes such as reducing aggressive weight bearing activities, losing weight, or taking arthritis medication can help, though non-operative methods may not provide a lasting solution because the joint itself is the wrong shape.

Once I feel a connection of trust with a patient, I can normally treat any painful hip with neuropathic overlay from L2/3 nerves to the hip with IMS and electroacupuncture, checking the core and muscle imbalance around the hip, and recommending exercises and magnetic resonance on a setting to help the inflamed labral tear to heal. Then, if it is severe, I would explain to the patient that the degree of dysplasia may need a surgical intervention. I understand that a strong bond between the current therapist and the patient should not be messed with, and on this occasion I felt no such strong bond. So, instead, I decided to text her people and suggest that I simply add in MRT to their treatment pathway.

Six weeks later, I reassessed this lady and to her amazement, the MRT had eased the soreness of the labral tear. Within three months the scan showed a lot of healing. As I understand, she went on to seek a surgical opinion about the angle of the hip joint and I suggested a full biomechanical assessment to help with the way she walked.

"You see," she said, "I am much better with your machine; it's a good job you didn't mess with me too much."

Taking a deep breath to calm myself down, I asked her, "Why did you come?"

She thought for a moment, looking rather confused. "Well, you come highly recommended as some kind of international expert in pain; why did you think I came?"

There's nowt so queer as folk, eh!

MANIPULATIONS AS SOFT AS SWISS CHEESE

Right, here we go in my time machine again, and this time we're heading back about six years, to when I was co-presenting the Z Factor in Switzerland. There was an American chiropractor demonstrating techniques, and it was then that I began to understand a little more about the art of chiropractic therapy.

There are different schools of thought within the profession – there is the softer touch of McTimoney and network chiropractors, and then there's the more traditional thrusting manipulating chiropractors. This is such a huge subject to cover in an eclectic volume on body work, so I will just give you several bite-sized pieces of information.

I remember Tony Robbins discussing how a chiropractor called Donald Epstein gently manipulated himself and his wife, and how emotional an experience it was. His description of the first consult under his glass roof – with the sun shimmering through his roof top pool – made it all sound very magical.

I have a book of Epstein's and in brief summary, the book *The 12 Stages of Healing* (1994) explains that Network Spinal Analysis is about wellness and body awareness. Gentle precise touch to the spine is thought to affect the brain and make it create new wellness-promoting strategies. Epstein talked about two unique healing waves that are associated with the spontaneous release of spinal and life tensions. Somehow, practitioners use existing tension as fuel for spinal re-organisation and enhanced wellness, combining their clinical assessments of spinal refinements with patients' self assessments of wellness and life changes. In some ways, this is like my team when they assess the four keys alongside the physical joint/muscle/fascial problem.

This kind of chiropractic work is very much a healing-focused practice. "Greater self-awareness and conscious awakening of the relationships between the body, mind, emotion, and expression of the human spirit are realized" (Epstein, 1994)." Dr. Epstein discovered 'twelve basic rhythms, or stages of consciousness,' and each stage of healing has a distinct 'rite of passage' – a chaotic experience or healing crisis – that helps us to reunite with aspects of ourselves that are traumatized, alienated, forgotten, abused, shamed, or unforgiven. Each stage also has a characteristic pattern

156

of breath, movement, and touch that can help us to reconnect with the natural, internal rhythms of our body and experience a greater sense of joy and well-being" (Epstein, 1994). Therefore, I made sure I paid more attention to Joseph McClendon's American chiropractor at the Z factor, as he also practiced a gentler chiropractic art.

Armed with this knowledge, a couple of years later I was visited by a network trained chiropractic lady at my practice. I was intrigued to discover that you lay fully clothed, and that after a couple of minutes of assessment, she knew with laser focus where to manipulate. Then, in 15 minutes, it was all over. I was impressed, although it was clear to me that this technique was only one part of a treatment that was needed to cure the problem. In my opinion, muscle memory, joint disease, posture, muscle strength, fascial release, and psychology would all need addressing.

CHIROPRACTIC CLUNK CLICK WITH EVERY TRIP

The following information is taken from the Thrive Clinic website (www. thriveclinic.co.uk):

"Chiropractic was founded as a health profession in the US in 1895 by a Canadian called Daniel David Palmer, who had no conventional medical training. Palmer argued that most human disease is caused by misalignments of the spine that apply pressure on surrounding nerves. He called these misalignments 'subluxations' and believed that they blocked the flow of a natural energy, or 'life force', through the body. Correcting [them] could restore the proper flow of energy, and so restore health."

In my opinion, he went overboard here, as he saw "chiropractic spinal manipulation as a treatment for 95% of all health conditions."

"Since its early days, chiropractic has fought for acceptance as a legitimate health profession. In the early 20th century, Palmer came close to declaring chiropractic a religion" – not very helpful to mainstream medical practice, and he struggled to obtain legal rights to practise in the US.

These days, chiropractic treatment is on a more "scientific footing through research to establish an evidence base for its principles and practice. Palmer's ideas do not always form the basis on which chiropractors practise, but this varies widely. The GCC (the statutory body for chiropractors in the UK) says the idea that subluxations are responsible for illness 'is not supported by any clinical research evidence' and that this idea should be taught as a historical concept and not a current theoretical model."

"Chiropractors, says the GCC, are 'concerned with the framework of the muscles and bones that support the body (the musculoskeletal system)' and with treating health conditions by helping the musculoskeletal system to work properly. Nonetheless, some UK chiropractors continue to claim that they can improve a range of health conditions by correcting subluxations," which is outside orthodox medical opinion.

1995 AND THE GOVERNMENT RECOGNISED OSTEOPATHS

Many years ago in 1995, I headed one of the first NHS hospital departments to employ an osteopath alongside physiotherapists – it was only in 1993 that the osteopath profession got a formal recognition. I had treatment from my osteopath due to a whiplash sustained in a car crash, and I can remember that his focus was very much on joint alignment and movement. He was strong but also very respectful of the recent trauma, and reluctant to mobilise a recently bruised neck, so I had a combination of osteopathy, physiotherapy, hydrotherapy, TENS (transcutaneous electrical nerve stimulation), and acupuncture in the NHS unit I ran.

I was known as Flipper at this hospital, as after a long, stressful day, I could often be found behind my reception desk, submerged in the hydro pool. At least I had progressed from my early days as a toddler, sitting in a sink of water to shut me up. I adore water and swimming – and all of its healing properties – and so do my head and spine.

After a good experience with this osteopath, I later employed another osteopath at my clinic, though it was difficult to get different therapists to gel and agree on treatment plans. This lady osteopath came to work with me for a few months, and again her knowledge of joint articulation was excellent. She also embraced a psychologically and nutritionally holistic approach – at least, up to a point; in my opinion, her huge resistance to employ other modalities of treatment, such as biomechanics, gait analysis, technology to repair damaged joints, shockwave to blast into calcified tendons and trigger points, and so on… was very self-limiting.

Now, let me explain my understanding of the history of osteopathy with a quick whistle-stop tour. Dr Still was a physician and surgeon – plus a founder of Baker University – and he came up with osteopathy back in the days of the American Civil War. In America, if you practise osteopathy you are a medical doctor, while in the UK you need a three-year degree and you are not a medical doctor.

I read that Still founded the American School of Osteopathy in Kirksville in 1892, and in 1898 the American Institute of Osteopathy gave DO degrees and started the *Journal of Osteopathy*. By that time four states recognised osteopathy as a profession. In London in 1917, John Martin Littlejohn – a pupil of Dr Still – started up a UK college, with the osteopathic profession in the UK finally being accorded formal recognition by Parliament in 1993 by the Osteopaths Act. So, to have an osteopath as part of my NHS team was a very new thing to do.

Osteopathy embraces the belief of innate healing in order to self-regulate and improve circulation. This includes looking at emotional patterns being responsible for poor breathing patterns, and beyond biomechanical issues, it also looks into responses to stressful incidents of the past or present. Osteopaths work on soft tissue and joint alignments, all of them evolving in their own specific blend of treatments, post-graduate.

In 1910, Dr Still said, "the body heals itself, and our primary role is to remove obstacles to the processes which allow this to occur. I do not claim to be the author of this science of osteopathy. No human hand framed its laws; I ask no greater honour than to have discovered it." He also said, "The me-

chanical principles on which osteopathy is based are as old as the universe"
(Andrew Taylor Still, 1828-1917).

I also like the following statement by Leon Chaitow: "the practitioner therapist should be able to recognize the least invasive therapeutic interventions
that can be a catalyst for self healing and repair" (in Myers, 2001).

WHAT IS WALKING?

When we swing the right leg forward, the right ilium – that is, the right side
of our pelvis – rotates back in relation to the sacrum. The sacrum is the triangular bone at the back that articulates both sides with our bucket-shaped
pelvic bones, and attached is our rudimentary tail, the remnants being the
coccyx, which my skiers keep bruising when they land on their arses. As the
leg swings forward, the tension increases in the protective elastic ligaments
around the sacrum, called sacrotuberous and interosseous ligamentous (see
the glossary). Just like a plane putting down the landing carriage/wheels to
soften the thump of the landing, in the same way the ligaments brace the
sacroiliac (SI) joint ready for the heel to land. The big muscles at the back of
our thighs – the hamstrings – fire up to tighten the sacrotuberous ligament
further and support the sacroiliac (SI) joint even more. Going through my
old notes, I have just read a study by Vleeming et al. (1999), describing the
essential role of the pelvis.

HOMEWORK:
Observe how you walk.

As your right heel approaches the ground, a slim bone called the fibula
moves downwards a little to pull on the outer hamstring and the sacrotuberous ligament. The big toe needs to lift like the nose of the plane on
landing, and this is the bit where my aerospace husband starts to talk about
the need for the fins on the wings of a plane to adjust in order to build wind
resistance so we don't crash when landing! And all this whilst I'm trying not
to think about how fast the ground is rushing up towards us. I was banned
from his flying lessons due to my rude comments.

Anyway, in my mind, the little wing flaps are the human equivalent of tibialis anticus, pulling up our big toe. Then, a network of fascial cabling links connect to a muscle called the peroneus longus running under the foot and along the fibula (the outer side) in order to pull the foot up and out (everting it). This clever sequence of pulleys and cables then tense the outside part of the hamstrings by pulling the fibula bone down a touch and bracing the sacroiliac (SI) joint for touch down – here I think of the undercarriage lowering its wheels. When the sole of the foot has rolled forward, this myofascial sling releases its elastic support on the SI joint, and you can just feel this if you place a hand on your right pelvic bone – the iliac bone – subtly rotating forward.

As physiotherapists, we often assess how your pelvis moves, and if it's complex, David Paling – one of my experienced physios at my midlands clinic – has a sixth sense with palpating this movement. I call him up to my office to slide a hand over an unsuspecting patient's bottom to see how they bump and grind. All in the best possible taste, you understand.

HOMEWORK:
Feel what's happening as you slowly step forward – do a 'bionic man' slow speed walk and bring awareness to the way you move and balance. Do you sense any tightness, weakness, lack of balance, or pain?

So, how does your right foot land? Can you feel your left arm moving forward as this happens? Your bottom muscle – the large one, gluteus maximus – fires to stabilise your SI joint on the right, and at this moment, the thoracolumbar fascia (bubble wrap) transmits the force, firing latissimus dorsi on the left. A winding-up mechanism of counter rotation of the trunk on the pelvis stores kinetic energy.

HOMEWORK:
Can you feel this rotation?

As your foot is placed on the ground, the hamstrings can relax and the right sacroiliac (SI) joint is less pressured. You are now in a stable double leg support stance, and with your next step, the left iliac bone rotates forward, as once again you go into single leg stance as the left leg swings forward. With the leg swing, the nutation (see glossary) of the left SI joint starts.

This ability to step forward is a micro-managed series of myofascial ligamentous effort. Within this complex gait cycle, these 'slings' form an elastic framework, and this can be subjected to a multitude of errors. This energy-storing fascial network is often overlooked, so my team of biomechanical/structurally-orientated physiotherapists routinely look for postural imbalances, bony alignment, poor balance reactions, and muscle weakness and tightness in these fascial networks.

I see a lot of patients with all kinds of issues, and here, briefly, I want to give you a handful of examples:

A weakened bottom/gluts can be due to SI joint or hip osteoarthritis. The hamstrings overwork to compensate, getting tight, and your step length becomes less. The hams can then tear.

Osteoarthritis in the knees weakens the inner quads (vastus medialis), meaning that knee lock-out is less strong and elastic, and the kneecap maltracking causes more accelerated wear and tear in the back of the knee.

A torn lateral ankle ligament means that the fibula pull down is less effective, and the whole sequence and effectiveness of the elastic sling is lessened in stepping.

Flat feet and lots of walking on tarmac in poorly cushioned footwear can lead to policeman's foot. This is where the sling of plantar fascia under the foot gets irritated where it attaches to the calcaneal heel bone. This lack of elasticity transmits up through the leg.

MY KNEE

Right, now it's back in my time machine to my early twenties when my right knee locked up. It was my first year of physiotherapy – when it's all fresh and exciting – and I was having fun working on hospital wards and finally earning a wage at long last. One morning, my knee locked so badly I could not straighten it out, and my friends – a mixture of newly qualified, fun-loving physios and doctors, including a recent ex-boyfriend orthopaedic registrar – took it upon themselves to fix me. Lucky me… not!

One moment I was wrestling with my leg, standing up and falling down, and then Victor (a South American student doctor) had a mask on my face, giving me laughing gas with the mask upside down! What can I say? He was still learning. In no time at all my crazy friends had me in theatre, as I had torn the lateral cartilage in my right knee. These cartilages are shock absorbance cushions and are there for a reason, but surgeons cut, so there we are. My ex was learning knee surgery at the time and made a few surgical errors, he and Victor had a fight in theatre, and they apparently gave me so much anaesthetic that I peed myself… lovely! The latter piece of information was woven into an after dinner speech at the medics ball by a thoughtful colleague – grrrrr.

I took a long time to come around after surgery, so all my dear friends kept visiting me –I'm sure the other patients thought I was dying! My knee remained swollen; it just would not heal up properly, and it took a long time to settle. I was told to give up running and tennis for life – which I did until four years ago – and I was also told not to get involved in dangerous sports, so I took up deep sea diving around the world!

HOMEWORK:
Were you told to give up sport because of an injury, and would you reconsider getting fit if you knew treatment existed to reduce the damage?

So, let's head forward in my time machine now to just four years ago, when I decided to push my knee as I was due to present the Z factor and the idea was to powerwalk or jog the audience around the lake each morning. Joseph McClendon was not able to do this, as he had a knee problem himself and a lady had also dropped her suitcase on his foot.

Let's just say that my new fitness regime had not exactly gone to plan; I hobbled into work on a stick with a badly swollen knee. Vinod – my friend and in house clinic surgeon – MRI scanned my knee and consulted me in my own clinic. 20 years on from my surgery, I had post surgical changes, accelerated osteoarthritis due to a chunk of the cushioning lateral meniscus being cut out, and moderate kneecap changes with hooky calcified stalagmites of bone (osteophytes). This was due in part to surgery, in part to leg length difference, and in part to being flatfooted, which further affects the articulation of the patella femoral joint.

I had a course of MRT for osteoarthritis of my knee and never looked back; I started running everyday – though never more than four miles. I didn't do marathon running as I figured there was still damage there even though there was evidence of new cartilage, but most importantly there was no pain and no swelling, hooray!

Dean put me through my paces on a treadmill and Gaitscan, as well as advising me on trainers and orthotics. He watched my walking and running style while the computer translated the pressure signals – the contact phase is when 3 to 5 times my body weight of force gets absorbed in a shockwave up through my body. I now know from a recent scan that my running style could have been better, and that now it has to be, due to the bony end plate changes and disc degeneration at the base of my spine. Depending on your personal biomechanics, you can contact more on your heel, or your midfoot, or your forefoot. I needed to know how to soften my contact to the floor; as my heel hits the floor, my pronating foot absorbs some of the force. My propulsion through the ball of my foot is different in my right compared to my left, due to a diving trauma to my right toe and a stiffened right toe joint. My flat feet do not exactly help my old stiff toe either.

> **HOMEWORK:**
> If you run, have you checked out anti-aging, anti-arthritic exercise?

I have flat feet, so good shoes and wearing good insoles at times both help to reduce the uneven rotational forces going up through my shins, knees, pelvis, and spine, leading to arthritic skeletal issues.

Running is high impact, so cushioning and rigidity in the right measure is needed according to your foot biomechanics. For instance, I have to have strong padding, midsoles, and good support and motion control. If you have a medium arch then neutral cushioning and all over support is good, and you are perfect for running, whereas high arched feet need high cushioning and shock absorbency padding to protect the arch. In my case, Dean went on to order bespoke orthotics for my feet from Sub-4.

> **HOMEWORK:**
> Check that your running shoes are correct for you. If you're running two to three miles a day, make sure you replace your trainers every six months.

There are many, many possible problems when it comes to your biomechanics. Those psychologically-driven therapists look for mind in body issues, and treat the dysfunction between psychosocial and emotional triggers. Those specialising in the theory of trigger points hunt them down with shockwave, deep massage, and dry needling. A belief in bones being out of place leads to joint adjustments, whereas a belief in anatomy trains would result in myofascial massage and muscle energy work. Podiatrists/ foot specialists – as well as biomechanical experts – may well use Gaitscan analysis to look for pressure transmission through specific places in the feet, plus analysing the gait on a treadmill in terms of walking and running. They would prescribe the correct footwear for the foot posture, and often bespoke orthotics to correct the poor foot posture. Movement therapists, Feldenkrais, Alexander, Tai Chi, yoga, and Pilates would correct dysfunction through specific repeated movements in the correct posture.

My team all have their specialisms, however, they also incorporate a blend of treatment approaches, cross-referencing between them. All of these different approaches involve a connection between patient and therapist, and the ability of the detective to listen and piece together the evidence, identify the cause, and call in the relevant experts, can only grow with experience and learning. When our patients walk into the clinic badly, they present a confusing assortment of soft tissue issues, poor inflexible or hypermobile degenerate joints, psychological baggage, and postural dysfunctional habitual patterns, not to mention poor diet and obesity issues.

As the saying goes, problems walk in on two legs.

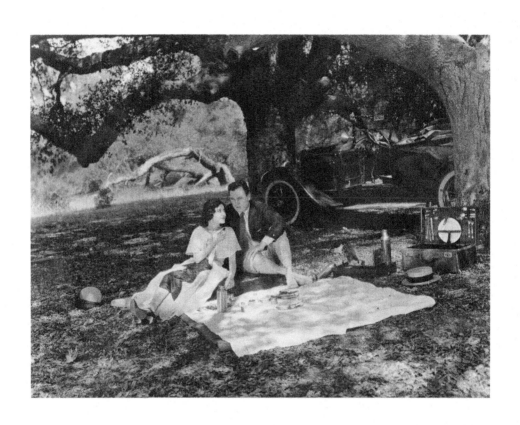

Chapter Five

"Wisdom comes with winters"

– Oscar Wilde

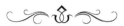

Anti–aging secrets and food, the elixir of life

WHEN THE SOUL BURNS WITH PASSION, THE BODY IGNORES OLD AGE

In this chapter I look at information taken from a lot of nutrition and health experts, as I value their knowledge and advice. References can be found in the bibliography if you'd like to read more from them.

"By the time we are fifty, we have learned our hardest lessons. We have found out that only a few things are really important. We have learned to take life seriously, but never ourselves."
- Marie Dressler

I couldn't agree more, Marie. Agelessness means not buying into the idea that a number determines your health, value, usefulness, fitness, and value to society. Agelessness means to engage fully in life without the nagging fear that you could fall apart at any moment. Centenarians are the fastest grow-ing segment of the population – there are currently 53,000 in the USA, with a predicted 66,000 by the year 2050 – although I'm not sure I believe that unless lifestyles change. I have, however, seen a video clip with my own eyes taken last year of a 105-year-old Japanese runner 'Golden Bolt', achieving the 100m record for his age group (Patel, 2015). Incredible.

I believe it is a driving, enthusiastic passion that gives our bodies the lon-gevity we crave for – a burning need to leave this planet a better place for having been here, a need to impart knowledge, love, art, music, and any-thing creative in order to make a difference. Here's a list of just a handful of names that had this type of passion in common:

Goethe was 82 when he completed Faust. Picasso was painting into his 90's. Vanda Scaravelli was busy practising yoga till her death in her 90's. Wagner composed Parsifal at age 80. Giuseppe Verdi wrote the Falstaff opera at 79. Les Misérables was an idea that started with Victor Hugo when he was in his 60's. At 80, Toscanini conducted his orchestra with amazing vigour. Look at Tina Turner at 76, touring and singing and dancing. Wayne Dwyer died recently in his 70's whilst still lecturing and writing. One of my dear professors, Prof Gunn, is treating patients in his 80's. Hay House founder, Louise L. Hay, set up a wonderful international publishing house in her 60's and is still actively involved. Rudolf Serkin played piano passionately well into his 80's. Pablo Casals' cello was seductively stroked until his 90's.

Focused, attentive minds drove these human bodies beyond what they could normally be expected to achieve at their age, so start planning what you will do in your old age now.

LIKE A WICK (TELOMERE) ON A CANDLE, WE HAVE A SHELF LIFE

"Regret for the things we did can be tempered by time; it is the regret for the things we did not do that is inconsolable."
- *Sydney J. Harris*

I love candles; the candle wick reminds me of the human spirit, and in the genetic material in our cells there is a telomere – just like a candle wick – which is believed to be a measure of our longevity. This protective tip sits on top of a chromosome (genetic material), and as we age it grows shorter and shorter, until it glows too dim and can no longer tell the cell to divide again. At this point, we die. Science is now starting to become convinced that lifestyle could influence the wick's life, and this is done by stimulating the release of a body juice/enzyme called telomerase. I have an abundance of papers scattered on my desk regarding this subject, and one by Jaskelioff et al. (2011) caught my eye: they showed that degenerate mouse tissue was made youthful with the reactivation of telomerase.

WHAT ACCELERATES AGING?

Due to my research for this book, I have piles and piles of papers in front of me, stacked up in my room and piled high on the floor; hundreds of hypotheses and theories from dozens of universities all around the world. Mostly they discuss consequences of aging rather than causes of aging, and as we all age differently and so uniquely, this surely points to differences in our lifestyles. One of the aims of my first book on the 4 keys was to flag up to my patients how a lack of exercise, poor diet, lack of purpose, toxic chemicals, and stress can all steal their healthy aging.

Over time, why do we have less vitality and more pain? Well, part of this is because our physiology changes as we age. For instance, for us ladies, our hormones change in our 40's to 50's as we go through the menopause. Men, on the other hand, have andropause; often delayed to age 60 or so, this involves a lack of male sex hormones that reduces sexual drive, as well as muscular physique and ambition. Both men and women have less growth hormone as we age, which makes us fatter and which means we have less physical endurance as we get older. The thyroid is also less, so again we have a slower metabolism and become more rotund... and on and on... On top of this, our intelligence gives weaker signals to the nervous, endocrine, and immune systems. But why?

Could these protective tips – the telomeres at the ends of each strand of DNA that control aging – really alter all these physiological effects we experience when we age? These telomeres shorten as we age, and at the same time, our cells are producing fainter photocopies of themselves. Could it be that these telomeres are acting like a control switch to play out the drama of aging? Certainly, papers by Harley et al. (1990), Sahin et al. (2011), and Horner et al. (2011) all back this theory up. Could these structures be receiving messages in order to create an older or younger version of ourselves? Could the age difference between our metabolic/physiological age and actual earth years be down, in part, to telomeres? Could this be what the Chinese hinted at with their views on Chi and having a finite reserve of energy to draw down on until death? The Indians talk of Prana in a similar way to Chi – this is echoed in the rate of loss of photons of piezoelectric energy (see glossary) lost from our bodies. Research suggests that this form of energy loss from the body accelerates during times of rapid aging, stress, and when we're near death, especially through our fingers and toes.

At times I feel very old these days, and especially when allowing the stress of a busy life to affect me. My hands are cold, my bones ache, and I feel that I need to distance myself from everyone around me in order to rekindle my energy. Are we pushing the control switch into the older part of our genome as we become stressed? Are we consciously accelerating the time of our programmed death?

I knew from my formative years as a biologist that stem cells in a foetus have a short time limit when cells can form into and become anything, such as muscle or bone or nerves. After this time, they become specific and mortal and unchangeable. IVF babies can only be made with the few cell divisions of the egg.

THE ANTI-AGING BODY JUICE, THE ELIXIR OF YOUTH

In 2009, Dr Elizabeth Blackburn, Carol Greider, and Jack Szostak all won the Nobel prize for finding the elixir of life: the body juice, telomerase. It was proposed that in order to rebuild time, you could rebuild the protective genetic chromosome tip – the telomere – with telomerase. In humans and animals, telomerase is thought to be switched off after birth, so – literally like an hour glass – as the last grains of sand fall through, we die. However, studies have not been able to prove all this, so more research needs to be carried out. Here I'd like to just briefly mention Dolly, the genetically-made sheep, as they were not able to work out how to reverse aging.

By 2005, one thousand studies had been carried out, and yet still the controversy raged – there was still heated debate about the amount of telomere involvement in aging and chronic disease. However, they did concur that the length shortens with age, with each cell replication losing between 30 and 150 nucleotide pairs of genetic material, DNA. Once a critical length is met, you have literally drawn the short straw, and you die.

MICE TIME TRAVEL

This idea was demonstrated in an experiment by Sahin et al. (2011), when mice were literally the stars of an aging time machine program. Scientists flipped control switches in their genes, causing the telomere to be artificially shortened, and the mice to age in response. This genetic trigger caused a loss of the cell's powerhouse, the mitochondria. The mice then lost their metabolic control, which in turn led to heart disease and blood sugar disasters.

The next experiment was for posh, privileged mice, with first class time travel to youthful times. Joking apart, in 2011 a professor of Genetics at Harvard did just this. He turned on the fountain of youth in the equivalent of eight-year-old mice, by lengthening their telomeres through the enzyme, telomerase. Within a month, brain neurons sprouted, hair darkened, sperm and eggs led to a litter, and key organs functioned better. The mice went on to have long, healthy lives.

There followed a lot of unsustainable claims, mixed in amongst good, sound research of telomerase activators. This elusive elixir of youth is believed to work by activating anti-aging genes called sirtuins, which are thought to signal cells in order to stimulate the DNA repair processes that otherwise would lead to decay and, ultimately, death. Since then, more gene switches have been named that are known to affect cell division and longevity – for example, M1 and M2 are a couple that can change the age of mice. Even with all these studies and all this knowledge, however, the whole picture still remains a mystery.

HOMEWORK:
Think about this: if man could live longer, what would you want to achieve? If this were possible, breeding would need to be controlled in order to avoid a population explosion. How would you feel about that if children were scarce?

WHY TANTRIC SEX?

On his show about longevity, Dr. Oz prescribed sex once daily – I wonder if he has a secret lover or two in order to achieve this! The subject of tantric sex was taught to me in theory, though sadly not in practice. I have to say it sounds a wonderful practice and one perhaps suited to a retired couple, or friends who meet and share the same spiritual and sexual energy and who can devote the time needed for such practice.

Tantric sex involves the practice of various meditations and exercises (including yoga) to arouse and channel tremendous energy throughout and within the body. Tantric sex is commonly associated with the *Kama Sutra*, the ancient Hindu texts of love. Shiva, the male Hindu God's energy represents bliss, whereas Shakti, the female Hindu God's energy represents wisdom. "The perfect pair is often depicted in statues and paintings in many entwined positions – embracing, sitting, standing, balancing on one leg, or dancing, with Shakti wrapped around Shiva's body or hiked on his hips" (Vample website).

The goal is to cycle that energy with a partner, and to send it out into the world with a prayer for enlightenment. It is intended for personal peace and fulfilment, interpersonal intimacy at the highest level, and connection to the entire world of beings. On top of this, the energy generated by tantric sex can be used for pleasure and blissful personal enlightenment, as well as anti-aging and healing – that must be why the yoga teachers I know always have big smiles on their faces! Sexual union is seen as a divine gift, honouring all beings, and this reminds me of Wicca and the horny god Pan – I mean, the horned god Pan. In the west, there is a growing interest in Eastern philosophies and their ability to ease depression and stress.

As we get older, due to modern day pressure we are told to downsize, to accept being less active, and to invest in a large drugs cupboard, especially with regards to pain meds. With technological advances, materialism, families living further apart, commuting being less enjoyable with busier roads, and less help with health issues due to increasingly busier doctors' practices and hospitals – not to mention world tensions, war, and terrorism; since writing this book, both Paris and Brussels have been hit in the last three months, and currently we are bombarded by footage on the news of destroyed cities and desperate refugees – the pressures and stresses of everyday life can be overwhelming. This, I feel, has fuelled a need to feel safe, trustful, and youthful. A meaningful life means every cell feeling nurtured, with the heart-head connection being strong.

Over my 25 years of clinical experience, there has been a slow increase in the acceptance of Eastern treatments, although only this week, NICE (government health) guidelines changed their minds on giving Acupuncture a gold standard for treating low back pain, revoking the research. However, beyond their drugs, they interestingly embraced yoga and manipulation, so all is not lost.

On the whole, there has been an increased awareness of the soul, which I will cover in my next book.

THE TANTRIC BREATH

Here I have selected a few breathing exercises you can do, and they can also help with back pain. I have no intention of writing about the *Kama Sutra* – not in this book, anyway – and besides, I would have to research it first. Wishful thinking!

HOMEWORK:
Try out the following breathing exercises.

Egg to eagle. For this you can be sitting at work or home, and it is a good exercise to do when you are feeling tired. Exhale as you crunch down into a ball, bringing your elbows in close to your body and resting your hands on the back of your head. Feel the stretch across and down your spine. Then inhale, lifting up slowly and stretching to bring your elbows as far back behind you as is comfortable. Feel the stretch in your chest, throw your chest out, and arch your back. Feel the air filling your lungs – like bellows – and connecting with your spine.

Now for the *Buddha breath*, which simply speaking is a big, slow, deep breath into the belly.

Fire breath, on the other hand, is shallow, rapid breathing. This is a strange one, as it involves you breathing into your naughty bits to fire up your sexual energy. For this, you need to bring awareness to the place in your body from which your breath is coming. Is it appearing from your throat, chest, or tummy? Make a deliberate effort to ensure it comes from deeper within your body. With each gentle, slow breath, trace the breath and bring your hand to where it stops before you exhale. Lower your hand and make the breath come from as low down as your naughty bits – this is supposed to be the key to firing up your sex energy, if you haven't fallen asleep by now.

Ecstatic breathing. To do this breathing technique, lie on your back and inhale long, slow breaths through the mouth. Count to five as you expand your tummy, creating an archway under the small of the back. Then you can exhale, allowing the air to rush into the chest and through your mouth. Allow the arch in your lower back to go as you move into slight flexion. Repeat rhythmically to create a wave-like motion throughout the body.

Circulating breath. Inhale, imagining energy/white light rising up from your second/sexual chakra (kundalini) – which is located just below your naval – and through your body (passing through all the chakras on the way, as listed in my 4 keys book), before travelling to the top of your head. Then imagine it going back down to the base of your spine, pausing at the second chakra of seven, on the exhale. Finally, picture tracing a loop inside yourself and then out to a partner. Practices can be called different names by different disciplines, but to the Chinese Taoists, this is known as the Microcosmic Orbit or the Golden Circle.

Synchronising breath. For this you need to find a partner, and if you haven't got one, you can practice with a cat! Breathe in and out at the same time as your partner so you can get on the same wavelength. Then, sit comfortably, cross-legged and facing each other, and on a pillow if necessary – just as long as your spine is straight. After a while, close your eyes to sense each other's energy pattern. Sitting up helps you not to fall asleep!

Reciprocal breath. For this, imagine that you are exchanging air, inhaling your partner's breath (or imagine breathing for each other). Inhale while your partner exhales, then exhale while your partner inhales. For this exercise, it is a good idea to avoid garlic and clean your teeth beforehand!

Well, I am now very bored of all that deep breathing, so let's move on.

SACRED SCIENCE – IS IT HIDDEN IN A JUNGLE?

"'Hope' is the thing with feathers
That perches in the soul
And sings the tune without the words
And never stops. At all."
- Emily Dickinson

I watched an online documentary recently by Sacred Science, that really stayed with me, and I'd like to talk about it briefly here. The video footage – taken in a jungle –fascinated me, as it looked at seven very different chronically ill individuals who had lived a much westernised life, and yet at the eleventh hour, they'd chanced it all to live closely with nature, taking plant medicine and experiencing Shamanic healings.

The documentary took place in a Peruvian jungle in October 2010, the purpose being to bring to our attention the fact that out of 44,000 plants, only 1% have been studied for medicine. The Shamans know their plant medicine, and they are judged by their ability to heal.

At times, the guests were placed in solitude in order to feel at one with the jungle, but help was always close at hand in the form of friendship, ritual meds, prayers, and shared rituals. By healing their physical conditions, they were able to get to know themselves and become aware of their inner strength. In solitude they could not hide from themselves; they learnt that they were not separate beings but a part of everything, and therefore they learnt to embrace nature and the sounds of the jungle.

Immersed in nature, they rediscovered the calling of their hearts, and they also learnt to stare into another man's eyes and see a reflection of themselves, their soul. They had to change every ritual of their lives and some of their beliefs, not to mention changing their diet and sleeping patterns. To stand the greatest chance of recovering from their serious illnesses, they were also encouraged to embrace an awareness of sacred medicine.

The physical diseases that these individuals suffered from included Parkinson's, neuroendocrine cancer, breast cancer, prostate cancer, alcoholism/depression, irritable bowel, Crohn's, and diabetes (see the glossary for definitions of all of these). After just 30 days, the most peaceful man – who had very advanced neuroendocrine cancer – had died, and the Crohn's lady and breast cancer lady needed much more help. On the other hand, the Parkinson's, prostate cancer, alcohol/depression, irritable bowel and diabetic patients had all improved tremendously.

I think that the study was very successful, as five out of the eight patients (that western medicine could not do anything to help) had been helped by the Shamans. These Shamans study plant medicine for years – passed down from grandfather to father to son – and walk many miles every day in order to collect the plants. They then work late into the night to prepare the medicines, administering them to the patients and praying over them as they perform rituals. All in all, they work really hard. Their driving passion is to help others and cure their sickness, and when the time comes, to ease their passage to death.

Should we rethink how sensible it is to destroy rainforests when ancient cures that can be found within are now becoming extinct?

REGROW YOUR BODY PARTS IN THE HUMAN GARAGE

Can you imagine going to the photocopier at work only to find that someone is reprinting their head? I can remember writing a story all about this at just 12 years old, stating that we would do this in the future, and consequently being laughed at for it. Fast forward to the present day, and custom-made, living body parts that function normally when implanted into animals are now being 3D-printed. This significant advance for regenerative medicine raises the hope of using living tissues in order to repair the body.

The team of scientists at Wake Forest Baptist Medical Centre in North Carolina developed a new technique that 3D-prints a tissue riddled with micro-channels – rather like a sponge – to allow nutrients to penetrate the tissue. "The Integrated Tissue and Organ Printing System – or ITOP – combines a bio-degradable plastic which gives the structure and a water-based gel which contains the cells and encourages them to grow. When the structures were implanted into animals, the plastic broke down as it was replaced by a natural, structural 'matrix' of proteins produced by the cells. Meanwhile, blood vessels and nerves grew into the implants" (BBC Website).

Professor Martin Birchall, a surgeon at University College London, said that "the prospect of printing human tissues and organs for implantation has been a real one for some time" but confessed that he "did not expect to see such rapid progress" (BBC Website). The question now is only *when* and not *if* we will see our first patients with a 3D-printed knee joint or ligament reconstruction.

KEEP A FOOD DIARY

If you want a healthy body, what you put in it is critical. You wouldn't put honey instead of fuel into your car and expect to get the engine started, would you?

"It's time to be truthful and conscious about how much and how often you are eating, and a food diary is an excellent tool for making dietary changes.

You can only change your habits with awareness, and writing things down makes you fully mindful" (Shimoff, 2015).

Of course, if you don't like the idea of having to write everything you eat down, you can always take pictures on your phone. Patients tell me time and again that they have no memory of naughty snacking; it's as if they do it in a trance, a kind of comforting sleep walk. Yet all these comforting sugary snacks are causing our cells to feel sick. If you snuck some brandy snaps into your car fuel pipe, the car would splutter, and probably do a lot more than that!

At home, I have a small cupboard full of comfort food that represents about a tenth of my total food storage, and I consciously do it this way so I understand that it means just that: it is comfort food, not everyday food. Unhealthy food and drink may be pleasurable for the mind, but not for the body, so take in moderation please.

I understand that Jamie Oliver – the well-known celebrity chef – eats very healthily for at least four days or five days a week, but then also partakes in wonderfully tasty, less healthy food as a treat. I had a pizza yesterday at his parents' pub and it was orgasmic –OK, so pizza is not the healthiest of foods, but my God my immune system soared with the pleasure signals my brain was making.

WHAT IS HEALTHY FOOD?

So, what do we actually mean when we talk about healthy food? We're talking *fresh* fruit, vegetables, eggs, some poultry, fish, nuts, seeds, and a few whole grains. I personally don't eat animals, though I do eat the odd bird and fish, and I make sure to cover up my tropical fish tanks if cooking fish, so as not to traumatise their inhabitants – just kidding. I am always reading about having less wheat, dairy, and sugar – if you want a flat stomach, and fewer bottom coughs, then some of these should go. If you are eating grains, again get the healthiest, freshest ones possible.

Make sure you stop having sugar-laden drinks, as that's a sure way to get a fat arse. Drink alcohol and fruit juices (yes, even fresh fruit juices), in moderation please, because of the sugar. For at least half of my fluid intake, I make sure I have a jug of still water –with a bit of lime in – handy at all times, plus some herbal teas. Keeping really well hydrated with water or healthy drinks helps to keep you more youthful.

Eat three moderate-sized meals a day – and I'm talking portion control here, guys. This means no snacking between meals, unless they are small, healthy snacks, as I find that leaving a long gap between meals makes my stomach sore. No second helpings, and minimise the comfort food – it's simple: if you want to lose weight and tone up, eat less.

"Breakfast kick-starts your metabolism and helps you to be alert and awake throughout the day. Make sure you always eat a nutritious breakfast. Make it wholesome and make it count" (Jamie Oliver website).

Don't try any fad diets, just good, old-fashioned cooking at Snazzy's house. Let go of all the confusion – it's time to eat real food in sensible portions and get moving. Prepare healthy, yummy, superfood meals several times a week. Grow some of your own herbs and veggies. Have pots of herbs both inside and outside the house.

On top of all this, you need a minimum of eight hours' sleep – and that's sleep in between meals, not during. Make meals so colourful and pretty that you want to stay awake to eat them.

As an example, here is what I typically eat for breakfast: soya or almond milk, crushed nuts, banana, and frozen berries. Plus variations on fruit, nuts, and seeds, and often a naughty slice of whole-wheat toast.

My dear friend Joseph McClendon wrote a book about changing your breakfast to change your life. "In 1986, Joseph met and teamed up with best-selling author and speaker Anthony Robbins. After mastering the technology, he became extremely proficient in assisting people in overcoming the fears, phobias and emotional challenges that hindered their lives. After working as a trainer and then master trainer, Joseph now serves as Head trainer and instructor at Robbins' acclaimed 'Mastery University', attended by business entrepreneurs, CEOs and people seeking a greater quality of life from 46 different nations" (Joseph McClendon III's website).

Wasn't I lucky to be invited to present Z factor with him, a seminar all about health? He always made sure that we all ate healthy food at his seminars and drank plenty of veggie juices and water. "It's that simple: what we put in our bodies and when we do it will determine the quality of our lives," Joseph says in his book about breakfast (*Change Your Breakfast, Change Your Life*). He also adds in his e-book that not getting nutrients "results in fat storing, energy depletion, emotional stress, and the acceleration of the aging process." Joseph explains that he is not a doctor but a wellness coach, however, he says: "Our company has over 20 doctors and scientists on the advisory and research board, including a Nobel Prize winner."

I was spoilt to have such a wealth of knowledge at my fingertips when I worked with him.

LUNCH

I use lettuce with most meals, as well as tasty, coloured baby leaves including rocket, grown fresh in season. Then I load up a small plate (or bowl or jam jar) with a handful of an assortment of the following: oily fish such as tuna, cherry tomatoes, spring onion, cucumber, herbs, red pepper, orange segments, watercress, mixed home-grown sprouts, quinoa, rice, beetroot, broccoli, sundried tomatoes, walnuts, avocado, spinach, red onion, apple, lemon juice, olive oil, and a partridge in a pear tree… good God, there's so much stuff when I list it all.

DINNER

Here are some of my favourite things to have for dinner:

◊ Fillet of fish (i.e. Salmon) with garlic, ginger, lemongrass, and herbs from the garden such as dill, tarragon, and coriander.

◊ Grilled chicken breast with baked potato and veggies.

◊ Veggie salad with avocado, apple, and feta cheese.

◊ Omelette and salad.

◊ Prawn/mushroom/bean stir fry – use ginger, Chinese 5 spice, lemon juice, lots of coriander, broccoli florets, and half a cup of cooked cannellini beans, then cook together with onion, celery, and garlic.

◊ Veggie soup done in the Vitamix blender. Sauté the carrots and the veg (like sweet potatoes) you want to use with onions. You can add vegetable stock and a touch of naughty crème, then blend it all together to make a thick, creamy, filling soup.

◊ Your drink can be a veggie and fruit smoothie – they're so healthy, but they're very filling, so they're probably best put in the fridge for a snack. Carrots, apples, and berries make a nice one, and mint or ginger can add a twist to the flavour. Or you can have a jug of water, or at the weekends a glass of red wine or a gin and tonic.

I read a lot of nutritionists' stuff, and I like Amelia Freer (a nutritionist celebrity dude) and her gentle approach to eating healthier: You can ease yourself into her healthy eating plan by giving just one thing up. I love her book, *Eat. Nourish. Glow.* (HarperCollins, 2015) – my husband Alan bought it for me for my birthday.

"Whether it's dairy, gluten, sugar, alcohol, or caffeine, start with your main diet weak spot. Once you've mastered that, you'll feel motivated to give up something else" (Amelia Freer website/blog).

KITCHEN DETOX

Throw away any food that's out of date, and more importantly, throw away any REALLY JUNKY FOOD. As I've mentioned, I do have a comfort food cupboard, and it is a blessing if used in moderation, as well as being a blessing for guests – especially my little nephews as they love Auntie's cake, and besides, they don't need to lose any weight.

So, if you want to put a naughty cupboard together, clear out any unhealthy food and put it in there: sugary breakfast cereals, chocolate, processed foods, crisps, biscuits, cakes, and sweets. For my healthy cupboards, in go the nuts, seeds, spices, pulses, olive oil, coconut oil, quinoa, brown rice, and pasta. Growing sprouts go into a dark cupboard. In the fridge there are veggies, fish, butter, yoghurt, and almond and soya milk. In the freezer, we have frozen veggies and fruit to hand for smoothies.

My main tools of the trade are as following: a greenhouse, good quality knives, a Vitamix blender, a Nutribullet, a juicer, a grater, a spiralizer, and lots of teapots. Not to mention lots of recycled jars to put food in out of plastic wrappers.

HOMEWORK:
Sort out your kitchen!

IT'S IMPORTANT TO FIGURE OUT WHAT KIND OF EATER YOU ARE

To really get to grips with a healthier eating plan, you need to figure out what kind of relationship you have with food. "Are you a comfort eater? Or a rushed eater? Perhaps you binge when you're drunk or hungover? Identify your eating behavior and start being more mindful with your food" (Shimoff, 2015).

Here I have included notes from Dr. Mosley's approach to matching a diet to the type of eater you are. Dr. Michael Mosley is a celebrity GP who has done TV shows on healthy eating and exercise. His well-known books, *Fast Exercise* and *The Fast Diet*, sit on my desk at home. Thank you so much for doing this documentary and for being so brave and honest about your own health concerns – may many of us health professionals follow in your footsteps.

As I was typing this, I had the munchies, and my inner voice just shouted at me, 'Put down the crisps and chocs, I'm watching you! You've got to stop unhealthy snacking, and it's all calories. Fat arse!'

You know that whole philosophy of eating little and often? Well, you have to be careful of heavy snacking. Have small, healthy snacks to hand, and have a drink first as sometimes you may think you feel hungry, but you might in fact just be thirsty. I minimise my baking, and when I do bake I freeze some of the cake or pie at once, as if it's in the house it will get eaten too fast. It's OK to be naughty sometimes, just cut down on the next meal to adjust the balance of calories.

HOMEWORK:
What sort of eater are you?

FAT IS YOUR FRIEND, SUGAR THE FOE

We need fat to keep our cells strong and healthy: avocados, coconut oil, milk, a little amount of cream, yoghurt, nuts, seeds, oily fish (salmon, mackerel, sardines, tuna), butter, and in moderation, poultry, are all healthy fat essentials (taken from the Marie Claire website). It's the devil Mr Sugar that you really need to stay clear of.

If you have consumed too many calories for your height, make sure you exercise and generally just move more; getting your heart pumping burns up the calories faster.

HEALTHY FOOD WILL MAKE YOU HAPPY

Your diet can affect your mood, your sleep, your sex drive, your motivation, your thinking, your digestion, and your skin – I can tell a lot about a patient's diet just by looking at their skin. Picking up some healthier eating habits is a no-brainer. Now, if you associate being happy with comfort food such as pizza, you can prepare some healthy options that will also excite you. For this, Jamie Oliver's *Everyday Super Food* book is orgasmic – I love the colourful pages and delightful recipes. Also, I enjoy Amelia Freer's food blogs, recipe ideas, and her book *Eat. Nourish. Glow.*, which again is full of colourful food.

"'Don't equate healthy food with deprivation or misery,' says Amelia Freer. 'Add vibrant colours and flavours to your meals, enjoy the process of making them and eat with friends and family. Don't starve yourself or make eating a joyless experience'" (Amelia Freer website/blog).

I am far from perfect when it comes to healthy food, and if I am away from home I find it so much harder. I am, however, consistent in that I eat well most of the time. As we age, we need healthy food even more as our digestion often gets more fragile. There's a quote from an American holistic health expert and author called Ann Wigmore that goes, "The food you eat can be either the safest and most powerful form of medicine or the slowest form of poison." And it's absolutely true: healthy eating tends to be cultural and often goes against the flow of the western busy life of processed, ready-made meals. Obesity with diabetes is affecting more and more people.

Manufacturers have hijacked our ability to put work into preparing healthy food. I love cooking from scratch, and I can remember at just four years old helping my grandma to cook in her Devonshire kitchen. I guess I was clumsy – as I seem to remember stories of pasties being dropped all over the floor – but at least I was trying, and I grew up understanding the importance of cooking and growing some veg. For those of you who didn't have that education, I think it's best to ensure consistent changes, say, 80% of the time, and then you are not setting yourself up for failure. Big changes are hard to make; small ones are easy. I swap my Sunday croissant for a healthy smoothie in the weekdays. Then, for at least five or six days a week, I make my own meals from scratch rather than buying the shop-bought, processed ones or eating out. Eventually, all these tiny tweaks will result in a low sugar diet, and each change will bring about a health boost that will spur you on to make the next subtle change, and so on, and so on.

With everyday food, I store as much as I can in recycled glass jars to avoid using toxic plastic packaging – plus, it looks cool. I always have mostly raw food at every meal, and I use colourful turmeric when I can due to its anti-inflammatory properties. I sometimes cook in coconut oil as an alternative to olive, as it does not denature so much at high temperatures.

Now, let's talk about bread and possible bread substitutes. I love bread, but it does make my stomach bloat, so instead I grind up nuts, adding them to smoothies and salads to fill me up more and minimising the portions of bread I eat. I will also deep-freeze sliced loaves and toast to avoid temptation to finish fresh loaves, and I rarely cook my own bread.

SUPPLEMENTS

Supplements should never be taken in place of healthy food, but when taken correctly, they can make a huge difference to your well-being. If you have any health problems it is good to see a qualified nutritionist first, but as a generalisation, my in-house nutritionist says that most people need probiotics, omega-3, and Vitamin D, as well as good minerals and antioxidants if possible. Personally, I take USANA Essentials (vitamins and minerals) every day, Procosa for my joints, healthy oils, and occasionally Nature's Sunshine smoothie protein mixtures.

PASTA AND FLOUR

We don't eat a lot of pasta at home but I still have a wide variety to hand for when we do. So many people are now gluten intolerant that I always bear this in mind, and I have all sorts of types and colours of rice. In terms of flour, for baking moments, I have whole meal flour, plain flour, brown rice flour (which is great for making pizza bases, although mine come out tough), coconut flour, and I nearly bought some chick pea flour in a little health shop in Norwich yesterday, but I'm not sure I would use it; I do tend to get carried away and don't use everything. You know, ladies, sell-by dates are a bit of a giveaway in my kitchen.

Now for sugar alternatives: I like to use honey, dark chocolate, and dried fruit.

Where do the celebrity nutritionists shop? Amelia Freer says that she "buys her goods from a variety of health food shops and farmers markets, and for clients recommends Goodness Direct as well as places like Whole Foods and Planet Organic" (Get The Gloss website). Jamie Oliver grows some of his own food; he has a place up the road from his parents' pub and supplies them with delicious fresh veg.

I CAN SING A RAINBOW, SING A RAINBOW

Eating a rainbow of colour is like painting your meal – it makes it so appetising to both the palette and the eyes. This is a big theme this year in celebrity restaurants and blogs. Vegetables and fruits are SO colourful – especially raw – though eating colourfully is not merely about vitamins, minerals, and fibre, all of which are essential components of our health, but is also about other essential proteins. I always want to make colourful food; it's the artist in me. Metaphorically speaking. Haha.

Celebrity nutritionist Amelia Freer loves colour and discusses this a lot in her book and blogs. I love the way she talks about plants communicating and surviving with colour. Plants use colours as their protection from the sun's rays and pests, as well as to attract birds and insects for pollination and seed dispersal. Even though I am a biologist, I hadn't really understood that colours are the sources of powerful phytonutrients – which is a name to describe thousands of different chemicals that studies show reduce the risk of chronic diseases such as diabetes, heart disease, and cancer, and oestrogen levels (Amelia Freer's website). Thank you for pointing that out, Amelia. They do this by boosting cell-to-cell communication and the immune system in people who eat a diet high in plant-based foods (United States Dpt. Of Agriculture Research website). Though sadly this is not supported by the papers selected by the NHS, as you will read later.

The wonderful colours in vegetables and fruits represent over 100,000 different phytonutrients. When eaten, they stimulate enzymes that help the body to get rid of exhaust fumes/toxins, as well as boosting the immune system, promoting a healthy woman's hormone levels (oestrogen metabolism), supporting cardiovascular health, and killing off free radicals and cancer cells. These plants' protective properties – if grown naturally in mineral-rich soil – are believed by nutritionists and Shamans to be powerful allies of our health.

HOMEWORK:
Make an effort to learn about the food you're eating – we all need to understand where our food comes from and how it affects our bodies. Make sure that the majority of your energy intake comes from nutritious calories that ALSO provide your body with nutrients like vitamins, minerals, protein, fibre, and good fats. Study nutrition and avoid empty calories (calories from unhealthy food).

"It's important to read packaging correctly. Be aware of the recommended portion sizes, and the sugar, salt and saturated fat contents. Remember that not all E-numbers are bad, but too many is often a bad sign," (Jamie Oliver website). Jamie also says: "Aim to eat a balanced diet that contains each of the food groups in the correct proportions, cook from scratch." I remember Joseph McClendon showing me his fist... no wait, I can explain... to say, "This is the size of your stomach, Nicky, do I make myself clear?" I was probably trying to make the food on my plate look smaller at that moment.

Water is also an essential part of your diet, as only hydrated cells replicate healthy cells. Drink plenty of water and avoid empty calories from things such as fizzy drinks, energy drinks, or juices with added sugar. Eat your calories – don't drink them.

THE COLOURS IN PLANTS HEAL US

Each different colour of the rainbow – red, orange, yellow, green, blue, indigo and violet – represents different families of healing chemicals. Back when we were hunter-gatherers, we ate over 800 different types of fruit and vegetables, of all different shapes, sizes, and colours. The anthropologist, biologist, and chef in me all meet to agree. Yes, 800 varieties – crazy, eh? That could make shopping a lengthy hobby! Also, we could eat six pounds of food for the same calorie input as two pounds of food today.

These days, we have selectively bred the colours we eat into very narrow ranges, whereas in nature, plant foods come in a painter's palette of colours. There are red carrots in India and purple potatoes in Peru, but being British, we eat orange carrots and white potatoes. I once bought my father a box of veggies of different colours – such as purple carrots – but he didn't seem very impressed, so I just bought him chocolates the next time. "Phytonutrients aren't just limited to fruits and vegetables; you can get them from legumes, herbs, spices, nuts, seeds, and teas" (Shimoff, 2015) as well.

HEALTHY TRAVEL SNACKS

When I travel between clinics, I take a smoothie with me, adding things like chia and ground nuts to give extra protein, as well as fruit, yoghurt, and nuts. When buying snack bars at the service station, the ones with the fewest ingredients are usually the most natural. Almonds, pumpkin seeds, walnuts, fruit, banana, and dried fruit... these are all healthy snacks. Choose a selection of interesting nuts and seeds.

Think, shop, and cook with health and colour in mind – pack as much unprocessed colour as you can get into your fridges and onto your plates and then sit back and watch the magic happen. As a guide, try and include at least three colourful veg and one fruit per meal.

Ignore the next section if you are colour-blind.

PAINT PALETTE FOR YOUR MEAL

Thank you, Amelia Freer – I cross-referenced your list of colourful food for the following groups of food listed by colour, for those of you who are not colour conscious:

Red
Tomatoes, beetroot, watermelon, strawberries, red peppers, raspberries, apples, plums, adzuki and kidney beans, blood oranges, cranberries, cherries, goji berries, red grapes, red onions, pomegranate, radishes, rhubarb, rooibos tea, red rice, red quinoa.

All of these foods have reported anti-inflammatory, anti-cancer, gastrointestinal, heart, hormonal, and liver health benefits.

Yellow
Banana, lemon, yellow peppers, pineapple, ginger root, squash, corn on the cob, apples, yellow courgettes, honeydew melon, yellow tomatoes.

These foods have anti-cancer, anti-inflammatory, cell protective, eye, heart, skin, and vascular health properties.

Orange
Carrots, mangos, apricots, pumpkin, winter squash, sweet potatoes, red lentils, turmeric, oranges, peaches, nectarines, orange peppers.

These foods contain anti-cancer, anti-bacterial, immune supportive, reproductive, and skin health benefits.

Green
Broccoli, green peppers, olives, Brussels sprouts, courgette, cabbage, Chinese cabbage, bok choi, kale, asparagus, avocado, bean sprouts, melon, celery, cucumber, green beans, green peas, green tea, chard, lettuce, spinach, limes, pears, watercress, herbs.

Anti-inflammatory, anti-cancer, neurological, hormonal, heart, liver and skin health.

White, Brown & Beige
Leeks, garlic, onions, celery, pears, white wine, dates, cauliflower, mushrooms, nuts, ginger, cocoa, coconut, coffee, tea, sauerkraut, seeds, quinoa, chickpeas, butter beans, hummus.

Anti-cancer, anti-microbial, gastrointestinal, heart, hormone, and liver health.

Blue, Indigo & Violet
Blackberries, blueberries, blackcurrants, figs, purple grapes, red wine, plums, prunes, raisins, purple broccoli, aubergine, purple potatoes, cabbage, onions, kale, olives, rice, carrots, cauliflower, aubergine.

Anti-cancer, anti-inflammatory, cognitive, heart, skin, and liver health.

Colour your shopping list: Find some colouring pencils, or if you have children, get them to colour code your shopping list, or play with veg and fruit puppets and talk about the colours. However you do it, get that rainbow into your shopping basket.

Drink colour: Shake up your smoothie or juice routine and opt for different colours each day. The green smoothie with chlorella was a big mistake; it looked like mould! We want rainbow smoothies!

Plate up colour: I fill at least half of my plate with salad/vegetables at every meal. Enjoy fruits, but eat less than your veggies because of their fructose content.

Freeze the rainbow: If you have too much fruit or too many vegetables or herbs on the go, freeze them in bags to use for smoothies or soups at a later stage. I have carrots, spinach, broccoli, chopped onions, garlic and ginger, fresh herbs, loads of different berries, mango slices, banana slices, melon cubes, lemon, and limes. There is also a naughty lemon cake for my nephews in the naughty drawer in my freezer (along with the ice cream).

Create art with food: Food is so much more than nutrition – it is our earliest, deepest, most emotional relationship: as a baby, we screamed for milk. How can we survive and achieve optimal nourishment? Is it compatible with our modern 'don't cook in it' kitchens? Eating phytonutrients does require kitchen time, but creating rainbow meals can be fun and joyful, creating deliciousness for your loved ones and yourself. It doesn't have to be gourmet, but if it's made from scratch, it's one of the most powerful things you can do for your health: it really is food for the soul.

GARDENING TIPS FOR BETTER GUT HEALTH

I liked an article/blog post sent to me by my friend Lucille who is big into nutrition, where Amelia Freer talked about the stomach/gut microbiome being like a garden. It was along the lines of adding some fertiliser for the fresh organic vegetables and fruit, and sprinkling on some seeds – these are probiotics (or 'friendly bacteria') and can be bought in fermented foods such as sauerkraut. Avoid feeding the weeds (i.e. unhelpful bacteria that can contribute to poor health and even obesity), which thrive on sugar. "Cancer loves sugar, so reduce your sugar tastebuds by eating less sugar" (Jamie Oliver website/blog).

Get rid of smelly weed killers – think garlic, onions, and horseradish. Lastly, we need to water our 'garden' daily and generously. Thanks Amelia, I liked that analogy – it made a nice change from cars.

EAT YOUR WAY TO HEALTHY HORMONES

Do you have balanced hormones (body juices carried by blood to the organs in order to carry out functions)? Hormones stimulate cell growth, mood, and so on, yet common symptoms such as unexplained weight gain (around the middle), fatigue, skin problems (including acne), severe pre-menstrual symptoms, or insomnia, could be influenced by a hormonal imbalance. There is so much to say on hormones and a good, comprehensive start for anyone who wants to address a possible imbalance is Marilyn Glenville's book, *The Nutritional Health Handbook for Women*, or Patrick Holford's book, *Balance Your Hormones*. I must have about twenty of Patrick's books and have been to many of his lectures, but it was when he showed me how to use Heartmath that I really understood the problems with my connection with stress hormones (fight and flight) and getting a sore stomach. Thank you Patrick for that winter's day in the midlands about five years ago, when you showed me how to use Heartmath (a device to show how the heart reacts to stress) – it was an inspirational lightbulb moment.

For hormone balancing, I am told to eat the right fats. Choose organic butter, coconut oil, and olive oil over man-made fats (such as margarine and vegetable oil). Balance your blood sugar. Reduce your sugar intake, eat protein at every meal, and follow a low-glycaemic-load way of eating (see Patrick Holford's books on this). Buy organic fresh fruit and veg. Avoid xeno-oestrogens (the hormone disrupters found in plastics, household chemicals, and pesticides). Use natural cleaning products and Pyrex glass food stores. Avoid microwaving food in plastic containers. Makeover your make-up bag – we absorb up to 60% of what we put on our skin so I try to use the cleanest products I can. Sleep more – a lack of sleep raises hormones that trigger hunger and it affects learning, growing and behaviour, not to mention healing, and all the maintenance repair checks. Cut back on coffee, especially before going to bed. They say coffee in moderate amounts is healthy, but too much can increase your stress hormones, causing high insulin levels and inflammation in the body.

ANTI-AGING SKIN SECRETS

Ladies, each year we spend millions of pounds on creams and serums – and countless other beauty products – in an attempt to recreate that radiant-looking skin of our youth. It's crazy to imagine that you can eat rubbish and still glow with health. Think of a plant: its shiny leaves reflect the soil it is in. However, if you want glowing skin, there's an easier, cheaper, and longer-lasting solution.

If you suffer from dry skin, it's imperative that you make sure you're getting enough water. I can tell if a patient is hydrated by the feel and look of the skin – it's a very aging look, dry skin. "Diet can play a huge role in your skincare regime, and can even help to manage conditions such as acne or dry skin" (The Sunday Telegraph blog/website, March 2014). Health expert Sara Stanner (the Sunday Telegraph Health Coach) goes on to say that while "genetic factors and hormonal status do play a significant part in determining your skin type, dry skin can be caused by a poor diet that lacks the necessary amount of fluids." My patients nearly always say they hate drinking water so I suggest they eat wetter food. So, as well as drinking as much as is comfortable and enjoyable, try and eat wet food, such as cucumbers, melons, oranges, lettuce, and smoothies. Most people get around 40% of their fluid from food rather than water. My cats get much more than that as they will not eat veggies.

Almonds: If you suffer from acne, you might want to try a handful of almonds. Tony Robbins, a well-known American Celebrity and presenter, loves his pocket of almonds to munch on. "Almonds are rich in Vitamin E, an antioxidant that, according to the NHS, helps to maintain healthy skin, eyes and the immune system" (The Telegraph website). They have also been known to help control cholesterol levels, protect against diabetes, and also boost brain power. I have some on my desk, but I'm still waiting on that last bit.

Onions: Sulphur is often called the 'smelly face lift nutrient' thanks to its skin-strengthening properties and its ability to reduce wrinkles and sagging. Onions have a very high sulphur content and studies have shown that sulphur-rich foods have the ability to improve acne. They are also packed with Vitamins A, C and E; all the antioxidants you need to help fight against the damage caused by the sun. Great to eat in moderation, but make sure you have a mint to suck on afterwards!

Mangoes: The beta-carotene and Vitamin A found in mangoes can help to rejuvenate your skin, as well as reducing dark spots, blemishes, and acne.
Oily fish: Nutritionist Dale Pinnock (the medicinal chef) swears by oily fish when it comes to overall skin improvement: "With skin issues like

acne, eczema, and psoriasis, the redness and irritation you see is caused by inflammation" (Pinnock, 2012). "You may have taken Ibuprofen in the past to fight against inflammation, but the body has its own natural anti-inflammatory compounds."

MAKE HEALTHY FOODS FUN, ESPECIALLY FOR KIDS

"Eating healthily is all about balance. Every now and then it's perfectly OK to have pie for dinner or a nice slice of cake at teatime – treats are a part of life – but it's also important to recognize when we're pushing things too far. Indulgent food should be enjoyed and savored, but only occasionally – it's important to remember that the majority of our diet should be made up of balanced, nutritious everyday foods. Make healthy food a priority in your life and allow it to bring your family and friends together. Learn to love how it makes you feel, how delicious it is and remember that a healthy balanced diet and regular exercise are the keys to a healthy lifestyle" (Jamie Oliver website).

In order to protect your family's eating habits, celebrity chef Jamie Oliver has suggested the compulsory reformulation of high-sugar products (read more at //www.jamieoliver.com/news-and-features/features/jamies-plan-to-combat-childhood-obesity). Having four children of his own, this project is very much in Jamie's heart, the idea being that a watchdog COBRA-style committee within parliament could keep an eye on the marketing of food – such as the labelling of the food being more honest and detailed as to what is in it. A simple traffic lights system to labelling was suggested. He also thinks sugary kid's products should be banned from adverts and supermarkets, and that they should work with poor families to make healthy food more affordable and easier to understand.

Jamie also wants obesity at schools tackled as early on as possible, with full support from teachers. Well done, Jamie, thank you for empowering the health of future children.

I bought my little nephews the COLOURFUL superfood cuddly toy gang, and we did stories together with them. It is important that healthy food is seen as being fun.

SUPERFOODS, OR ARE THEY?

Recently, the NHS joined forces with the British Dietetic Association in order to examine their evidence behind the health claims of 10 of the most popular so-called celebrity superfoods. I have reviewed their report in detail and summarised it for you here. If you're interested, the complete report can be found at:

www.nhs.uk/Livewell/superfoods/Pages/what-are-superfoods

I thought I had better include a measured argument for and against the superpowers of superfood, though if you are happy with the results you get from eating healthily, you can skip this bit. For those of you who are sceptic scientists out there, here goes.

The National Health Service and association of dietitians kick off with, "there is no official definition of a 'superfood' and the EU has banned health claims on packaging unless supported by scientific evidence". Personally, I thoroughly enjoy the colours and tastes of these foods, and I feel healthier for eating them, but I also feel that I have to put across a balanced view.

Many food brands fund academics to research the health benefits of their product, as well as hiring marketing companies to push the virtues of their foods. The superfood trend in particular "exploits the fact that healthy lifestyle choices, including diet, can reduce our risk of chronic diseases like heart disease, stroke and cancer" (NHS website). It's becoming all the rage these days, with many celebrities – including Jamie Oliver and his latest wonderfully colourful book on superfoods, plus his chain of Italian restaurants – pushing this. And very delicious it is too, I may add. I like going along with the hype on this type of food, because I am pleased that healthy food is being embraced, which I personally enjoy a lot. I just have to shop more carefully, as it can be a license to print money!

'SUPERFOOD' OR 'SUPER DIET'?

NHS dietitians – rather than nutritionists – avoid the term 'superfood' and prefer instead to talk of 'super diets', where the emphasis is on a healthy balanced diet. The food industry wants to persuade us that eating just a little bit of some foods can slow down the aging process, lift depression, and boost our physical ability and even our intelligence. It suggests that certain anti-oxidants or enzymes within certain foods will target diseased cells.

The problem is that most research on superfoods tests chemicals and extracts in concentrations not found in the food in its natural state. Sadly, the soils are badly depleted, the mineral and vitamin content is far from high enough, and with the shelf life and pesticide usage, the nutrient dosage isn't high enough for the food to be effective medicine. I understand that.

I remember discussing with Professor Wentz – CEO of USANA – how we now need to eat a crate of spinach or broccoli to get enough nutrients to combat chronic disease. For vitamin E, we need to eat 33 spinach heads a day, for B6, 41 medium bananas, for vitamin D, just 22 eggs, for vitamin C, 160 apples or 16 oranges, for folate, 4 cups of black beans, for riboflavin, 16 cups of yoghurt or 9 dozen eggs, for thiamine, 64 cups of peas, and so on… get my drift? It would be a massive food bill. Wentz always advocated supplementing. I wonder why?

Yummy foods that have been elevated to superfood status in recent years include those rich in antioxidants (such as beta-carotene, vitamins A, C, E, flavonoids, and selenium) and omega-3 fatty acids. It depends, however, on whether the word 'rich' really means just that. In the right amounts, these nutrients are all very important for optimum health. Antioxidants are chemicals that protect against the harmful effects of free radicals – naturally produced in cells and known to cause damage – and they are believed to be responsible for aging. Oxygen is a paradox, as it has a dark side – too much and it's deadly; it is responsible for 70 chronic diseases.

When I researched nutritional papers in the States, I came across over a thousand double blind, placebo-controlled trials on nutritional supplements. Time to get your seat belts on now, folks: the majority of those studies showed a SIGNIFICANT HEALTH BENEFIT in patients taking nutrients at OPTIMUM LEVELS (well above RDA levels). This is why I supplement.

In 2011, the NHS chose a damning review of this scientific evidence: "the European Food Safety Authority (EFSA) found no evidence that the antioxidant action on free radicals observed in the lab was of any benefit to human health" (NHS website).

To make matters worse to us supplementers, they also highlighted research to suggest that "certain antioxidant supplements may be harmful" (NHS website). I beg to differ, and so do some 1,300 excellent research studies. The EFSA were not very enthusiastic about healthy food either: "While the concept of a 'miracle food' remains a fantasy, it's pretty well-established that obesity and alcohol are the two most common causes of major long-term illness and increased risk of premature death" (EFSA, 2011).

I disagree with such a negative press, as there is so much research out there to discuss the need for vitamins and minerals in order to enable cells to function. I do agree that our food is not grown at source in healthy soil, and that it is not brilliant and has few nutrients in it. However, if we make the best choices with what we have available to us, I believe that it at least helps with anti-aging and health from all the articles and books I've read on the subject – all of which is far beyond the scope of this book.

According to the NHS website, "'No food, including those labelled 'superfoods', can compensate for unhealthy eating,' explains Alison Hornby, a dietitian and spokesperson for the British Dietetic Association (BDA). 'If people mistakenly believe they can 'undo' the damage caused by unhealthy foods by eating a superfood, they may continue making routine choices that are unhealthy and increase their risk of long-term illness."

I agree of course that if you eat a lot of rubbish, then you have still polluted your body, however, the biologist in me says that any amount of good stuff will help. In my greenhouse, if my plants get a little of the vitamin or mineral they are deficient in, they change in leaf colour and strength – plants don't lie.

If you want to know about the healing power of food and supplements, just ask any vet. One of my recent patients was a vet who was involved in the type of feed given to animals that were going to slaughter, and he said they had very specific food supplements in order to control circulatory and weight issues. He said that only a fool thinks that food is not medicine. Furthermore, if a fool thinks that this fast-grown and stored food has enough nutrients in it to avoid degenerative disease, why do you think animals – especially those going to slaughter, poor things – need a massive amount of supplements in order to combat disease?

Interestingly, the 2016 NHS/dietitian league buys into the healthiness of the Mediterranean diet, saying that "there is good evidence it can reduce the risk of some chronic diseases and increase life expectancy" (NHS website). This diet includes plenty of fruit and vegetables, olive oil and legumes, and less meat and fewer dairy foods than the typical western diet. The food is grown in better soil and is also eaten fresher.

From the BDA point of view, Alison Hornby states: "When it comes to keeping healthy, it's best not to concentrate on any one food in the hope it will work miracles. All unprocessed food from the major food groups could be considered 'super'. All these foods are useful as part of a balanced diet. You should eat a variety of foods, as described by the Eat Well Guide, to ensure you get enough of the nutrients your body needs. Focusing on getting your five portions of fruit and vegetables a day is a perfect way to start" (Hornby, What Are Superfoods? Article, NHS website).

Of course, we know that RDA (Recommended Dietary Allowance) is not optimum nutrition, and that it's not enough to combat disease – perhaps someone should tell them this. We only have to look around to know that Dr Oz (a TV celebrity doctor) is working with USANA in order to get the research to deaf ears via the media.

Now, here is my summary of the NHS dietitians' and BDA's lengthy report on the 10 most popular superfoods.

BLUEBERRIES

The report cited a handful of studies, the first one being a study in 2012 called 'Heart Health and Blueberries' by Cassidy et al., which found that of the 93,000 women studied, those who ate three or more portions of blueberries and strawberries a week had a 32% lower risk of a heart attack compared with those who ate berries once a month or less. Great news! However, sadly, the study could not prove that these fruits definitely caused the lower risk.

CAN BLUEBERRIES CLEAR OUT OUR FUEL PIPES?

The report found the evidence they looked at inconclusive, however they did say, "It is thought that blueberries may relax the walls of the blood vessels, which may help reduce this risk of atherosclerosis – hardening of the arteries" (NHS website). I think this is positive, as a hardening of the arteries can increase the risk of a heart attack and stroke. It's a very positive thing to have medicine in the form of food.

A small study in 2015 by Johnson et al. – involving 48 post-menopausal women – found that "women who were given blueberry powder supplements over the course of eight weeks experienced a small, but clinically significant, drop in blood pressure" (NHS website). Again, a positive conclusion. A study from 2015 by Stull et al. – this time involving 44 adults with metabolic syndrome (a combination of diabetes, high blood pressure, and obesity) – were given yummy blueberry smoothies, and had less promising results as there was no effect on blood pressure. A similar finding of inconclusive evidence was presented in a 2013 study by Ana Rodriguez-Mateos et al., which involved 21 healthy men.

The Shaman in me says they needed a stronger dose of them, especially as they had such complex medical histories.

BLUEBERRIES AND CANCER

Regarding cancer, the report stated that in their opinion, there was so far very little evidence that blueberries could help protect against cancer. In laboratory studies on cells and animals, blueberry extracts (such as anthocyanins) have been shown to decrease free radicals, the dark side of oxygen causing damage that can cause cancer, which is really good news for animals. However, it is not clear how well humans absorb these compounds from eating blueberries, and whether or not they have a protective effect.

CAN WE IMPROVE OUR MEMORY WITH BLUEBERRIES?

"A number of small studies have found a link between blueberry consumption and improved spatial learning and memory. However, most of these studies relied on small sample groups or animals" (NHS website). The BDA concluded there was currently no evidence of a link between eating blueberries and improved memory.

THE DIETITIAN'S VERDICT ON BLUEBERRIES

Alison Hornby (dietitian and BDA spokesperson for this superfood report) concluded her verdict with: "While research on the health claims of blueberries is inconclusive, they are a fantastic choice as one of your five portions of fruit and vegetables a day. They are low in calories and high in nutrients, including phenolic compounds with an antioxidant capacity significantly higher than vitamins C or E" (NHS website). So, even if research is controversial as to how much this superfood could change our health, there is agreement that it is a healthy, tasty food choice.

BROCCOLI

I find this little chap not very tasty, and it is certainly an acquired taste in a smoothie! But can eating broccoli prevent cancer?

The conclusion on this is very promising. We know that eating non-starchy vegetables, such as broccoli, is associated with a reduced risk of some cancers (including mouth, throat, and stomach cancers), and according to the evidence on cancer prevention provided by the World Cancer Research Fund, "It is highly likely some of the compounds in broccoli may help, but before claims can be made clinical trials are needed to investigate this further" (NHS website).

DOES BROCCOLI STOP OUR GASKET FROM BLOWING?

In a 2010 study by Christiansen et al., it was concluded that there was no evidence to suggest that broccoli can help lower blood pressure. "40 patients with high blood pressure who ate 10g of dried enriched broccoli sprouts for four weeks saw no improvement to the health of their blood vessels and did not reduce their risk of atherosclerosis (narrowing of the arteries)" (NHS website). Personally, I think that four weeks is not long enough, and hey, guys – you only talked about one study.

CAN BROCCOLI HELP TO KEEP OUR ENGINE GOING?

In a small study from 2012, Bahadoran et al. monitored 81 people with diabetes who ate 10g a day of enriched broccoli sprouts powder for four weeks. Bear in mind that's not a lot of veg, but they still saw a reduction in their levels of cholesterol and triglycerides (a type of fat found in the blood). Very promising news.

DOES BROCCOLI HELP WITH FUEL CONSUMPTION?

In a lab study from 2008, Xue et al. applied the antioxidant sulforaphane from broccoli to human blood vessels incubated with sugar. They found that sulforaphane appeared to prevent the damage to small blood vessels caused by high blood sugar (which can happen if you have diabetes), which is a plus for broccoli fans. However, it is unclear from this study whether sulforaphane would protect a person who already has diabetes from damage.

This was the verdict by Alison Hornby, BDA: "Broccoli may not live up to the hype, but nevertheless it contains many nutrients, such as folate, soluble and insoluble fiber, vitamins C and A, and calcium, which are needed for numerous functions in the body. It is a member of the family of cruciferous vegetables along with cauliflower, bok choy and cabbage. These all contain compounds that are linked to improving the body's ability to impede the growth of cancer cells" (NHS website).

GARLIC – DOES IT KEEP THE REVS DOWN?

The report picked for studying garlic was by Stabler et al. in 2012, and the study suggested that 200mg of garlic powder, taken three times daily, reduced blood pressure. However, the review also concluded that there was insufficient evidence to say if garlic was an effective means for treating high blood pressure and therefore reducing death rates.

CAN GARLIC CLEAN OUR FUEL PIPES OUT?

Good news now from a 2009 review by Reinhart et al., which looked at 29 good-quality studies involving a combined total of 1,794 participants. This review concluded that garlic powder gave 'modest reductions' in total cholesterol levels – such a promising result.

CAN GARLIC PREVENT THE COMMON COLD?

Their chosen review regarding the common cold was Lissimen et al's study in 2012, which is not to be sniffed at – ha ha. This concluded that there was insufficient evidence regarding the effects of garlic supplements in either treating or preventing colds. Most studies that claimed this, however, were deemed as poor quality, and the review said that one reasonably good study suggested that garlic *may* prevent colds, but that more research was needed in order to back up this finding.

WILL GARLIC PROTECT AGAINST CANCER?

The evidence for this is mixed: "A 2007 World Cancer Research Fund review concluded that garlic 'probably protects against' bowel and stomach cancers. A more recent review from 2009 [by Kim, JY and Kwon, O] concluded there was 'no credible evidence' with stomach, breast, lung and womb cancers, but that there was 'very limited evidence' that eating garlic may lower the risk of colon, prostate, oral, ovary or renal cell cancers" (NHS website).

Here is the dietitian's verdict: "Studies using high concentrations of garlic extracts have been associated with improved blood circulation, healthier cholesterol levels and lower blood pressure, all of which reduce the risk of cardiovascular disease. However, current evidence does not support the use of garlic supplements to improve health" (Alison Hornby, NHS website). I can't say I agree with this going by what I've heard from experts I've met around the world, but it is useful to hear what this report concluded.

CAN GOJI BERRIES IMPROVE IMMUNITY, FUEL EFFICIENCY, AND LIFE EXPECTANCY?

The BDA said that there was "no reliable evidence to support these alleged health benefits. Most of the research into these conditions are small-sized, of poor quality, and performed in laboratories using purified and highly concentrated extracts of the goji berry" (NHS website). Ouch! Mind you – the scientist in me says it's still good news if a concentrated amount has an impact.

DO GOJI BERRIES AID PERFORMANCE?

"One small study from 2008 [Amagase, H and Nance, DM] found a daily drink of 120ml of goji berry juice for 14 days improved feelings of wellbeing, brain activity and digestion. However, the study involved only 34 people and was attempting to measure the effects of goji berry juice on a variety of conditions. The results of the study were inconclusive" (NHS website) – due in part to sample size, and the concentration of the juice – though the results were mainly positive.

CAN GOJI BERRIES PREVENT CANCER?

One important study on goji berries is a "1994 Chinese study [Cao GW et al.] conducted on 79 patients with various advanced cancers. It found those treated with immunotherapy in combination with goji polysaccharides saw their cancers regress. Information on the study and the goji berry compounds used are lacking, so it is difficult to fully assess the significance of the results" (NHS website), though it could be very good news.

THE BDA/NHS VERDICT ON GOJI BERRIES

"Various goji berry products are sold as health foods, but the evidence of their health benefits so far comes from scientific studies using purified extracts of the fruit at much higher concentrations than the products contain" (Alison Hornby, NHS website). Perhaps if the soil was healthier, this would not be such an issue.

GREEN TEA – SUPERLEADED PERFORMANCE FUEL?

We know that "green tea has been used in traditional Chinese medicine for centuries, to treat everything from headaches to depression" (NHS website). I just love tea, and have a wide collection of teapots!

The leaves of green tea are said to be "richer in antioxidants than other types of tea because of the way they are processed. Green tea contains B vitamins, folate, manganese, potassium, magnesium, caffeine and other antioxidants. All types of tea – green, black and oolong – are produced from the Camellia Sinensis plant using different methods. Fresh leaves from the plant are steamed to produce green tea, while the leaves of black tea and oolong involve fermentation. Green tea is alleged to boost weight loss, reduce cholesterol, combat cardiovascular disease, and prevent cancer and Alzheimer's disease" (NHS website).

So what did the British Dietetic Association – those party poopers – say about these health claims?

DOES DRINKING GREEN TEA PROTECT YOU FROM CANCER?

The BDA concluded that in their opinion, there is "no evidence drinking green tea protects against different types of cancer" (NHS website). Ouch. "A review from 2009 [Boehm et al.] involving 51 studies, with more than 1.6 million participants, looked for an association between drinking green tea and cancers of the bowel, prostate, breast, mouth and lungs. The authors of the review concluded evidence of a link between green tea and cancer was weak and 'highly contradictory'" (NHS website).

A more recent 2014 study, researched in Singapore and Harvard, "looked at the cancer-fighting effects of a compound found in green tea when combined with a drug called Herceptin, which is used in the treatment of stomach and breast cancer. Initial results in the laboratory were promising and human trials are now being planned" (NHS website).

CAN GREEN TEA LIGHTEN THE CHASSIS?

"It's thought the antioxidants catechin and caffeine found in green tea may have a role in helping the body burn more calories [speed metabolism] which can help weight loss. Green tea preparations used for losing weight are extracts of green tea that contain a higher concentration of catechins [antioxidants] and caffeine than the typical green tea beverage prepared from a tea bag" (NHS website). Sadly, the BDA quoted a review from 2012 [Jürgens et al.] "of 18 studies involving 1,945 people who found no significant effect of weight loss from drinking green tea" (NHS website).

CAN GREEN TEA STRIP OUT THE SLUDGE IN THE FUEL PIPES?

The selected study from BDA's review was a paper from 2013 (Hartley et al.) where "11 studies involving 821 people found daily consumption of green and black tea could help lower cholesterol and blood pressure thanks to tea and its catechins. The trials were short term and more good quality long-term trials are needed to back up their findings" (NHS website). The limited evidence suggests that tea has favourable effects on stroke and heart attack risk factors, but due to the small number of trials contributing to each analysis, the results should be treated with some caution and further high quality trials with longer-term follow-up are needed to confirm this.

Another review in 2011 (Kim et al.) found that "drinking green tea enriched with catechins led to a small reduction in cholesterol, a main cause of heart disease and stroke."

CAN GREEN TEA HELP PREVENT THE CPU/BRAIN BREAKING DOWN?

The BDA chose one study to review, stating evidence that a positive link between drinking green tea and Alzheimer's disease is weak. "A 2010 laboratory study [Okella et al.] using animal cells found a green tea preparation rich in antioxidants protected against the nerve cell death associated with dementia and Alzheimer's disease" (NHS website).

"Whether these lab results can be reproduced in human trials remains to be seen. As such, the findings do not conclusively show green tea combats Alzheimer's disease" (NHS website) in humans. To me, this means there is a positive angle to it. "A cup of green tea a day appears to protect against Alzheimer's disease and other forms of dementia," reported The Daily Telegraph in 2011.

CAN GREEN TEA LOWER THE REVS?

"A 2014 survey of data [in the European Journal of Nutrition] from previously published studies looked at the evidence of whether drinking green tea could help lower blood pressure. There was evidence of a modest reduction in people with high blood pressure who consumed green tea" (NHS website).

CAN GREEN TEA GIVE US A STRONGER BITE?

A small study (from Neturi et al., 2014) "looked at how effective a green tea mouthwash was in preventing tooth decay compared with the more commonly used antibacterial mouthwash chlorhexidine" (NHS website). The results were not what I was expecting: they "suggested they were equally effective, though green tea mouthwash has the added practical advantage of being cheaper" (NHS website). Although it does lack that minty fresh feel!

So what is the verdict on green tea? The BDA spokesperson (Alison Hornby) says: "the evidence about green tea's health benefits is inconclusive" (NHS website). Short and sweet.

FISH

"Eskimos, who mainly eat oily fish, had fewer than average heart attacks and strokes" (NHS website). This could be because they live in igloos or play in the snow, but researchers looked to the fish.

"Oily fish such as salmon, mackerel and sardines are said to help against cardiovascular disease, prostate cancer, age-related vision loss and dementia" (NHS website). Oily fish are smelly and slimy but rich in "vitamin D, protein, some B vitamins and selenium. It's also a rich source of omega-3 fatty acids [healthy fat]" (NHS website).

The British Dietetic Association and the NHS have been examining the evidence on oily fish, as follows.

OILY FISH PROTECTS OUR PUMP

"The UK Scientific Advisory Committee on Nutrition reviewed the evidence on the health benefits of fish in 2004. It said 'a "large body of evidence" suggests that fish consumption, particularly oily fish, reduces the risk of cardiovascular disease'" (Independent Public Health report, 2004). This is not good news for fish wanting to live to an old age! "Studies have found eating oily fish can lower blood pressure and reduce fat build-up in the arteries. The evidence is strong enough to warrant a government recommendation that we eat at least two portions of fish a week, one of which should be oily" (NHS website).

PROSTATE CANCER

The BDA concluded that "evidence for oily fish's effect on prostate cancer is inconclusive" (NHS website). I think they mean eating it and not rubbing it on your naughty bits! Also, that "some limited research suggests that eating fish may reduce the risk of prostate cancer" (NHS website). So make of that what you will.

DEMENTIA

"A 2012 review [Sydenham et al.] looked into whether consuming more omega-3 in oily fish, could reduce the risk of dementia. The review looked at healthy 60-year-olds who took omega-3 capsule supplements for six months. The review concluded that there is no preventative effect of decline in brain function and dementia when healthy older people take omega-3. The review suggested that longer-term studies would offer researchers a better opportunity for identifying the possible benefits of omega-3 in preventing dementia" (NHS website)

FISH HELPS OUR HEADLIGHTS

The NHS dietitian advice quoted a review in 2010)Senior et al.) where there was "some evidence that eating oily fish two or more times a week could reduce the risk of age-related macular degeneration – a common cause of blindness in older people" (NHS website). However, they mentioned weaknesses in the research.

"A further review carried out in 2015 looked at whether fish oil supplements could reduce the progression of macular degeneration in people who already had [it]" (NHS website), and this review found no evidence of any benefit.

RHEUMATOID ARTHRITIS – CAN FISH OIL HELP THE OLD SUSPENSION?

A 2013 study (Giuseppe et al.) looked at 32,000 women, middle-aged and older, to see if oily fish had any impact on them developing rheumatoid arthritis. "They did find that women who ate one or more servings of oily fish were 29% less likely to develop rheumatoid arthritis than women who never, or very rarely, ate oily fish" (NHS website). So that's encouraging for potential RA suffers, but not so much for fish hoping to reach the old bones stage themselves.

SCATTY DRIVING

"In 2013, the National Institute for Health & Care Excellence (NICE) reviewed the evidence about whether medication based on omega-3 fatty acids could improve the symptoms of schizophrenia. The results were mixed. Four out of the eight studies showed some modest benefit when compared to placebo (a dummy treatment). The other four showed no benefit" (NHS website).

Based on these results, it was decided there was not enough evidence as yet to use omega-3 fatty acid-type drugs as an alternative treatment. Now, it's time to get your seat belts on again, folks: the overall BDA and NHS report findings for oily fish were positive – bloody amazing, in fact: "if there's one food that's good for your heart, its oily fish" (Alison Hornby, NHS website).

WHEATGRASS

"The discoveries in the 1930s by US chemist Charles Schnabel, dubbed 'Mr. Wheatgrass', have inspired a body of scientific research into wheatgrass that continues to this day" (NHS website). Wheatgrass is said to have a higher nutritional content than any other vegetable, protects against inflammation, builds red blood cells, and improves circulation. Wheatgrass is known to contain "chlorophyll, vitamin A, vitamin C, vitamin E, iron, calcium, and magnesium" (NHS website).

NUTRITION CLAIMS FOR WHEATGRASS

Now this surprised me! "Despite claims that a 30ml (1oz) shot of wheatgrass contains as many nutrients as 1kg (2.2lbs) of your finest veggies, tests show that, pound for pound, the nutrient content of wheatgrass juice is roughly equivalent to that of common vegetables, such as spinach and broccoli" (NHS website).

CAN DRINKING WHEATGRASS TURN NORMAL FUEL INTO SUPER FUEL?

"Fans of wheatgrass believe that because chlorophyll and haemoglobin (a protein that carries oxygen) are similar in structure, taking wheatgrass juice enhances haemoglobin production," but the BDA stated that "there is no scientific proof to support this claim" (NHS website).

DOES WHEATGRASS SOOTHE OUR TANK?

"A small study from 2002 [Arya et al.] found patients with ulcerative colitis (inflammation of the colon) saw their symptoms improve after they were given 100ml of wheatgrass juice daily for a month" (NHS website). This is a really good outcome, but such a small sample size makes it a weak study: it only involved 21 people.

The BDA/NHS verdict says: "There is no sound evidence to support the claim that wheatgrass is better than other fruits and vegetables in terms of nutrition" (Alison Hornby, NHS website).

POMEGRANATE

Used for medicinal purposes for thousands of years, "the Middle Eastern fruit is claimed to be effective against heart disease, high blood pressure, inflammation and some cancers, including prostate cancer. Pomegranate is a good source of fibre. It also contains vitamins A, C and E, iron and other antioxidants (notably tannins)" (NHS website).

CAN POMEGRANATE STRENGTHEN OUR CHASSIS?

"A 2013 study [Spilmont et al., in the European Journal of Nutrition] found evidence that pomegranate strengthened bones and helped prevent osteoporosis. The catch was the study involved mice, not humans" (NHS website).

DOES POMEGRANATE JUICE SLOW DOWN PROSTATE CANCER?

"One small study from 2006 [Pantuck et al.] found that drinking a daily 227ml (8oz) glass of pomegranate juice significantly slowed the progress of prostate cancer in men with recurring prostate cancer. This was a well-conducted study, but more are needed to support these findings. A more recent study from 2013 [Freedland et al.] looked at whether giving men pomegranate extract tablets prior to surgery to remove cancerous tissue from the prostate would reduce the amount of tissue that needed to be removed. The results were not statistically significant" (NHS website).

CAN POMEGRANATE UNFUR OUR FUEL PIPES?

A good study from 2004, by Aviram et al., "on patients with carotid artery stenosis (narrowed arteries) found that a daily 50ml (1.7oz) glass of pomegranate juice over three years reduced the damage caused by cholesterol in the artery by almost half, and also cut cholesterol build-up" (NHS website).

"A well-conducted trial from 2005 [by Sumner et al.] on 45 patients with coronary heart disease [so a small number!] demonstrated that a daily 238ml (8.4oz) glass of pomegranate juice administered over three months resulted in improved blood flow to the heart and a lower risk of heart attack" (NHS website). This is a nice, positive study for pomegranates, even if getting them prepared can be a pain. Jamie Oliver cuts them in half, then thumps them to make the seeds come out easily. Well, for him they do!

Of course, here comes BDA's opinion to burst our bubble: "Research suggests there may be a benefit, but we've not shown it yet. The studies that have found an improvement in existing health conditions were very small and more investigation into the role pomegranate plays in these improvements is needed" (Alison Hornby, NHS website).

BEETROOT

Beetroot's "deep, overpoweringly red juice" has earned it the reputation of giving the plate an incredible purple blast of colour, and has the added benefit of being super healthy too. "Although the leaves have always been eaten, historically the beet root was generally used medicinally for fevers, constipation and skin problems" (NHS website).

"Beetroot is a good source of iron and folate. It also contains nitrates, betaine, magnesium and other antioxidants. More recent health claims suggest beetroot can help lower blood pressure, boost exercise performance and prevent dementia" (NHS website).

CAN BEETROOT GET A BETTER PERFORMANCE OUT OF OUR ENGINE?

"Beetroot is rich in nitrates. When ingested, our body converts nitrates into nitric oxide, a chemical thought to lower blood pressure. A well-conducted review of the current evidence from 2013 [Siervo et al.] concluded that beetroot juice gave a modest reduction in blood pressure" (NHS website). Hooray!

DOES BEETROOT GIVE US MORE MILES FOR OUR FUEL BILL?

"Another well-conducted review from 2013 [Hoon et al.] looked at research linking beetroot juice to improved exercise performance. The review found that inactive and recreationally active individuals saw 'moderate improvements' in exercise performance from drinking beetroot juice. However, the review noted there was very little effect on elite athletes" (NHS website).

CAN BEETROOT HELP PREVENT BRAIN/COMPUTER DYSFUNCTION?

This 2010 study was carried out by "researchers from Wake Forest University, Winston-Salem in the USA. One of the researchers is also listed as co-author on a patent for the use of nitrite salts in the treatment of cardiovascular conditions. The study was published in the journal Nitric Oxide: Biology and Chemistry. The press release [in the Daily Express] reported that the university is currently looking into ways of marketing the juice" (NHS website).

They suggested that a diet high in beetroot juice *may* increase blood flow to certain areas of the brain. "This news story is based on a small study in 16 elderly people. The participants were given either a diet that was low or high in nitrates over a four-day period. Nitrates are present at high levels in beetroot and other vegetables, and converted into nitrites in the body, a chemical that is thought to increase blood flow. The participants' blood flow to different regions of the brain was measured on a scan" (NHS website).

"This was a small study conducted over an extremely short time span. Its findings suggest that adults who eat a diet high in nitrates may experience an increased blood flow to certain areas of the brain within a short interval, compared with eating a diet low in nitrates" (NHS website). Exciting! However, the BDA moaned about it being a small and short-term study, which is not considered robust enough evidence to show that a diet high in nitrates aids cognitive function.

Muggeridge et al. (2004) "looked at the effects of beetroot juice on cyclists, who were cycling in a chamber designed to mimic the effects of relatively high altitude (2,500 meters above sea level). Researchers found that cyclists given the juice had a modest but significant increase in terms of their time trial scores; on average there was a 16 second improvement" (NHS website).

So, what is the UK BDA/NHS dietitian's verdict on beetroot? "Beetroot and beetroot juice, along with green leafy vegetables, cabbage and celery, are very useful as part of a balanced diet as their nitrate content may help to reduce blood pressure" (Alison Hornby, NHS website).

THE RIGHT DIET FOR YOU

The BBC did a recent program on the right diet for you; you can go online to the *Horizon* home page where you can watch the program and do an online test to see what sort of dieter you are. I liked the approach of discussing the mindset of the people who were too heavy for their height and shoe size! In the programme, several scientists divided 75 overweight individuals into three teams, or 'tribes' as they called them.

I have read Dr Michael Mosley's books on fast exercise and fast diet, and fasting for two out of seven days is very popular. My sisters-in-law did two different diets this year – one did the 2:5 while the other did Slimming World – both with amazing results. They have different approaches to eating and that is so important when deciding how to tackle being overweight.

THE TRIBES

These are the tribes set out in the *Horizon* program, and are not of my own invention.

The Constant Cravers: those that just seem to graze all the time – personally, I think of sheep grazing on grass. These people have genes that put them at greater risk of becoming obese. It takes a lot for these people to feel full, and they enjoy the pleasure of snacking.

The Feasters: people whose bodies produce low amounts of a gut hormone called GLP-1 in response to food. This hormone tells the brain "you have eaten enough", but feasters will go on eating because their gut takes much longer to say to the brain, "you're full". You know the ones, those who just go on and on eating… In the *Horizon* documentary, these individuals were the ones who ate the most at a buffet. When I think of this group, I think of Labradors, eating too much and then throwing it back up. An old flame of mine had a golden lab called Buster, who in seconds could completely empty my fridge, then do huge elephant poos (the dog, that was, not my old flame), nice!

The Emotional Eaters: these individuals were selected on the basis of their responses to a psychological questionnaire, and are typically the sort of people who turn to food when stressed. I know a few people who comfort eat to fill an emotional need, and it's very difficult for these folks to diet. The diets that focus on healthy eating and counting calories often fail these folks, as they need an emotional fix – praise, love, or something more. They can also get easily upset if they put weight on. Others take it a step further and make themselves sick afterwards, and this needs a counselling approach. In a few cases, this behaviour can be a cry for help, and is sometimes linked to self-abuse.

I think of my cats with this group, as they are emotional mammals and they didn't get fed very much when they were kittens (they were underweight when I got them). Even now, on occasion, if they get stressed they will eat all of their food at speed, resulting in having too much food and sicking it all up again – usually over white quilts or carpets!

THE DIETS

Each tribe was given a different diet to try. The Emotional Eaters were put on a standard low calorie diet, and were given psychological support. The Constant Cravers, on the other hand, were given the 5:2 intermittent fasting diet – like the diet Dr Michael Mosley writes about – whereas the Feasters were put on a high protein, low GI (glycaemic index) diet, which controls the blood glucose release to a steadier, slower supply.

"I was pleased that Professor Susan Jebb, one of the UK's foremost diet experts, had chosen 5:2 intermittent fasting as a solution for the Constant Cravers. They are probably the toughest group to help since their genetics make them particularly susceptible to over-eating" (Mosley, TheFastDiet. co.uk), and it is always tougher if your lifestyle has to drive your genetic predisposition away from its program.

Dr Mosley's reaction was as follows: "I think it is a novel way of approaching dieting and the dieters do impressively well on their allocated programs. The reality, of course, is that most of us are a mixture of the three tribes (I am mainly Constant Craver, with some Feaster and Emotional Eater thrown in). I also think that most of us would benefit from all 3 solutions" (TheFastDiet.co.uk).

He goes on to say that for "a diet high in protein and in low glycaemic carbohydrates, the advice given to the 'Feasters' will keep you fuller for longer, whatever your tribe". He also added that "most people would benefit from doing the Fast Diet, whether they are Constant Cravers or not". As for the Emotional Eaters, he realised that "most of us would relate to that" (TheFastDiet.co.uk).

When we are stressed, or really tired and burnt out, comfort food is lovely and comforting to engage with. Losing weight is tough, and we need all the psychological support we can get, whether this comes from family, colleagues, or friends.

STICKING THE DIET OUT FOR A YEAR REPROGRAMS YOUR NAUGHTY GENES

A recent article in the Times (April 14th, 2016) stated that a breakthrough experiment proved it takes 12 months of dieting before the body's chemicals change and a new weight can be maintained permanently. Unhelpful powerful defence mechanisms within our body stockpile calories if we feel hungry.

Researchers in Denmark (the results can be found in the European Journal of Endocrinology, April 2016) showed that if dieters lost, say, an eighth of their weight and kept it off for a year, the chemicals controlling their diet made a step change. Associate Professor of Biomedical Sciences at the University of Copenhagen, Signe Sorensen Torekov, stated: "It's very difficult to fight the hunger. It's like a drug you're fighting against" (The Telegraph website). She went on to say that after a year, it becomes so much easier.

Three important gut juices/hormones are GLP1, PYY, and Ghreline. The first two are increased in order to reduce appetite, whereas the latter is reduced in order to satisfy appetite. Big people have these juices shouting in their ear to eat more, the opposite to what you need when dieting. They shout: 'just one more slice of cake, just another bun, just a few more chips on my hips!' After a year of being monitored on a strict diet, 20 Danes had lost an average of 28lb, which is like a small child, or a dozen bags of sugar. Most importantly, however, from a hormone point of view, their set point (the weight their bodies strive to maintain and protect) had changed.

Giles Yeo – a hunger expert at Cambridge – made a good point on this research, saying that he was more interested in the changes in brain juice. From my point of view, the most interesting thing is how the change in motivational drivers connecting the gut and the brain get hardwired. Giles Yeo believes that the brain will never stop fighting to keep a fat person fat, much like a so-called 'recovering' alcoholic cannot recover if he tastes alcohol, as the addiction once the alcohol hits the stomach is still there. I mentioned in my Mind book a brain juice called Leptin, and in a study published in the Journal of Endocrinology (April 2016), Dr. Yeo looked into giving doses of this to overweight people to trick the mind into thinking you have eaten more than you have. I wonder if hypnosis could do this – if so, I should try it on the cats. It would certainly save on food bills.

Anyway, early results say it could well help. The mind and the power of desire is a strong drive, and this was echoed in Professor Paul Fletcher's work in neuroscience at Cambridge. In some brains, not only is the decision-making process centre smaller in size, but it is also wired in such a way to find resisting temptation difficult, so knowledge of healthy food is not strong enough to say no to a slice or three of Snazzy's homemade coffee cake. Therefore, the jury is still out on how much time is needed to stay thin and stay thin happily – and I'm sure that for those of us who are larger than others, it will always be a battle as long as unhealthy food is present.

Long-term solutions, I think, can only reside in food containing less sugar. At the turn of the century, however hungry we were, we would eat maybe a couple of bags of sugar a year at most, as processed food did not exist like it does today. Get my point?

FOOD BROUGHT ME BACK TO LIFE

This true story really inspired me to eat rainbow food. Ella Woodward ('Deliciously Ella') is a celebrity nutritionist, and the biggest thing in nutrition since Jamie Oliver's campaign for better food in schools. She has POTS (postural tachycardia syndrome), where the sufferer experiences an "abnormal increase in heart rate after sitting of standing up" (NHS website), which she was diagnosed with in 2011. Symptoms for POTS include extreme exhaustion, dizziness, bloating, and weakness, and lots of forced bed rest is needed due to the person not being able to walk. It is rare and poorly understood, and there is no known cure. Medication failed to help Ella, however, using food as medicine greatly reduced her symptoms. Overnight, Ella took up a whole foods, plant-based diet and gave up all meat, dairy, sugar, wheat, and anything processed, not to mention all chemicals and additives, which was a pretty drastic change to say the least.

Eating this way allowed her to take control of the illness, stopping the constant pain, restoring energy, and giving her life back to her. "It really has healed me, and just eighteen months after starting this lifestyle I've been able to come off all my medication and I feel so incredible, better than ever really! I'd never have believed that I could come this far simply through diet; it is just incredible – better than any drug ever. I've learnt more on this health adventure than I could have possibly imagined too" (Ella Woodward, MindfullyBliss.com).

SNAZZY'S TIPS FOR EATING CHEAPLY WITH HEALTHY FOOD

Overhauling your cupboards to stock up on a new pantry could – and probably will –result in a big spend. Whenever I go into health food shops I come out shocked; little bags of stuff are so expensive! However, after an expensive experience in a darling little shop in Norwich, I learnt my lesson, and my subsequent shopping bills have now been dramatically reduced.

Just keep an eye out for bargains, and don't get everything at once – you'll only end up throwing it out. Buying new things keeps cooking fresh, though it's a good idea to buy dry ingredients such as nuts, seeds, and grains in bulk. Online stockists like Amazon are a good place to look and the price is always better when you buy more. Cooking larger quantities of food is an effective way of saving money, especially when it comes to using fresh food. My eldest brother, Rich, is a darling – he cooks up stuff when he gets a bargain, and freezes it for future use. It has in part been his love of healthy cooking that has given my sister-in-law her figure back. It's a shame he's no longer chatting over the BBC airwaves; I would have had fun discussing healthy living with him on the radio.

If a recipe calls for half a bag of vegetables for your favourite soup, but you know that you won't use the rest of an enormous bag in another recipe, then make double the recipe and freeze the other half. I do this all the time, especially if it's to take up north to my nephews. You save time, food, and money, plus you have a freezer full of goodness to enjoy when you don't have the time – or the patience – for cooking.

Seasonal produce tends to be much cheaper than anything imported, however, you have to swot up to know what's in season. If you are fortunate enough to have local produce available nearby, make sure that you base your meals around what's local to you now. If you were going to do pea soup and you have bucketloads of spuds, just change the recipe. Try farmers' markets, or farm shops – some produce will be cheaper than in supermarkets, but even if it's not it will probably be healthier, especially if in odd shapes and grown locally. This helps support locally grown supporters, plus the produce almost always tastes better. Why would you buy a vegetable grown in a foreign country when you can source it locally? Food from other countries will be older, with fewer nutrients left in it due to shelf life, and it does absolutely nothing to support our local farming infrastructure. Also, talk to your neighbours; if they have surplus produce in their allotments, buy their extra food or swap. If you have space and time, fill up pots with herbs and have a veggie patch.

You can mix and match plants and veggies in your flower border. I had a new greenhouse built in my garden and I love it; it extends the time I can grow stuff for. Food always tastes better with fresh herbs, and these can grow throughout the year, even in your kitchen. For out-of-season foods – such as blackberries in winter – try buying them frozen, which will again save lots of money. I blitz a handful of berries in my smoothies to give that yummy flavour all year round; I just use my frozen ones out of season.

The things I eat day-to-day can be expensive if bought in supermarkets or health shops, so be careful to buy those items only when the price is inexpensive. You can bulk up salads with balls of colourful black rice, beans you have soaked and cooked, quinoa (it takes just 20 minutes to cook), pulses, or home-made hummus, and then you can drizzle some olive or coconut oil on some tired veggies and roast them for a warm salad. Roast veggies and fresh salad are one of my favourite savoury meals when it's cold. After all, a fresh salad on its own is far less inviting.

I grind nuts to a fine powder – especially if I find some bargain ones – and then add these to my salads, smoothies, and soups. Add your home-grown herbs as well: basil, mint, and coriander are my favourite to add, due to their soft texture for salads, though of course, there are so many you can blend them into everything you cook. I let them marinate for a while first to infuse their flavour, then I may grind them up a little with a pestle and mortar, before adding a drop of olive oil. I will then place a small pretty pot of the herbs I have added to the meal near or on the table so the fragrance of the leaves further blesses the food with its fragrance.

I will have a jug of water with either lemon or lime, and mint leaves imbibing the flavour of the fruit. Then I'll add ice before serving, making for a very inexpensive drink that stops the boredom of plain water. Again, if the same herb is used, it enhances the olfactory and taste experience even further.

If we have wine or spirits at the weekend, I will have large water glasses and a much smaller collection of glasses for the sugar-laden alcohol. On occasion I may put a salad or smoothie in a glass jar to remind me of portion control, as your tummy is the size of your fist, and once on a plate, the 3D size of food just disappears. Also, if you can bring out most of the servings at once, you can see how much food will be consumed in one sitting – oink oink!

I use my late grandma's pretty crockery, as well as my modern plain white plates, as shabby chic is in. I think food should look artistic, and different crockery helps to frame this. Food presentation is important to me, and I have always been emotional about food and meals; to me, to prepare good food with care and love is like sharing your soul. Food is medicine, and it needs to both look and taste good. Tricks like drizzling a dark-coloured dressing onto a white plate transforms the whole look. I also have a thing about tea; I love the whole ritual with fresh tea in little pots and milk or lemon in little jugs. Tea or coffee can be delicious and reasonably inexpensive, and it is a very social thing to do that doesn't necessarily have to involve food.

LADIES' ANTI-AGING COSMETICS/FASHION

As we all know, age is so much more than just a number. However, no matter how confident you feel, it only takes a visit to the opticians (I was recently told I needed varifocal glasses), or a trip to the hairdressers ("Are you sure you don't want a colour today?"), or to catch your reflection in a shop window with your shoulders bent over like... well, like a little old lady, to take the shine off your day. But all of these things can be easily helped. Here's how:

SNAZZY SPEC APPEAL

My friends have some really cool frames for both sunglasses and reading glasses, and you can tell just by looking at them that they feel positively snazzy. When I next get a prescription for my glasses, I will look for something less boring too.

SAY YES TO COLOUR, A GOOD CUT, AND STRAIGHTENING

I'm a big fan of glossy long hair and subtle, natural colours. A bit of grey looks OK, as long as your hair is shiny and healthy-looking. I changed hairdressers last week and she did a really nice cut. It was kind of an emergency as I had been nominated for an award, and I had a small bump and cut on my head. Thank God for fringes – everyone said, "You look younger!"

TIDY UP YOUR WARDROBE

I was sent for a wardrobe makeover last month, at John Lewis, Norwich, and it was a real eye-opening insight having someone different pick my clothes – this is a sure-fire solution to sharpen up your look. Did you know that the age you look (and your body shape) determines what length of skirts and dresses you should ideally wear?

TRY A NEW COLOUR PALETTE

During this recent style and colour profile they gave me the colour chart that best suited me, and in fact, it already included all of the colours I generally wear a lot. As you age, your choice of colour may change, and fashion consultants talk in terms of spring, summer, autumn, and winter colours. I am autumn, apparently.

HOMEWORK:
Do you know what season you are?

SOFTEN YOUR MAKE-UP

Last month I had another make-up lesson with a delightful Russian lady. I am very slap dash and don't wear a lot as a rule, as I am either with patients, out exercising, working in the house/garden, or writing in my office. However, on the occasions where I present or do a video, it's quite shocking to see how crap you can look if everyone else is made up and you're not. Bright lighting can also make you look washed out.

Some of the secrets to looking good include moisturising well before applying a gentle foundation, using lip brushes, and using eye shadow in four shades, having been brushed on with about 25 strokes and blended a lot. Highlight your eyes with a darker line above the eye and then smudge. Clever make-up can match your whole complexion, and along with the clothes you wear, it can make you appear more youthful.

GOOD POSTURE PUSHES BACK THE HANDS OF TIME

There is one small thing you can do to make yourself instantly more youthful, and as I write, I am doing it myself. It's very simple. Pull in your stomach – gently firming your core – and sit or stand or walk upright. Keep your shoulders and head back, and your spine straight. You will immediately look slimmer, taller, more interesting, and confident. Celebrities are big into body posture and how aging it can be, and when they act, they embrace the body language of the person, including their mood and age.

Now, how young did you say you were?

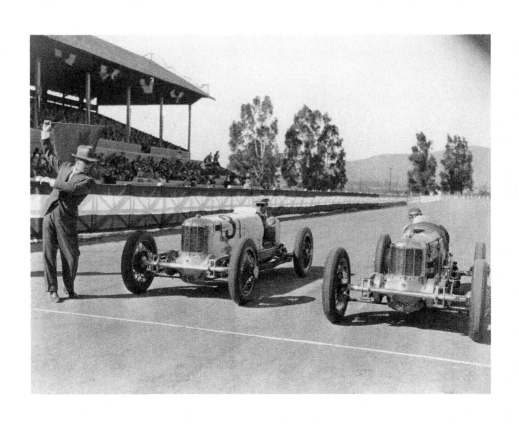

Chapter Six

"I want to grow old without facelifts... I want to have the courage to be loyal to the face I've made. Sometimes I think it would be easier to avoid old age, to die young, but then you'd never complete your life, would you? You'd never wholly know you."

– *Marilyn Monroe*

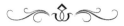

AGELESS FITNESS

There is a lot of physical homework in this chapter, so you may want to read this when you're feeling energetic, and preferably when you are wearing a tracksuit or yoga pants so you can stretch out comfortably.

I've just returned from collecting a painting from a local artist who trains hard with my father, and I felt that his story was a perfect example of what this chapter is all about. Just a few years ago, Michael went to university full-time, and he regularly works out with heavy weights and intense cardio sessions. He tells me that 'just' a cool two-hour workout suits him fine, and keeps him injury free as long as he stretches. He was in good spirits when I saw him as he was going out later with some of his university chums. Did I mention that both Michael and my father are in their eighties?

As we age, it becomes ever more necessary to avoid injuries and keep exercising – and, ideally, to still really enjoy fitness. One of the key secrets lies in the core muscles of the torso, and the importance of keeping a good posture and strong core is well known by Yoga, Chi Kung, Tai Chi, and Pilates instructors. It's interesting to me that running gets such bad press as we age. It is not the running, but the *way* we run and what we run *on* that damages us

TAI CHI

Now, back in my time machine we go, to about ten years ago. I remember learning Tai Chi on Sunday nights in a draughty village hall, which was part of my getting ready for a trip to China. I say 'learning', but in truth I was so crazily busy and so under practiced at the complex moves that I was just trying to get through the classes; Tai Chi classes in particular require more time than my busy schedule back then allowed. The beauty and grace of my classmate's movements, however, were truly breath-taking to see, and very inspiring. The key message I carried from Tai Chi was that my arms and legs were just an extension of my spine. Also, that my arms could float effortlessly – like water through pipes – and yet appear to be working really hard at the same time. I still practice a handful of movements, and I try to remind myself that being so busy 'doing' and not 'being' can be bad for our health.

WHY THE SNAZZY CHI JOG?

So, I hear you ask: "why run, especially at 50?" Well, I run as it fits in with my crazy schedule. It burns up the calories of food and gin overindulgences, and it helps strengthen my heart, lungs, muscles, and bones, not to mention easing my troubled mind.

I find that when patients get problems with their back, it is nearly always linked to poor posture at work, or poor biomechanics whilst running. This made me think about how running may be irritating my own poor back. In the east they talk of centering your chi, by focusing on a point called the Dan Tien just below your tummy button, so I read up on Chi running and put it into practice. I'm afraid that when *I* was running, however, I bore a strong resemblance to Mr Bean.

Reading up on Chi running advice from Danny Dreyer reminded me of my puppet presentations on stage: with my hand up their bum, their spine is straight and their flailing arms simply float around.

HOMEWORK:
Try doing the above (though not the first bit about a hand up the bum – ha ha), and bring awareness to how tight your shoulders really are. Lower them down and gently pull those rounded shoulders back. Then rotate your body so your arms flail around. Can you feel how much tension you carry in your body under the radar?

Now, do I put enough quality time aside to sprint, jog, and walk? Quite simply, no. I grab half an hour to run when I can, and I remind myself to slow down when I start panting; it's not very dignified to be breathing heavily, especially if you already look like Mr Bean. I remind myself to use a Pilate's style breath. Ideally, you should be able to talk to someone whilst jogging or cycling; it's only when sprinting to maximum heart rate that you can be forgiven for not being able to hold a conversation.

> **HOMEWORK:**
> Breathe out – pulling in your tummy button – and empty your lungs. Then refill the lower lobes of your lungs, feeling your tummy expand again as you relax. Breathing correctly means you can sing, swear, shout mantras, and enjoy yourself.

DRIVING MY BODY WHILST LEAVING MY MIND AT THE TRAFFIC LIGHTS (ON RED)

Relaxing is not all about sitting still and staring at a candle; it can also be about focusing on your body's needs and wisdom whilst being actively engaged in an activity. Sensing what these needs are and responding to them – not to mention breathing well – are magic keys to relaxation and longevity.

I see so many patients with tense postural muscles that are accelerating body rot, and there are many simple relaxation exercises you can do in order to improve body awareness. For example, let's try something now:

> **HOMEWORK:**
> Close your eyes and concentrate on your breathing. Then, as you tense some specific, individual muscles – say, in your foot – you can draw your awareness into those muscles in your foot. Relaxation classes go through the body from your head down to your toes or vice versa, and it is important to bring awareness to feeling tense, before relaxing. Have a go at tensing as many muscles as you can, and then let go. This 'letting go' technique brings awareness to hidden tension and unhelpful posture, and many relaxation classes use these kind of techniques with good results.

Having a good posture is so important, especially when it comes to therapists. When I'm working clinically, and am therefore positioning my body to manipulate a client's body, I have to be in the correct place, and use the correct force. I focus, check my body posture, and sense any unhelpful tension. Then I wind the joint up, and with minimal physical force, I employ a small, gentle movement – a specific nudge navigated with both my Chi and my positioning.

I attempt to apply this body awareness to all my fitness routines as well as my running, and it is helpful in that it quiets my chattering monkey mind. Most importantly, it helps to minimise injury, as I am now at an age where I am privileged to still be able to run, and I need to cherish my joints so that I may be like my friends and parents (who are also still able to run) should I live till my eighties.

I will admit that stretching is a weakness of mine – I rush it – and it is important for your muscles, ligaments, and tendons to feel elastic. There is new research questioning how useful it really is at preventing injury, and several new ideas use dynamic movements in order to stretch, and only after warming up with activity first. With a sprinting run, it really is necessary to walk, then jog first, with a stretching session afterwards. I tend to quickly have a stretch whilst dashing to the shower. Experts say that the constant coiling and uncoiling in a rhythmical action (for example, when running) can only work properly with your healthy, elastic, energy efficient rubber bands (your tendons and ligaments) doing this for you.

CRAWLING WITH OUR L PLATES ON

Whenever our body experiences pain, we have to remember to return to our basic movements. For instance, prima ballerina Margot Fonteyn took a beginner's class every day, explaining that taking the class kept her extraordinary performances sharp, even after 20 years. If she didn't take the class, she believed that both her choreographer and her audience would be able to tell.

HOMEWORK:

Do you go through beginner's steps and classes regularly in your sport or hobby? If not, why not give it a try?

HOMEWORK:

How heavy are you really? Here are four exercises for loosening up your spine – why not give them a go?

1. Kneel down next to the bathroom scales, then press your hands hard down onto them as you read what the scales say. Next, bring your tummy button closer to the scales. Move your knees further back until you are in a crawling position, then straighten your arms and spine, and smile. See how much heavier you are, and how much more force you can generate as you stop trying.

2. When you feel tired, lean on your partner and feel supported. Here, you are in 'being' not 'doing' mode.

3. Crawling – now I bet you haven't done this for a while! This is an important movement that is studied in an eastern adaption of shiatsu called Ohashiatsu. Basically, it is a cross patterning move-ment (moving the arm with the opposite leg) that is excellent for back pain suffers. Can you feel the relaxation in your spine? Also, it means you can find dust and lost socks more easily.

4. The figure of 8. On all fours, move your tummy button (or Hara, the centre of Chi) in a figure of 8, feeling the weight transferring around your body, then relax. This is great for horse riders as this infinity movement works wonders for the spine.

THUNDERBIRDS ARE GO

You need to stop crawling around and get some fresh air. As I type this, I've just got back from a cold, wet run around my village (in the Staffordshire countryside). I did my Pinocchio puppet run because I was tired. This is a

Chi style to relax you, as they say that in order to avoid injury, you need to stop being so tense. I imagined my spine as a lot of cotton reels, all lined up. I hold a neutral pelvis by scooping back slightly, as if my pelvis is a cup of tea and needs to be level. I pull in my tummy, imagining strings holding my feet and hands up, and let my arms and legs go as floppy as possible. I must look like an episode of *Thunderbirds* gone weird.

RIDING ON AN IMAGINARY HORSE

I remember reading a book called *Running With A Mind Of Meditation* by a Tibetan Lama called Sakyong Mipham. Just like a lot of my patients, I find it difficult to sit quietly and meditate – I either fall asleep or start to get distracted by my chattering mind. Personally, I like to still my mind in a meditative way whilst swimming or running, and I was glad that Sakyong agreed with this. Jerry Lynch – who wrote *Thinking Body, Dancing Mind* – commented in his book that Sakyong's lessons "are like spiritual vitamins that will nourish the runner's soul."

Whilst we know that activities such as running (in moderation) can strengthen bone integrity, our muscles, and blood vessel resilience, it also very importantly builds a relationship with our breath, the most elemental aspect of being alive. This, in turn, stills our mind.

I enjoy the Tibetan imagery of the breath being the horse, with the rider sitting on a saddle that is made from a jewel – the jewel, like the mind, is clear and reflective. Whilst researching this I was heard neighing and saying giddy up – to remind myself of this image, that's all. Building a close relationship with your mind and imagery (such as the Tibetan horse) improves your mental health as well as your general oxygenation levels. Mind you, it is rather questionable if you start thinking you really are riding a horse! If we learn to breathe better, that gives us 21,600 happy, healthy breaths a day.

A QUICK RECAP ON MEDITATION

If you have no experience with meditation, just sit comfortably and focus on your breath. Concentrate on how it is normally, and then – should you wish to – you can learn how to gently soften and deepen it. I talk more about meditation in my Mind book if you want to look deeper into it. Once familiar with this breathing lark, you can then go on to focus on a theme, gently caressing your wandering mind back to the subject as it drifts away, as this will strengthen focus. It also strengthens your ability to drive your mind in useful directions, and it increases longevity for your body.

I find that running is a good time to use mind-breath techniques.

HOMEWORK:
Look up meditation and see if you could combine it with a hobby such as running.

DON'T SKI LIKE A CRUMPLED NEWSPAPER

I still remember one cold winter – when I was skiing and thinking about my posture – I was imagining I was skiing like an angel in my furry hat and gear, when a Bridget Jones moment interfered with this illusion. I heard my French ski instructor say, "She skis like a crumpled newspaper!" Had I gone through my postural exercises, I could have avoided that comment.

HOMEWORK:
Put your hand on your sternum (above your heart), and one hand on your tummy. Move your chest up towards your top hand, and inwards, away from your lower hand. This gives you a straighter spine and the ability to breathe better.

HOMEWORK:
Sit with your head correctly on your shoulders – every inch you move forward doubles your head weight through the neck. Place your thumb and middle finger of one hand on your collarbone. Extend the pointing finger and rest your chin on the tip.

I have flat feet. When I was an infant ballerina, I was taught to pick things up with my toes and imagine that I was walking on a tight rope, which helped to reduce the problem of pronated (flat) feet. Check if you can see your feet clearly when you look down, even where the shoelaces go. If you can't, check your pelvis position or lose weight!

Do you have any body sense of where your bucket-like pelvis should be in relation to your spine? OK, no problem – let's take a few minutes out together to have a play.

HOMEWORK:

Lie on your back with your knees bent and your heels touching your butt. Press and raise your lower back into and off the floor, feeling the gap come and go. Then, gradually move your feet further away, so you can repeatedly do this action with your legs straighter. Hold for ten seconds, with your spine against the floor and your tummy button pulled in. This is very useful if you stand without any curve in your back. You can finish with your legs straight, then repeat the whole thing through.

Then, in standing, you can lift up your pubic bone and pull your tummy in again for ten seconds. This should give you the gift of good posture – the key to reducing backache.

TO PLAY OUR SPINE LIKE A VIOLIN

The spine has always been a fascination to me – in India it is referred to as a 'lute' or 'violin'. The 33 bones and nerves can be thought of as a string instrument that can be tuned by movement to a higher vibration of health. Gravity pulls us to earth through our feet as we walk, compressing our spinal discs throughout the day, so when you sit and walk, you should have a soft curve in your lower back that then changes direction to house your ribcage and lungs. The waist – where, in effect, your spine moves in two different directions – is a delicate point. So many exercises around the world concentrate on protecting this area, including stretches and strengthening combined with breathing. Chi Kung, Tai Chi, Pilates, and Yoga are just a few of these.

My embryology (the study of the tiny human in the womb) professors would tell me that the spine is the first thing to be formed in the womb. All the limbs and organs extend from it, hence all movements should start in the spine. All physical treatments should also include assessment of the spine, as the spine's function is to elongate and be elastic and youthful. Exercise, therefore, is not a battle against old age, but a resuscitation of neglected body parts that have stiffened over time.

Gentle arts such as Chi Kung, Tai Chi, and Yoga involve the discipline of listening to the body's wisdom, as well as stretching, balancing, and strengthening every day in order to bring back youthfulness to our aging bodies. In this context, when I say 'aging' I mean that as soon as we stop growing and become adults, we start rotting. Correct posture and exercise, however, slows the degeneration (rot). We have 31 pairs of spinal nerves all going through bony tunnels widened by our spinal discs. With poor posture, the spine ages faster, and the nerves get damaged, influencing the nerves they connect with as well as the target tissue.

When the spine is locked down by small muscles in tension, tight ligaments, and frayed discs, osteoarthritis moves into the little joints and further stiffens the spine. This is bad news for our sensitive, insulated nerve fibres firing messages to and from every part of the body. Nerve impulses are specific electrical discharges consisting of a delicate balance of potassium ions inside the nerve, and sodium outside the nerve. Even mild compression due to poor posture can cause the spinal nerve roots to be neuropathic (damaged) and even a mild temporary compression can change the sensitivity of the nerve until treated. Normal, nice sensations can be sent incorrectly as pain signals.

HOMEWORK:
STOP SLOUCHING! Grrrrr...

You can get little biofeedback devices that vibrate when you slouch... and no, you don't sit on them! I asked that question, and let me tell you, it did not go down too well. These devices are strapped onto your back, the idea being that the habit is broken by bringing conscious awareness to your posture.

Did you know that we can shrink by up to an inch a day? So that's why we adjust the car's rear view mirror at night! Imagine if your tyre pressure changed that much throughout the day – you would be pumping it up on the way home every night. Also, at night, our spine drinks water – though 'imbibes' is the posh word for it – and elongates. Spinal extension stretches and good posture can all help with its thirst during the day (echoed in a paper by Ressel, 1989). A medic called Batmanghelidj wrote extensively about the importance of water not only for your spine but also generally in your body, and I talk about this in my *4 keys* book.

WALK AGELESSLY

Do you people watch? I watch my patients walking down the path between my flowerbeds as they approach the clinic; in doing this, you can tell a lot about that person's chattering mind, and their life's purpose – about whether they feel loved and connected and needed, or in love, or dejected. Whether they are connecting with their body's wisdom or just driving their vehicle/body with little awareness.

HOMEWORK:
Lift one of your feet and move it slowly forward. Concentrate on it, let your heel make contact first, then roll forward through the arch and push off through your toes. Feel gravity controlling it, and feel your weight transfer across to the other foot.

The arch is in our foot for a reason; its ligaments and tendons need to be elastic in order to shock absorb our steps on tarmac, up throughout our knees and our hips and our spine, eroding away with every thoughtless jolt. When we gracefully walk and run with focus, the arch becomes a great big softening lever, and our body thanks us for it.

"The true man breathes with his heels."
- ***Vandi Scaravelli.***

This quote is from a lovely illustrated book about the philosophy of Yoga by Vanda Scaravelli entitled *Awakening The Spine* (2012).

The feet were worshipped in ancient Buddhist times. The Chinese and then the Japanese would depict a Taoist principle, telling you to lead with your left foot, as that was the spiritual one. They also believed that the cycle of Qi is expanded again and again from the crown of your head to the soles of your feet during exhalation, and back up through the spine during inhalation. The centre of breath and energy/Qi is the waist of the spine/lower abdomen, dating back to ancient scripts of Buddhism and Shintoism in the 6th century.

The heel of the foot has important muscles attached to the calf muscles – Gastrocnemius and Soleus – via a thickened tendon that transmits a strong contraction to push off the ground. The tendinous attachment is very susceptible to being damaged, and heals badly due to a poor blood supply.

Body anatomy was often taught through stories, and several Greek stories have survived to tell us about this vulnerable part of our body. One of those stories is the well-known tale of Achilles: Achilles was dipped in the river Styx to protect his body, but his mother held him by his achilles whilst she dipped him, meaning that part of his body was left unattended. This Achilles was later shot at by Paris in the heel, and the Trojan enemy died.

In another story, in order to avoid a nasty prophecy, King Laius of Thebes pierced his baby son's feet with spears, binding his ankles and leaving him to die. Oedipus (he who limps) survived, limping throughout his life, and ended up killing his father and marrying his mother (what a sad prophecy). I think this story was about the disconnect between the mind, body, and soul, as it was believed that a damaged foot could not connect the soul to the universe. Not a bedtime story I would choose for my nephews and niece!

DRVING DOWN THE WHITE LINE WITH CHI AND GRAVITY

When you go from walking to running, you create a counter rotation between your hips and shoulders, causing your spine to gently twist. Like rubber bands, they store energy in order to whip the spine back in counter rotation, back to its neutral position.

Your core abdominal muscles are crucial; if you want to go faster in your car, you press on the accelerator by leaning further forward, not by bending. Gravity then does a lot of the work for you so your achilles (the tendon in your heel) doesn't have to work so hard in propelling you forward. If you don't place your body weight forward from your feet, you break with every step, shoving six times your body weight through your worn knee joints. Imagine your feet forming a big wheel just behind you, your stride length being the gears. At slow speed (the low gears), you have less upper body lean and shorter strides. When you get faster, there is more upper body lean forward and with a longer stride, and then you're into a higher gear change.

What's slow and fast in terms of running, you may ask? Well, I read a book called *Chi Running*, and the author (Danny Dreyer) stated that 85 to 90 steps per minute is a good tempo to aim for, landing mid-foot. A pocket-sized metronome could help with this (Dreyer, 2008). He also states that the arms should do 50% of the work – though I'm not entirely sure how – and also that the elbows need to swing behind the body, fingers to ribs and forward. Learn to run again, mindfully.

> **HOMEWORK:**
> Place your feet side by side as if standing normally, then, engaging your lower abdominals, fall forward a little in front of a wall, placing your hands onto the wall. You should be leaning forward, with your feet still in contact with the floor and your back straight. Do it repeatedly, then – if you're a smarty-pants – try one leg at a time. My skiing 'like a crumpled newspaper' wasn't quite this position, but almost.

> **HOMEWORK:**
> Scatter books around your office and step over them. You are pick-ing your feet up, not pushing off the ground – do you feel the differ-ence in your feet? Feel relaxed in the calf of the leg you picked up, and give it a shake. Do this exercise often to remind you. Ladies: if your husband is annoying you, use anything of his that is fragile.

Good posture and regular stretching – perhaps incorporating yogic poses – will lengthen your spine and ease your mind. By spending time concentrat-ing on the body with various yogic poses, you will switch on the connection with your body's innate wisdom and this process will keep you healthier.

The Kenyan national team of long distance runners switch off completely after a run in order to heal. Westerners find it difficult to train in this way – they think resting means watching TV, eating out, seeing friends, and fiddling with their phones, whereas rest actually means stillness, peace, and emptiness.

THE COILED SNAKE, THE SPORT BUTTON ON YOUR GEAR STICK

When I heard that we had a Kundalini Yoga expert co-presenting at Z fac-tor, I thought to myself, 'that's a brave lady, demonstrating orgasmic yoga! This will be fun'. If you haven't read my *4 keys* book, Z factor is Joseph Mc-Clendon's Health Seminar, and yes he is crazy enough to let me present on it. Did I hear you say, "Who is Joseph?" Only Tony Robbins' co-presenter of a worldwide show called UPW (Unleash the Power Within)!

Kundalini is all about training your mind whilst getting a more flexible spine, and it became fashionable to westerners when an Indian chap called Yogi Bhajan brought it to the hippy Californians in 1969 – no pun intended on the number.

The typical Yoga pose of sitting with the legs crossed is not easy for every-one, so I suggest starting gently, with a little cushion under the bum, and your legs gently crossed, as able. Just to add insult to injury for those who are less flexible, this is known as the EASY POSE. The hand position you're meant to do in this pose – with the first finger to the thumb – is a big thing, and it's called the Gyan Mudra. It is important to remember this part of the pose, as it stops you from reaching for snacks whilst doing Yoga.

Now, we have the same old same old pulling in of the tummy button, which is universal throughout Pilates, Tai Chi, and Yoga, and is so important. Ensure that you also tighten up your naughty bits, your bum and the pelvic floor; this area in particular is very important to work as we age… in my dreams… This is said to be where the Kundalini energy is curled up, and contracting these muscles wakes it up. It is called performing a 'root lock'.

YOUR EVENING WORKOUT

HOMEWORK:
The Naam bread pose or root lock. This is called Sat Kriya, and it's a simple exercise said to work on 72,000 nerve endings in the naval area. This will wake up the Kundalini, making you more creative and giving you a stronger core. For this you can sit on a chair, on the floor cross-legged, or on your heels. Put your arms above your head, with your hands together, your fingers interlocked, and your two index fingers pointing upwards. Your shoulder blades should be together with your shoulders relaxed. Those who are good at imagery, think of looking through an eye between your eyebrows called the third eye. Chant "SAT" while pulling your tummy button in suddenly with the pelvic floor, then slowly release it as you say, "Naaaaaam". Do this for several seconds or minutes. This is great for lumbar spine stability.

DEAD BODY POSE

Whenever you want a break, this next pose is easy: the corpse pose. Except, unlike a corpse, you keep breathing and have a pulse, and you just lie on your back and relax. This one I can do easily, tee hee!

HOMEWORK:

Breathe with your spine.

Sit either at your desk or in the cross-legged position. If on a mat, hold your ankles – obviously, don't if you're at your desk, ha ha. The spine extends easily with exhaling (breathing out exhaust fumes) – it's wired this way – so breathe in and curl inwards, then exhale and extend your lower back, arching it. Repeat this several times to get a good rhythm, then, after three minutes, return to the upright position and apply a root lock. Start with three sets of 10 seconds, then work up to 30 seconds. Do not try too hard, and keep the contraction less than 90%. If you've been sitting for an hour or more, repeat this to help your spinal discs and concentration.

The mid-back often stiffens up and cries out to be turned and stretched, whereas the thoracic vertebrae are chiselled to allow twisting.

HOMEWORK:

Spinal twissle stick. Mid-back and lower back stretches are essential if you work at a desk a lot. Sit on the floor – or at your desk – in the Easy Pose, then place your hands on your shoulders with your elbows at 90 degrees. Twist at a good speed to your right and left, then inhale in one direction and exhale in the other.

Place your fingers in the Gyan Mudra position (with the thumb and first finger touching), then raise your arms like Greek dancers and twist at different levels of elevation. I like the way this movement stretches different bits of the spine. I imagine the spine like a ladder, and I am twisting around at higher and higher rungs. Raise your arm up as far as you can reach, with your hands together, and then bring them down in a prayer hand position, staying still for a minute. I find that three minutes of moving your arms around is more than enough.

HOMEWORK:

The Sufi Grind. Sitting in the Easy Pose with your hands on your knees (or at your desk), move your spine and pelvis in big circles, in both directions. Inhale as you move one way and exhale as you move the other. A variation on this pose is the Infinity – a figure of eight movement I was taught in Shiatsu – which, although it is a little trickier in terms of breath coordination, it is great for the back. Again, in between your horse riding manoeuvres, sit still and apply a root lock to strengthen your core, and – in eastern terms – the Kundalini energy.

HOMEWORK:

The Pelvic Lift. For this pose you need to lie on the floor, with your knees bent up and your heels near your buttocks. Inhale as you gently lift your bottom off the ground, then exhale and lower it down.

HOMEWORK:

The stiff neck stretch. Gently, with breath, roll your neck back when inhaling and go forward when exhaling. Do not do this if you suffer from dizziness issues, or if you have a very stiff neck or any known problems with your neck. If this is the case, gently tilt your head from side to side for the upper neck stretch, then turn it horizontally (and slowly) left and right, inhaling one way and exhaling the other. Then you can repeat the turning with your chin tucked in, scooping right and left.

HOMEWORK:

Strong arms. Sitting down, put your arms in front of you then out to your side at 90 degrees. Breathe deeply and slowly, pull your shoulder blades back together, and hold your arms, rotating with your palms up and down. Start with 10 seconds and go up to three minutes. This is good for posture and for strengthening the arms. You can add in your root lock here if you wish.

HOMEWORK:

This one is good for your arms, lymph drainage, and releasing frustrating emotions. Sitting down, stretch one arm up in front of you, whilst the other one stays at your side, with the elbow at 90 degrees – then rhythmically alternate, inhaling as the first arm goes up.

HOMEWORK:

This one is good for anger release. Sit down with your elbows at 90 degrees, then extend your arms parallel to the ground and criss-cross across the body in front of the diaphragm (just above the tummy button), with your fists tight as you shout, "HAR!" (or "F***!"). These are strong movements, just stopping short of hitting the body.

HOMEWORK:

Lift your bum. Here's another arm strengthening exercise for you now, as long as you don't have shoulder problems. Sit down with your legs out in front of you, then push your palms down to raise your bum – I have to say, mine doesn't lift far! Inhale as you attempt to raise your bum and legs, then exhale as you come down. Eastern medicine says this helps with kidney function. Be very careful if you have weak wrists, and only attempt a few at a time.

HOMEWORK:

If you are fit and flexible, you can add in hip stretches with the spine by sitting with your legs apart and your knees straight out in front of you. Stretch down to the middle with each leg in turn as you exhale. Take care if you have any kind of sciatica or stiffness in your spine.

HOMEWORK:

Lung workout. All this can make you a little light-headed, so let's just have a brief play with breathing exercises (some of these are also mentioned in other chapters). During a Z Factor seminar, my friend Goedelle went through the following panting exercises.

HOMEWORK:

'Breath of Fire' is breathing loud and hard, in and out through your nose, while pumping your tummy muscles. Get into a sitting position with your hands in front of you and your little fingers interlocked. This helps with tiredness; it's a breath of caffeine! The Cannon Breath is all about the mouth and consists of loud in and out breaths through your open mouth – with an equal effort for both in and out. Be careful of too much garlic and smelly breath! Both of these breaths are said to be good for the adrenals.

If you're a Yoga expert, you can do the Fire Breath lying on your front, with your arms behind you, your fingers interlocked, and your legs raised, with your forehead still on the floor. This is said to stop you worrying about money; I should think in that position you would be so uncomfortable that money would be the least of your worries!

Another crazy tough one is to use the Breath of Fire whilst lying on your back, with your head and legs six inches off the floor – less than a minute and I am a jelly with this one. Do not attempt unless very skilled at Yoga. This pose is said to build trust and belief in yourself, to help with grief and forgiveness, and to improve your immune system.

HOMEWORK:

Anti-anxiety breath. Sitting in the Easy Pose, extend both your arms up and out, creating a V-shape. Keep your elbows straight and criss-cross your arms in front and above your head. Synchronise this movement with Breath of Fire. If you suffer from anxiety, try this pose.

HOMEWORK:

Sitting in the Easy Pose, hold your arms up to the left and extend your elbows, with your palms together at about 60 degrees, then hold. Breathe in through your nose powerfully, and out through your open mouth.

HOMEWORK:

Calming breath. If you feel nervous, inhale through your nose, then exhale powerfully through your mouth as you're saying the 'shhhhh' sound. If you do this in a crowded room, you will make everyone *else* feel nervous and you may have a giggle. This pose is for helping relationships and self-love.

HOMEWORK:

Sat in the car chant. Sit in the Easy Pose and chant the following mantra. Say "SAT" as you press your hands into the prayer pose, and say "KAR" as you start extending your arms out sideways, level with your shoulders. Then, when saying "TAR", fully extend. Practice this for up to three minutes. If you are experienced in Yoga, you can do a pose called Kundalini Lotus – if it doesn't give you a rupture, it is said to improve your sex life.

HOMEWORK:

Crippling pose! Sitting in the Easy Pose, stretch out your legs, hold your toes, and put your legs up and out at about 45 degrees. This is NOT for the faint-hearted. If by this point you haven't fainted, progress onto Fire breathing – sounds very dragon-like!

HOMEWORK:

Stop the pee! Ladies, this is an exercise for your undercarriage. Kegels involve pulling up the pelvic floor – for this, imagine a lift gently going up – and holding for 10 seconds. If you have a weakness, doing this for up to 50 times a day over several weeks should help, and if not, seek out a physio who specialises in women's (gynaecological) issues.

HOMEWORK:

Humping. The Child's Pose is said to be relaxing if you are flexible, and it is also said to stimulate the pituitary (a gland in the brain). This pose involves sitting on your heels, spreading your knees a little – or a lot – to make room for your tummy, and then leaning forward until your head is on the floor. From here you can go back onto all fours to do circular hip movements, figure of eight pelvic movements, or the Cat stretch – all of which are great for the spine. The Cat stretch involves kneeling on all fours, inhaling as you curl back, and exhaling as you arch your back. We call it 'humping and hollowing' in the clinic, which are perhaps not the wisest of words.

HOMEWORK:

Down dog to lions paws. To help with meditation, you Yoga experts can push up into a V-shape called the Downward Dog, and without breaking anything, you can even go onto lifting one leg straight back. This is good for the core, and – in eastern terms – the Crown chakra. It allows you to prepare for meditation. Sitting in the Easy Pose with your arms swept out and up at your side, make sure your hands are clawed – this is called Lions Paws. You can do a Cannon Breath to this. Also, sit in the Easy Pose for meditation with your hands cupped, or your elbows in at your ribcage and your hands out at 60 degrees – or Gyan Mudra, whatever feels right.

CORE, A BRIEF SUMMARY OF MODERN DAY DISCUSSION ON THE CONCEPT OF CORE IN MOVEMENT

There are all kinds of research studies from all around the world exploring how we should improve our skilled, dynamic movement in sport, though I believe that it only emphasises the importance of cultural differences in the interpretation of movement. I remember Prof Gunn saying to me in a Korean hospital that before some of his eastern patients could read or write, those farming the land knew how a goat or a tiger moved, so their concept of movement was to copy an animal form.

I just want to mention an article here (*Injury Prevention and Movement Control*) by sport movement specialist, Lincoln Blandford, as he summarised one of his projects over 15 years to see where core strength training was taking us (Blandford, 2013). Thank you Lincoln for such a detailed report, and I hope my brief summary of it does it justice. Lincoln Blandford was operating within a performance outcome arena, which is always surrounded by conflicting and confusing information, not to mention big egos.

From the late 90's onwards, CST (core stability) gained worldwide recognition, and it was adopted on a global scale, with a huge variance in the way it was taught. Back in the early 90's, I remember going on my Mark Comerford courses about which muscles should contract in what sequence. This was my first introduction to specialist core work beyond Pilates and Yoga.

Blandford reviewed lots of research studies, and was particularly interested in how therapists adapted to suit the training bias of the specific movement discipline's own cultural take on 'effective' training. Strength and performance-focused sportsmen developed core strength training in order to match the forceful, strong, endurance activities. Physios and sports therapists saw the western evolution of 'motor control' – a low intensity version of core stability – and both camps, in confusing conflict, thought, 'do I teach fast, functional muscle recruitment or low-threshold, gentle, small amplitude postural muscle recruitment?' As physios, we were trained more in a low-threshold, pain free approach before progressing onto high-threshold performance work. The old core stability debates of low or high, hollow or brace, are slowly resolving themselves out of necessity for what works. Low-threshold was back on the menu.

"The Performance Matrix movement analysis system has supplied many answers, a systematic, evidenced based approach, acting as a lighthouse in the CST-functional training storm. The system's ability to assess and retrain movement at both low and high intensity solved the question of motor control or core strength; both are required, but we need to know when [the timing of each is important in rehabilitation]. The specificity of the system allowed the performance of seemingly non-functional exercises to be easy to defend" (taken from ThePerfomaceMatrix.com).

As each exercise addresses a specific problem before it's put back into an improved, working whole – like cleaning up the carburettor before switching the engine on and getting the car moving – the cognitive testing of movement control allowed for the development of different unique concepts of movement health. That's like checking the car's CPU (brain) to make sure it's telling the parts to engage at the right time, speed, and orientation.

It may seem crazy to have to relearn how to lift your knee up to work a little muscle called VMO (vastus medialis oblique), whilst gently pulling in your stomach, but relearning the memory of this skill is critical if you want to function optimally after, say, a knee injury. If you can't prevent a wrong movement occurring during a test, you have lost movement options/control – it's a bit like taking a driving test. The core's hardware is made 'smart' by a 'controller'; the nervous system wiring into your brain. In good movement, your joints – and active hardware/muscles – operate effectively under the control of this software (Panjabi, 1992).

Providing a constant internal conversation, the software allows all components to 'talk and listen' to one another, in order to meet the challenges of activity. And just like the hardware, this software and its language are also open to programming faults, though it can be upgraded through effective training (Tsao & Hodges, 2008).

Software biased training – often called 'motor control' – has been typically favoured by those from a rehabilitative background, and one function of the software – and central to movement health – are effective patterns of 'recruitment' (Briggs et al., 2004). The 'controller'/your brain must efficiently choose which particular muscles to employ at which point in time, as well as how much each will contribute to any given task. Hodges & Richardson (1996) have shown that training can change the sequencing of the software, selecting some muscles preferentially to others.

Prof Gunn would say that if nerves are neuropathic, then the correct muscle recruitment cannot occur without treatment. This discrimination of muscles requires a 'software biased' training. The internal conversation also allows for a virtual body to be 'mapped' out within regions of the brain, which is the software's interpretation of the hardware's form (Wand et al., 2011). In good movement health, each section of the hardware is accurately charted, allowing for efficient movement control – that's why you need to think through your sport or daily activities before moving your muscles, and it's also why eastern exercises (where you focus on repetition of movement) are so clever for gaining pose and balance.

In poor movement health, certain regions can become over-represented, becoming the 'squeaky wheel' and demanding excessive attention from the software's controller. These regions of the body – the ones that are constantly 'moaning away' – may change this map, altering efficient navigation/negotiation of movement challenges as the individual makes their way through the world. In such cases, a software upgrade is required, redrawing the map and taking the internal spotlight away from those attention-seeking players.

The movement control concept is wonderfully summarised by Blandford's 2013 article that I've already mentioned, as it can be seen to have evolved out of numerous schools of thought. Spinal and trunk 'stability' were once the extent of its limits, whereas now the whole body can be seen through the viewpoint of movement control at varying degrees of intensity. Pain, and neurological diseases such as motor neuron, multiple sclerosis, Parkinson's, and strokes, to name a few – and, to a lesser extent, neuropathic nerves – are all both a software and hardware disability.

GET UP OFF THAT FAT BUM OF YOURS – IT'S KILLING YOU!

In terms of moving around, kids do it naturally – watching my nephews and niece (all of whom are under five), they are always moving. They have a youthful aerobic system and the concentration span of a gnat, which is perfect for keeping slim. Do you realise that you may sit for 12 hours a day, then sleep for eight? Ladies, when we did housework the old-fashioned way, we burnt up to 1000 calories a day.

Professor Jim Levine at the Mayo Clinic, USA, is an obesity specialist in movement, and he says that movement is the secret of longevity – though he calls it 'non-exercise activity thermogenesis' (NEAT). This is the calories we burn up with the activities of daily living. In general, we need to move every half an hour in order to keep our fuels moving through our body efficiently. As I type this, I am bouncing on my fit ball.

Sedentariness is a killer: the lipoprotein lipase enzyme drops on being still, so fewer blood fats are available for fuel and you end up getting unhealthy sugar spikes in the blood after eating. If you wear fidget pants, you can find out how much you move: NEAT pants have multiple sensors and accelerometers in to measure this. Just take them off if practicing tantric sex, please – think of the poor researchers analysing the data! Dunstan et al. (2012) looked in-depth into the physiology of sitting, and they concluded that short bursts of activity are enough to help blood sugar levels keep you in a healthier state.

WHEN IS THE BEST TIME OF DAY TO EXERCISE?

When should you exercise? They usually say first thing is a nice mood elevator. However, in terms of physiology, they say mid-day till 7 p.m. is best. In 2005, some research carried out at Liverpool John Moore's University looked at doing exercise at 5 a.m., 11 a.m., 5 p.m., and 11 p.m., and they confirmed that mid-day to 7 p.m. is the best time.

ME TARZAN, YOU JANE

Us Homo sapiens have a long evolutionary history; we are the products of thousands of generations of our species, a species that for most of its existence has lived briefly and in danger. Life for a caveman or woman was generally nasty, horrifically scary, and short.

To keep in shape they didn't 'exercise' in their Pilates classes, wearing the latest caveman fur thong; they simply had to do a wide range of different activities to help ensure that they survived and passed on their genes, eventually, to us. Our bodies and our genes were forged by the demands of the environment in which they – the hunter-gatherers – lived. As you'll discover if you read *Fast Exercise* by Michael Mosley, there is compelling evidence that a hunter-gatherer approach is also good for our more cosseted bodies.

LATEST STUDIES TELL US TO GET OUR BODY OUT OF THE GARAGE AND GET MOVING

We need to be active, but not *too* active; we benefit most from short bursts of intense activity, and we need rest days to recover or we'll undo all the good work. As the authors of 'Achieving Hunter-gatherer fitness in the 21st Century', a paper in the *American Journal of Medicine*, point out:

"Hunter-gatherers would have likely alternated difficult days with less demanding days when possible. The same pattern of alternating a strenuous workout one day with an easy one the next day produces higher levels of fitness with lower rates of injury... The natural cross training that was a mandatory aspect of life as a hunter-gatherer improves performance across many athletic disciplines" (O'Keefe et al., 2010).

So what are the characteristics of a prehistoric hunter-gatherer fitness program? Well, they include short bursts of moderate to high intensity exercise (20 seconds to a minute) interspersed with rest and recovery, 2-3 times a week. I suppose for some that could be sex? Just as long as they're regular sessions of strength and flexibility-building. Hunter-gatherers had to chop wood, gather veg and nuts, climb trees, and carry children, or a dead animal for food.

Their 'exercise' was all done outdoors, as their caves were likely to be dark and cramped, so they were regularly exposed to sunlight, which gives the skin a chance to generate vitamin D, a hormone. Many of us – particularly those who live in the northern hemisphere – are chronically short of vitamin D. Some people, like our ancestors, find it much easier to do in a social setting, as self-motivation can be poor – and by 'it' I mean exercise, not sex. We are intensely social creatures, and doing exercise together is a good way of ensuring that we do it at all. Having said that, I personally enjoy exercising on my own.

SLAM YOUR FOOT ON THE ACCELERATOR PEDAL, HARD, FAST, AND BRIEFLY

All around the world, research has been looking at the extraordinary impact that ultra-short bursts of HIT (high-intensity training) can have, whatever your age or level of fitness. Fast Exercise is for those who don't enjoy exercise, but want to lose fat and stay healthy, as well as those who love exercise and want to get the most from it. I first came across HIT through Dr Mosley's social media and TV documentary. His mentor was Dr Jamie Timmons, professor of systems biology at Loughborough University, and he wrote a UK guide about the world of HIT. Jamie Timmons was also professor of aging biology at Birmingham University – I wish I'd met him when I was studying biology there. I would walk two to three miles and swim every day to keep fit, and would always have long wet hair throughout my afternoon lab session!

I have to say that Jamie's work fascinated me, as I simply could not get my head around how only three minutes of exercise could make a difference. You know what I mean, ladies – in my opinion, it's just not enough. The research papers, however, assured me that by doing just three minutes of HIT a week for four weeks, I could expect to see significant changes in a number of important health indices. Of course, this would be partly dependant on my genes – and no, not the denim type. On that subject, I would buy mine from a charity shop around the corner from the university labs, and always seemed to end up with baggy ones, hence my nickname, 'Droopy Drawers'. I suppose this made a change from 'Flipper' due to my wet hair, always going swimming, and having big feet.

Jamie Timmons worked out of labs at Loughborough, which is home to the Centre for Olympic Studies and Research, one of the leading sports research centres in the UK. He worked with Dr Mosley on the documentary, telling him that if he was prepared to give it a go, he was confident that in just four weeks he would see significant changes in his biochemistry. "So," says Mosley, "I got myself properly tested and then I went for it. The results were a revelation" (Mosley, FastExercises.com).

"Since 2011, HIT has really taken off but the principles remain simple [and time-efficient]: do 3-10 minutes of exercise a week, take lots of rests but pushing yourself hard enough to get your heart pumping" (FastExercise. com). It is said to help with getting slimmer, strength, fitness, and insulin sensitivity. The concept is simple, and in the *Fast Exercise* book, there are many workouts to play with (Mosley, 2013).

Whatever your age or level of fitness – and whether you prefer to cycle, run, swim, or walk – there is an exercise regime for you. Try jogging on the spot at speed for three minutes – it feels like forever! I just had a go now, and wow it doesn't half make your heart pump! The brain likes the number three; it's a nice sized chunk that also seems like an achievable goal. You can use your stopwatch setting on your phone. A word to the wise here: don't answer the phone straight afterwards – I frightened a friend to death as all they could hear on my end of the line was heavy breathing.

As well as Fast Fitness exercises – which will improve your aerobic and metabolic fitness in record time – you should also include Fast Strength exercises. These build muscle, make you look more toned, and can also be done in just a few minutes a day, requiring nothing more than a chair, a fit ball, or the floor.

Of course, there's a bit more to staying thin than that, as it also matters what you do when you're *not* exercising. Exercise, even with the HIT style, will just turn into a SHIT outcome if you're sitting down for hours, day in, day out. As has been mentioned earlier in this chapter, the concept of youthful activity and moving more is called 'NEAT' – non-exercise activity thermogenesis – and this is, as it says, the amount of energy you burn in everyday activities that are not considered exercise.

Think you don't have time to do some amazing training? You will see me running Snazzy-style, up a track behind the clinic, whenever I have a rare half an hour to myself – anything to exercise and get my heart rate up. I was cheered when I read about Roger Bannister's four minute mile training, and how he achieved this with – like me – only having half an hour to spare on his work days. Over 35 minutes, he would do 10 sets of one minute flat outsprint, then two to three minutes jogging. Seb Coe did 20 second sprints and 30 second recovery, alternating between the two.

SHOULD I STRETCH?

The jury is still out on this one. Whether it's a set of fast strength or fast aerobic exercises, a short one-minute warm up is kind to your body – it's just like giving your car engine a little kindness if she's been sitting still on the drive for some time. In 2005, Dr Ian Shrier wrote about stretches in the *Sports Medicine Journal*, stating that the evidence pointed to dropping stretches pre-workout. Peter McNair added in the 2004 *Sports Medicine Journal* that stop-start sports like football could well benefit from stretching, but that it made no sense for swimmers or joggers. Stretching is not evidence based at the time of writing this, as there is no proof that it stops injuries, especially with regards to swimming and jogging. It is deemed far more useful to start off with dynamic movements and stretches specific to the activity you are about to do.

Some of my older patients take anti-inflammatories to make them more flexible and more comfortable, forgetting that they could cause a stomach bleed.

I have talked at length about running, and you can see just how easy it is to put some sprints in to get your HIT. With swimming a 25m pool length, swimming at speed is equivalent to sprint running for 30 to 40 seconds. You could skip instead, or row, – though be careful of technique – use a cross-trainer, sprint on a bike, jog on the spot, run upstairs, do knee lifts or lunges… the world is your oyster.

For strengthening you could do the bear crawl, log lifts, bench push-ups, squats, step-ups, wall slides, side planks, or use Therabands or weights for limb strengthening. Most of these you could do at work, in the garden, or in the house. When I do knee highs in the clinic I feel guilty about the people underneath me – I work on the first floor.

HOMEWORK:
Write a list of your own exercises – examples below – and choose four different exercises each time you work out. Do five of each, then four, and then down to one rep, say, three times a week. If you are fitter, go up to starting at ten.

Bear Crawl: First, get on all fours. You can move the opposite arm and leg, or the same side to change it around. Keep your hips low, as in stalking, then raise your bum up for a high level crawl.

Log lift: I do this every day, getting logs into the wheelbarrow for the log burner. Get a smallish log, squat down with your back straight, then pick it up to shoulder height before carrying for 10 metres.

Bench push-up: Hold a plank position, with your hands on the front edge of a bench, your body straight, and the balls of your feet on the ground. Start with your elbows at 90 degrees, then straighten to push up, holding your body straight and bending your elbows again.

Squats: Stand with your feet shoulder-width apart. Bend from your hips, keeping your back straight, until your knees are at 90 degrees. Imagine you are about to sit, then stand up.

Step-ups: Place a foot on the step, then push with your body weight and stand on the step (or bench). Step back and down, then repeat with the opposite leg for 30 seconds.

Side planks: Lie on your side with your top leg over the bottom leg, slightly in front. With your body in line, rest on your elbow and lift your hips up, as if a rope is pulling them up. Keep them straight, and to start with, hold for ten seconds.

I know it takes about a three-mile run or a two-hour walk to burn off my morning banana smoothie, so I can't afford to be too sedentary. Every time I put a pound of fat on through enjoyable, delicious, intoxicating food and drink, it's a six-mile run or equivalent to pay it back – a sobering thought, eh! If we eat more after exercise because it stimulates our appetite, we simply get fatter, but HITs can stop this happening as much as our appetite is not raised so much after short bursts of exercise. We know from research that an unfit thin person is less well than a fatter fit person, so don't despair – it's all about moderation guys, moderation. We also know – from summarising lots of research studies that often feature opposing views – that very simplistically, up to an hour's exercise a day improves mortality rate, and more than this decreases it. Exercise instructors wear their joints out faster than the general public.

In a study by H. Sandmark in 2000, the hip and knee joints of 500 Swedish physical education teachers (who qualified between 1957 and 65, making them in their fifties at the time of the study) were assessed. Here we have slimmer, more health-conscious fitter people who are – guess what? – three times more likely to suffer with arthritis in their knees and hips. In fact, only 20% of the studied group could still work due to their joint problems.

HOW FIT ARE YOU?

At my clinic I have a fitness/nutrition expert to hand, should anyone want to check out their health before exercising. There are a few key measurements that need to be done in order to compute this, and VO2 max is a good predictor of health – literally, how much tiger have you got in your tank?

VO2 MAX

This is a measure of aerobic fitness – including how strong your heart and lungs are –and it is one of the most important predictors of future health. The most reliable way to find your VO2 max is to have it done in a lab or a gym, but you can use an estimate to get you started.

The simplest is the Uth-Sorenen-Overgaard-Pedersen estimation ($VO2_{max}$ = 15.3 x $HeartRate_{max}$/$HeartRate_{rest}$).

This shows the basal metabolic rate/fat burning potential, and I use our Quadscan equipment to measure it.

One way you can estimate your VO2 max is to do the Rockport One Mile walk test. Basically, time yourself walking a mile as briskly as you can, then measure your heart rate at the end. Then, you'll need to do a stupidly complicated bit of maths… I don't think so! Hence our darling Quadscan works it all out for us.

If you're interested, here is the equation: VO2 max=132.853-[0.0769x weight] – [0.3877 x age] + [6.315xsex]-[3.2649xtime]-[0.1565x heart rate].

Weight is in pounds, sex is not how many times you have it, but male is one and female is zero, and the time is in minutes and seconds.

BASAL METABOLIC RATE (BMR): This is the amount of calories you expend to survive just sitting down for 24 hours, doing nothing, at rest. Your BMR is relative to your weight, height, and age, and remember that men are regarded as needing more calories than women. Exercise, low temperature, stress, fear, and illnesses will all increase your BMR.

BODY MASS INDEX (BMI): I understand that BMI is still used a lot, however, the old-fashioned waist to height ratio was found to be better than BMI for predicting the risk of heart disease. So how does it work? Basically, measure your waist by putting the tape measure around your middle, at belly button height. Your waist should be less than half of your height. This is because the worst sort of fat is visceral fat, which collects inside the abdomen and coats your internal organs (liver, pancreas, and so on). The Fast Exercise and Fast Diet programs (which make use of a couple of days of low calories) are particularly effective at reducing this dangerous visceral fat.

BMI, on the other hand, is based on your height and weight, and it has several limitations: for instance, it's not accurate for pregnant women, people under five feet tall, the elderly, athletes, or people with very muscular builds. It also does not account for age, and the standard recommendations do not apply to children or teens. So, it's not necessarily that accurate for all of us.

BMI	Weight Status
<18.5	Underweight
18.5 – 24.9	Normal
25.0 – 29.9	Overweight
>30	Obese

DO YOU KNOW YOUR MAXIMUM HEART RATE?

"Many of the Fast Exercises require you to push yourself to 80% or 90% of your maximum heart rate. Alternatively, if you are not already doing strenuous exercise regularly or just want a quick number, you can calculate an estimate which will give you the average expected for your age, rather than your actual fitness level. Most calculations use a very simple formula: HR_{max} = (220 – age) for men and (226 – age) for women, but a more reliable estimate is: HR_{max} = 205.8 – (0.685 x age). We use the latter in our calculator" (Fast-Exercises.com).

In summary, consider these key factors that our nutritionist measures when looking at changes in fitness:
- Weight
- Waist circumference
- Body fat (%)
- Blood Pressure
- Fasting blood sugar
- Cholesterol (blood lipids)
- VO_2 max

IT'S IN YOUR GENES, NOT YOUR RUNNING SHORTS

From 22 separate studies – which followed one million people from Europe, North America, East Asia, and Australia – Woodcock et al. (2010) collated the data to show whether a sedentary person who started doing 2.5 hours of moderate activity a week (such as walking) could reduce their mortality by 19%. However, the fact is that people respond to exercise in very different ways. In a Finnish study by Karavirta (2011), 175 middle-aged humans of both sexes had set patterns of both strength and endurance exercise. The results reflected that regardless of sex or age, there were both super responders and non-responders to exercise.

In a big international study, "1,000 people were asked to exercise four hours a week for 20 weeks. Their aerobic fitness was measured before and after starting this regime and the results were striking. Although 15% of people made huge strides (so-called 'super-responders'), 20% showed no real improvement at all ('non-responders')," (BBC website) and also, 30% showed no improvement in insulin sensitivity. "There is no suggestion that the non-responders weren't exercising properly, it was simply that the exercise they were doing was not making them any aerobically fitter. [Scientists] investigated the reasons for these variations and discovered that much of the difference could be traced to a small number of genes" (BBC website).

This difference in response to exercise is believed to be a genetic code in just 11 genes. Prof Jamie Timmins' team in Loughborough have a DNA test to predict an individual's response to exercise, though this kind of genetic test is still in its infancy.

MICROLIVES – 30 MINUTES OF YOUR LIFE

David Spiegelhalter, a statistician from the University of Cambridge, developed the concept of microlives. Each microlife – or one millionth of an average adult lifetime – works out to about 30 minutes. *He designed a simple questionnaire on lifestyle, asking the following questions, then assigned a positive or negative balance of microlives against each question:*

- How many cigarettes did you smoke today?
- How many units of alcohol did you drink today?
- How many hours of TV did you watch today?
- How many minutes of exercise did you do today?
- How much red meat did you eat today?
- How many portions of fruit & veg did you eat today?
- How many cups of coffee did you drink today?
- Are you currently taking statins for a medical condition?

(1) Office for National Statistics. Interim Life Tables, 2008-2010.

A microlife is a unit of <u>risk</u> representing a half an hour change of <u>life expectancy.</u> Introduced by <u>David Spiegelhalter</u> and Alejandro Leiva, "microlives are intended as a simple way of communicating the impact of a lifestyle or environmental risk factor, based on the associated daily proportional effect on expected length of life. Similar to the micromort (one in a million probability of death) the microlife is intended for 'rough but fair comparisons between the sizes of chronic risks'. Similarly they bring long-term future risks into the here-and-now as a gain or loss of time" (Revolvy website).

"A daily loss or gain of 30 minutes can be termed a microlife, because 1 000 000 half hours (57 years) roughly corresponds to a lifetime of adult exposure" (D. Spiegelhalter). There are measures made against obesity, alcohol, being sedentary, watching TV, diet, coffee, statins, air pollution, sex, and geography – all of which are available to see on sites such as Wikipedia.

HOW MUCH EXERCISE IS NEEDED TO MAKE A SIGNIFICANT CHANGE IN YOUR HEALTH?

After reading up on losing longevity due to poor habits, let's tackle exercise. Even if you hate spending time doing exercise, a healthy change is still simple to achieve. For instance, you can get on a static exercise bike – these are great because you can put them anywhere in your house – and warm up by doing gentle cycling for a couple of minutes, then going flat out for 20 seconds. Give yourself a couple of minutes to catch your breath, then do another 20 seconds at full throttle. Another couple of minutes gentle cycling, then a final 20 seconds going hell for leather. And that's the job done – grab yourself a cup of tea and read on.

Active exercise is "needed to break down the body's stores of glucose, deposited in your muscles as a substance called glycogen. Smash up these glycogen stores and you create room for more glucose to be sucked out of the blood and stored" (BBC website). "Physical activity is a powerful lifestyle factor that on average reduces the risk for developing Type II diabetes. Further, a lack of fitness has been shown to be a better predictor of illness and premature death than some other factors that many people seem more concerned about, such as high blood pressure" (Metapredict website). Personally, I prefer the idea of doing HIT sprints within an aerobic workout; I think that combining both is a better idea – however, for you busy exercise haters, HIT could be the answer.

The objective of a group of researchers across several countries and universities (the Metapredict project) was to "discover if individualised lifestyle strategies can be developed to fight or prevent metabolic diseases such as obesity, diabetes and cardiovascular problems". By using "molecular profiling of blood/muscle samples" [in response to exercise], personalised lifestyle intervention tools could be developed (Metapredict website). The research is "supported by EU-funding of €6 million and is carried out by an international multidisciplinary research consortium of medical staff, physiologists, and experts in genetics, genomics, and metabolism" (Metapredict website). Several countries have done independent studies, including Martin Gibala in Canada at McMaster University, Niels Vollaard at Bath University, and Ulrik Wisloff in Norway.

"Gretchen Reynolds of the New York Times recently interviewed Metapredict participant Prof. Marty Gibala (McMaster University, Ontario) on the benefits of HIT: *'Instead of asking how much exercise we need, some scientists are looking into how little we can do and still get maximal health and fitness benefits. The answer appears to be a lot less than most of us think — provided we're willing to put in some effort. That's the secret behind high-intensity interval training, or HIIT, an approach to training that compresses all of your exercise into only a few minutes'"* (Metapredict website).

"Metapredict has set out to study how 300 people across the United Kingdom, Sweden, Finland, Spain, Canada and the United States respond to a 10-week supervised exercise-training programme. The study group will train for 15 minutes for three days a week. We will then conduct a number of physiological tests such as monitoring their appetite, body fat, fitness levels and metabolism" (Metapredict website).

"A major aspect of their current project will be High-Intensity Training (HIT), a programme developed during a previous study which took over eight years and involved hundreds of volunteers from the United Kingdom and Canada who cycled on an exercise bike for 20-30 seconds three times a week" (Metapredict website).

"Several years ago, the McMasters scientists did test a punishing workout, that involved 30 seconds of all-out effort at 100 percent of a person's maximum heart rate. After six weeks, these lacerating HIT (HIT can also be called HIIT, for high-intensity interval training) sessions produced similar physiological changes in the leg muscles of young men as multiple, hour-long sessions per week of steady cycling, even though the workouts involved about 90 percent less exercise time. Recognizing, however, that few of us willingly can or will practice such straining all-out effort, the researchers also developed a gentler form of intensive exercise. This modified routine involved one minute of strenuous effort, at about 90 percent of a person's maximum heart rate [subtracting our age from 220], followed by one minute of easy recovery. The effort and recovery are repeated 10 times, for a total of 20 minutes" (Gretchen Reynolds, New York Times website).

For years, the American Heart Association (and other organisations) have recommended that people complete 30 minutes or more of continuous, moderate-intensity exercise – such as a swim or brisk walk – five times a week, for overall good health. However, quick fast exercise requires little time.

The Norwegian study headed up by Meyer et al. in 2013 involved 4846 randomly allocated coronary patients trying out HIT or regular moderate exercise – very brave researchers! They concluded that HIT appeared to be safe and better tolerated by patients than moderate continuous exercise (called MICE).

"Despite the small time commitment of this modified program [of just 20 minutes], after several weeks of practicing it, both the unfit volunteers and cardiac patients showed significant improvements in their health and fitness" (Reynolds, NY Times website). It might seem counterintuitive that strenuous exercise would be productive or even wise for cardiac patients. But so far none have experienced heart problems related to the workouts, Dr. [Maureen] MacDonald [an associate professor of kinesiology at McMaster University] said. 'It appears that the heart is insulated from the intensity' of the intervals, she said, 'because the effort is so brief.' With HIT exercise, 'they showed "significant improvements" in the functioning of their blood vessels and heart,' said MacDonald" (Reynolds, NY Times website).

According to a preliminary study featuring a group of unfit but healthy middle-aged adults, with two weeks of modified high-intensity interval training there were positive changes (published in Medicine and Science under sports and exercise). The exercise prompted the creation of far more healthy cellular proteins involved in energy production and oxygen. The training also improved insulin sensitivity and blood sugar regulation, lowering their risk of Type 2 diabetes. Since then, the scientists completed a small, follow-up experiment involving people with full-blown Type 2 diabetes. They found that even a single bout of the 1-minute hard, 1-minute easy HIT training, repeated 10 times, improved blood sugar regulation throughout the following day, particularly after meals" (Reynolds, NY Times website).

On the other hand, for those of you who are fit, in 2008, Burgomaster et al. – part of the Canadian research team – came up with another recipe of four lots of 30 second bike sprints/hill running/swimming, with a three to four minute cool down gentler exercise – for instance, if swimming, cruise two lengths steadily – sandwiched in between. So, about a fifteen-minute workout in total.

COULD WE REALLY GET SUPER FIT AND REV UP OUR ENGINE SUPERFAST?

"Of course, this type of training is not ideal or necessary for everyone, said Martin Gibala, who's overseen the high-intensity studies. 'If you have time' for regular 30-minute or longer endurance exercise training, 'then by all means, keep it up,' he said. 'There's an impressive body of science showing' that such workouts 'are very effective at improving health and fitness.' But if time constraints keep you from lengthier exercise, he continues, consult your doctor for clearance, and then consider rapidly pedaling a stationary bicycle or sprinting uphill for one minute, aiming to raise your heart rate to about 90 percent of your maximum. Pedal or jog easily downhill for a minute and repeat nine times, perhaps twice a week. 'It's very potent exercise,' Dr. Gibala said. 'And then, very quickly, it's done.' Short bouts of very intense exercise improved muscle health and performance comparable to several weeks of traditional endurance training" (Reynolds, NY Times website).

In the *McMaster University Journal of Applied Physiology*, June 2005, Prof Martin Gibala looked at what happened to muscle with HIIT. The research states "repeatedly doing very intense [brief] exercise such as sprinting resulted in unique changes in skeletal muscle and endurance capacity, similar to training that requires hours of exercise each week. Sixteen subjects were used in the test: Eight who performed two weeks of sprinting at intervals, and eight who did no exercise training. The program had in it four and seven 30-second bursts of 'all out' cycling followed by four minutes of recovery time, three times a week for two weeks. Researchers found that endurance capacity in the sprint group increased whereas the control group showed no change. The muscles of the trained group also showed a significant increase in a chemical known as citrate synthase, an enzyme that is indicative of the tissue's power to use oxygen. 'Sprint training may offer an option for individuals who cite lack of time as a major impediment to fitness and conditioning,' said Gibala. 'This type of training is very demanding and requires a high level of motivation, however less frequent, higher intensity exercise can indeed lead to improvements in health and fitness'" (Metapredict website).

"A few years ago, researchers at the National Institute of Health and Nutrition in Japan put rats through a series of swim tests with surprising results". They had designer trunks to help aid water resistance, as well as tiny little goggles – just kidding. "They had one group of rodents paddle in a small pool for six hours, this long workout broken into two sessions of three hours each.

A second group of rats were made to stroke furiously through short, intense bouts of swimming, while carrying ballast to increase their workload. After 20 seconds, the weighted rats were scooped out of the water and allowed to rest for 10 seconds, before being placed back in the pool for another 20 seconds of exertion. The scientists had the rats repeat these brief, strenuous swims 14 times, for a total of about four-and-a-half minutes of swimming. Afterward, the researchers tested each rat's muscle fibers and found that, as expected, the rats that had gone for the six-hour swim showed preliminary molecular changes that would increase endurance. But the second rodent group, which exercised for less than five minutes also showed the same molecular changes" (Reynolds, NY Times website). Interesting news for rat Olympics!

'The potency of interval training is nothing new', I hear you say, and you'd be right; "athletes have been straining through [aggressive] interval sessions once or twice a week along with their regular workout for years. However, could we be as fit in less time exercising differently, like that second group of rats, and could we really "increase endurance with only a few minutes of strenuous exercise, instead of hours? Could it be that most of us are spending more time than we need to trying to get fit?" (Reynolds, NY Times website). This seems to be the latest thinking, although we forget the importance of exercise on our mind and social needs.

"'There was a time when the scientific literature suggested that the only way to achieve endurance was through endurance-type activities,' such as long runs or bike rides or, perhaps, six-hour swims, says Martin Gibala, but ongoing research from Gibala's lab is turning that idea on its head" (Reynolds, NY Times website). Busy lives need a short cut to fitness, or do they?

HOMEWORK:
Think it through like rats on a wheel – should we exercise super-fast?

HOW MUCH SHOULD I DO IF I DRIVE AN OLD BANGER?

I am forever hearing from fearful patients that they hate exercise, saying that their physio's exercises made them worse, not better, so they stopped going.

Communication and honesty is so important in prescribing exercises, and I always ask what exercise my patients do. If it's Tai Chi, I select forms that are great for their problem, if it is Pilates or swimming, the same applies. Its seems silly to take someone away from a form of exercise they will comply with in order to just give them regimented exercises that will soon be forgotten.

Culture, upbringing, and partners will determine the compliance to any exercise, and if you only ever hobble 10 yards, being asked to walk half an hour a day will be disastrous. This means that no thought has been given to your exercise capability/capacity. Always think about how much work you can achieve before the pain comes on, and tell your therapist this. A good exercise prescription takes into account your tolerance, personality, and current capacity. Some people can hardly walk without pain, so they need to take several tiny walks a day, whereas someone else could go on three long walks a week. For those with little capacity, progression takes longer until you get to your specific goals of pain free activities.

WHY IS SNAZZY SO CAREFUL IN THE MORNINGS SINCE SHE FELL?

Eliminating spine flexion – particularly in the morning when the discs are swollen from the osmotic super hydration (water seeping back into disc) that occurs with bed rest – has been proven to be very effective with my patients who have damaged discs. Because of this, Snazzy's early morning run was frowned on by my colleagues. Spine discs only have so many numbers of bends before they become damaged, so save the bends for essential tasks such as tying shoes or feeding cats, rather than using them up in sit-up style abdominal training. Even though I keep fit, my 25 plus years of bending over patients has taken its toll on my poor old discs.

"Evidence of the process of [the damaging mechanism leading to] disc herniation, or prolapse, is repeated lumbar flexion requiring only very modest concomitant compressive loads (Callaghan and McGill, 2001)" (IdeaFit.com). Which, when translated, means your posture when leaning over patients, teaching little kids, or sitting a lot. This trauma accumulates, with little indication to the unsuspecting future patient that it could happen.

If I had a dollar for every time a patient said "I haven't done anything and my back went", I'd be very rich. I say to them that maybe the *lack* of 'doing' caused it. Primitive man walked miles every day, not in a flexed posture.

"With repeated flexion cycles [which means bending] the annulus [circular layers in the disc] breaches layer by layer with progressive delamination (separation of the collagen rings) of the layers (Tampier et al 2007)" (IdeaFit. com). This allows a gradual seeping of the nucleus material between the delaminated layers. "The location of the annulus breaches can be predicted by the direction of the bend" (IdeaFit.com). How we work and our posture at work will predict where our disc will wear and then tear. Specifically, a left posterior-lateral disc bulge will result if the spine is flexed with some additional right lateral bend (Aultman et al, 2004)" (Rehab Medical website). This has come about because of body mechanics, my posture with patients, and my writing set up at home. "Subsequent twisting leads circumferential rents in the annulus that tends to make McKenzie extension approaches for these clients useless, or even exacerbating (Marshall and McGill, 2010)" (Rehab Medical website). Hence I found push backs irritating to my back.

HOW SHOULD I EXERCISE IF MY BACK IS SORE?

If you have a sore back, you'll need to choose some specific exercises honed by experts, and here is the science behind some of the current popular exercises. A common aberrant motor pattern (like a carburettor misfiring) is 'gluteal amnesia' – or 'numb bum' to you – and this happens when we bend or sit too much (McGill, 2007). "True spine stability is achieved with a 'balanced stiffening' from all your postural muscles", including the rectus abdominis and the abdominal wall (your tummy muscles), quadratus lumborum, latissimus dorsi (the powerful muscles in your back), and the extensor back muscles, longissimus, iliocostalis and multifidus (TightenTheCore.com).

Focusing on a single muscle generally does not enhance stability, but instead causes less stability. That's why dry needling has to be in the hands of the experts, as changing the way a muscle contracts will affect all the other muscles around it. "It is impossible to train muscles such as transverse abdominis or multifidus in isolation – people cannot activate just these muscles (McGill, 2009)" (TightenTheCore.com).

It's insane to say to a patient just contract muscle A, please, as the brain does not work this way; you have to exercise them by association, hence adding in a breathing drill. Breathing works the diaphragm – that is linked by the neural networks to your brain – and simultaneously, your abdominals. This is known by all Yoga and Pilates gurus. I personally like the gentle Pilates approach to engage the stomach with hollow exercises. Controversially, research is saying to disc sufferers to avoid abdominal hollowing techniques as they reduce the potential energy of the spinal column, causing it to fail at lower applied loads (McGill, 2009). With irritable discs, bracing the stomach is preferable, though I teach both to patients depending on their pathology.

Interestingly, a clinical trial by Koumantakis et al. in 2005 compared many of the exercises published in *Physical Therapy* (McGill 1998), "with the same exercises combined with specific transverse abdominis isolation (hollowing etc.)". They said our favourite "specific transverse abdominis training [of Pilates, hollowing and zip up] reduced efficacy!" (*Designing Back Exercise*, McGill). Food for thought! "Instead, the abdominal brace (contracting all abdominal muscles) enhances stability". This bracing is done by imagining someone trying to move your arm, and you brace against it. In the same way, if you dig your fingers in between your ribs, you can push your muscles up against your fingers, bracing them. Many bracing and training techniques are described in McGill (2006).

This difference in opinion in back exercises has been raging for many years. NICE 2016 is currently in favour of prescribing exercises, and McGill's approach of bracing is currently back in vogue, so to be current, it's in my last chapter before going to print.

SHOULD I BALANCE ON A BALL?

My practice manager Dean does a mean fit ball/gym ball class, and although again it is quite controversial with spines, personally I like it for rehab as it tackles balance reactions and movement in 3D, though I agree with folks who have delicate backs that some of the extreme core work is risky. The training approach of curling the torso over a gym ball replicates the injury mechanics I have just been discussing, about the disc flaking with repeated bending, and it's a big price to pay for creating the athletic performance that this exercise is all about. For sore backs, change the spine-breaking curl ups to a plank, where the elbows are placed on the ball. This 'stir the pot' is not a cooking tip; it is said to enhance the spring and spare the spine – and is now in vogue for 2016. Exercise is very much in and out of fashion, just like clothes!

Gym ball ('Stir the Pot'): I like this one but it's not easy to do. "The 'stir the pot' exercise is an advanced task that aims to build athletic [toned] abdominals but spares the painful discs of motion at the same time. It is essentially a plank where the elbows are placed on a gym ball". The spine is still and stable and you can "exercise the spine in alignment with no additional load. This is a better way to build that abdominal armour without the risk of developing back pain from repetitive sit ups" (Exerstend website). Begin by performing three sets of 4-8 circle movements. Perform two to three times a week.

THE SCIENCE OF EXERCISE GIVES ME A HEADACHE

Bum – or 'buttocks' as Forrest Gump would say, and in medic's speak, the Gluteal muscle – activation retraining was based primarily on the original work of Professor Janda, a lovely old boy. I had the privilege of meeting up with him in Chichester and looking after him at Dr Tanner's pretty cottage when he taught a fascinating course. Prof Janda worked in Prague where neurological patients were treated alongside back patients in a holistic way. The Prof battled bravely with secondary Polio, and he had a lovely sense of humour – if I fussed, he would say "if I stop breathing, just tap my chest; that always works!" Prof Janda and McGill seemed to agree that a firm butt was needed to protect the spine, but that it cannot be accomplished with traditional squat training (McGill, 2007). They liked the back bridge workout, which I'll mention later on.

Chronic back pain makes us overuse our hamstrings (the muscles at the back of the thigh) when extending the hip. Like the song, 'all about the bass, no treble', this poor motor pattern is 'all about the hams, no buttocks'. "Spine stability requires that the musculature be cocontracted for substantial durations but at relatively low levels of contraction" (*Core Training*, McGill) and energy usage, so as primitive man, we could wander off into the jungle for hours without falling over. Janda and McGill talk about bad backs having endurance, being a motor control challenge – not a strength challenge. Simply pumping away at weight machines to get stronger is not the solution to a bad back.

There is increasing exercise research pointing to the importance of keeping the duration of holding a position under ten seconds, and building endurance with repetitions, rather than increasing the duration of the holds – this avoids fatigue. Near infrared spectroscopy of the muscles show that this is the best way to build up the endurance without the muscles cramping from oxygen starvation and acid build-up, not to mention tearing. The Russian descending pyramid is a system of sets and reps aimed to make bigger initial gains without fatigue. There are three sets, each with holds of eight to ten seconds. If, on your first set, you do six reps, the next set is four reps, and the next set two, reducing by two reps per set. Each should be held for eight to ten seconds, with two second rests in between, then with twenty second rests between sets. With this in mind, I currently do and teach these exercises and variations on them for back troubles, as they're not so provocative to pain.

SNAZZY'S BACK EXERCISE ROUTINE

After lots of research, my back exercises for this book comprise of the following. I do these with swimming and jogging, as well as sitting on a fit ball and going on the exercise bike. I still run several times a week – just not twice a day – and I do my HIT sprints. I just can't shake off the problem with spinal extensions as yet. I am working on it, and it feels just like Napoleon Hill said in his book, *Outwitting The Devil*: "Edison converted failure into a stepping stone to achievement while the others used it as an alibi for not producing results" (Hill, 2014).

Here are the exercises, and you can find descriptions of these everywhere, including on YouTube. The star * denotes the McGill Big Three exercises.

Cat-camel: Every session should begin with a nice, easy cat-camel exercise. The cat-camel is a gentle motion exercise to reduce spinal friction and 'floss' the nerve roots. This motion can be performed daily and 5-10 reps is enough to get rid of stiffness.

Modified Curl-Up*: The modified curl-up follows the cat-camel exercise, and it involves a lot less curl-up than the usual abdominal drill. It is included in Dr Stuart McGill's "big three" stabilisation exercises. This one focuses on the front tummy area, and when performing this exercise, it is important to try to remove any movement and strain from the lower back and neck area. I tell my patients to put their hands under their lower back and imagine lifting their neck enough for someone to remove a pillow. Put one leg out straight with the other one bent, with your foot on the floor. This exercise involves little curl compared to crunches or sit-ups, and remember that research suggests repeated spinal flexion/bending associated with crunches and sit-ups may predispose you to spinal disc damage.

Now, you should try and do this every day, though preferably not first thing. Begin with three sets of 5-10 repetitions, pausing for one second at the top. For the second set do fewer reps, and for the third, fewer again. It is not recommended that you hold the curl position for any more than ten seconds due to muscle fatigue.

Bird-dog*: The bird-dog exercise works the back extensors without overloading them. Start in the cat-camel position – great news for all you animal lovers! – then lift the opposite arm and leg at the same time, which is good for core and balance too. Your arm and leg should not be above 90 degrees, and your limbs should be swept along the floor with stiffened abdominals. Don't point your toes, and clench yours fist to maximise the effect. Hold each position for up to eight seconds, then repeat the sets as fitness allows.

Side Plank/Bridge: The side plank/bridge targets the lateral abdominal muscles (quadratus lumborum and abdominal obliques). This is a superior exercise when looking at muscle activation, low spinal load, and stabilisation, especially when compared to something like the Pilates' diagonal sit-up. Begin by lying on your side with your body straight, and bend your knees to 90 degrees. Rise up on your forearm for support, with your elbow also at 90 degrees – imagine someone pulling up your hips. You can progress by straightening out your legs, with your top leg placed slightly in front. If you are fit, you can roll onto your front and then to the other side. Start with 5-10 repetitions, holding for ten seconds at the top.

Back Bridge: A weak back may cause you to activate your hamstrings more than the bottom (gluteals) for hip extension. The back bridge is designed to increase awareness of glute contraction, reducing the hamstring input and building glute dominance during hip extension, which helps to support the spine. This exercise may also improve the active flexibility of your quads and hip flexors (psoas). Begin with three sets of 5-10 repetitions, pausing for two seconds at the top, and don't forget the 'stir the pot' bridge on the ball as mentioned above.

Dumbbell Asymmetric Carry: An asymmetric carry challenges the lateral abdominal musculature (quadratus lumborum) and oblique abdominal wall. These muscles are so necessary for many everyday tasks, and cannot be exclusively trained by exercises such as the squat. It's a great functional exercise for a worker who regularly has to carry a load. Use a log, full shopping bag, briefcase, or dumbbell – anything that is heavy enough to create tension in your abdominals whilst walking. Begin by performing 3-5 repetitions of lifting this object while walking 30-50 steps, and perform this twice a week.

This chapter could be many volumes in itself, but it is meant to give you a glimpse of the current worldwide research into exercise, and how I determine the exercises that my team teach. If you've been doing some of this chapter's homework, go take a shower and have a well earned rest.

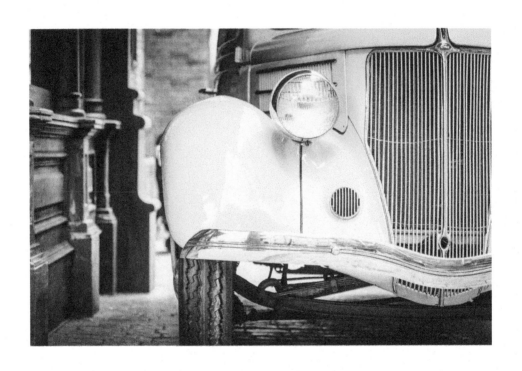

Summary

"It's paradoxical that the idea of living a long life appeals to everyone, but the idea of getting old doesn't appeal to anyone."

– Andy Rooney

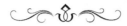

Dying too long

"That which fills the universe
I regard as my body,
And that which directs the universe,
I see as my own nature."
- Chang Tzu

"In order to live, man must believe in that for which he lives."
- Huston Smith

Y
ou have now read whatever parts of the book that have called to you, and ideally, I want you to keep this as a reference book. Dip in and out of it when you need to, looking up ideas to keep you youthful and healthy. Do some research into the different therapies I mention and see if they resonate with you. Hopefully what I've done here is share my clinical experiences with you in a light, amusing way; personally, I find it difficult to absorb information if things are too serious, and reading about health can certainly be boring at times. I've had 'homework' scattered throughout the chapters to enable you to change your life as you read, and in the appendix you can find more detailed clinical knowledge should you wish to read up on a problem either you suffer from, or a member of your family suffers from.

I have talked about how my training was disease-orientated, and that it wasn't until I studied alternative medicine that the penny really dropped – we should really be studying wellness, not illness.

Prevention should be the first step, but with just one percent of the World Health Organization's spending going on this, don't hold your breath! GPs are drug solution orientated: a specific disease is diagnosed, and a coloured pill follows. Why do vets know that nutrition is critical to the health of the animal, when doctors don't even get taught nutrition? Now, it's time to get those seat belts on again: less than 6% of doctors receive *any* education on this subject. I have discovered so many references to placebo-controlled double blind trials showing that high levels of nutrients tackle illness, and yet we don't come across them in our UK training at all.

In this book I have summarised in detail the tiny bits of evidence used to debate nutrition in the UK, as well as touching on the worldwide references that embrace fresh organic food and supplementing. I agree with the concerns of food not being fresh and lacking nutrients – there is a close correlation with healthy, older people, fresh food, and healthy soil, as echoed in my discussions of Japanese islands and studies in remote Russian villages.

I mentioned that oxygen was once a poison to the planet, and in high concentrations, it still is. There is the old oxygen paradox: too much causes oxidative stress and is responsible for not only aging, but about 70 chronic diseases. It's not only our cars that rust up; poor food, lifestyle stress, and pollution all increase the inefficiencies in the way our powerhouses (mitochondria) convert oxygen into energy and water. When hiccups occur, the dark side of oxygen ravages our cells. Like in *Star Wars*, Darth Vader is fuelling up.

Don't you find it strange that your GP reaches for his prescription pad – and your physiotherapist for an exercise prescription plan – without finding out what you are eating and thinking, and how you are moving? Hence my 4 keys drill with my patients. Having the good fortune of being a biologist before becoming a physio, I knew that the mind and lifestyle would affect the number and outcome of my treatments. I also knew that our lifestyles would affect antioxidant behaviour, perceived pain, the immune system, and ultimately, our healing potential. My training was injury/disease management driven, and I'm always arriving after a 'car crash' – when the accident has already happened – needing to know how best to mop up the arthritic knee or how best to help the stroke victim.

I enjoy writing these books, as I believe they will help protect readers from 'crashing' their 'car'. If only we could really time travel to a point in our lives before the arthritic cartilage destruction started, or before the blood vessel became blocked.

I would like to add that I am not anti-drugs – some are so clever and save so many lives and a lot of suffering – but what concerns me is the way they just get dished out to unhealthy bodies. Drugs are alien to our body, and create more free radicals that age us. The liver especially has to step up and work hard to eliminate the drugs we give ourselves. On top of all this, we never know how our bodies are going to react to medicine. Get your seat belts on again: in the USA, the 4th leading cause of death is properly prescribed and administered drugs – that's 100,000 deaths, and two million hospital admissions due to complications every year. This is, in part, due to oxidative stress, or Darth Vader – the dark side of oxygen.

Dr Bruce Operand in the *Journal of American Medical Association*, April 15, 1998, stated: "The medications we prescribe cause over 100,000 deaths a year and 2.1 million have serious complications because of meds. Nutrients carry no such dangers."

Healthy patients over the age of 70 take on average 3.5 pills (and ill people over 10), which is pretty concerning. We know that the brain can create new brain cells even into our eighties, so why aren't we using our heads?

"It is our own responsibility, and not our practitioner's, to keep as healthy as we can, so should we need drugs or surgery, our body may cope."
- N. Snazell

"Medical science is now just showing us that we must have to optimize these natural healing systems that are already present. We must take advantage of humanity's most tremendous asset in healing, 'the host', which is our body" (Strand, 2002).

Our bodies are constantly being attacked by negative thoughts, pollution, viruses, oxidation, and lifestyle stress, and we stay alive by regenerating our cells – every year, all our atoms will become different ones. The stomach lining is replaced every five days, the liver every six weeks, and the skeleton every three months. As we age, we all slowly unravel and unhinge, and all at our own unique rate. Our stamina falters, our eyesight and hearing weakens with our muscles, our bones harden, and our skin wrinkles.

"At a certain age it is our nature to wear out, to come unhinged, and to die, and that is that."
- **Lewis Thomas**

CAN WE THINK ANTI-AGING THOUGHTS?

Yes is the simple answer to that question. You should constantly refocus on your body's wisdom, and ask what is consciously flowing through your body. If you feel pain, ask your body how you can soothe it. Captain your bodily functions, rather than simply handing them over to autopilot. Senility creeps in under the radar for those of us awakened to listening to our bodies, and aging hinders the intelligent flow between the nervous, endocrine (hormone), and immune system. If we left our car to rust in a junkyard, we would not expect to see it self-repair, would we?

"People don't grow old.
When they stop growing,
They become old."
- **Anon**

30% of my patients get pain relief from a sugar pill – if only we could harness that kind of mind to accept an anti-aging pill! By the way, did you know that those of us who meditate will have a body 5 to 12 years younger than those who don't?

"To challenge aging at its core, this entire worldview must be challenged first, for nothing holds more power over the body than beliefs of the mind."
- **Deepak Chopra**

THE AGING GENE

In this book I have also discussed telomeres and the quest for geneticists to find longevity. After Watson and Crick decoded DNA, the hunt for the switches that control immortal genes began – and is still ongoing today.

There are believed to be many more secret genes and switches to do with aging, as well as an infinite intelligence responsible for flipping those switches. Genetic engineering still claims that one day it will give us immortality – though I'm not sure how new babies would fit into this. Michael West at the University of Texas found two of the mortality genes – M1 and M2 – that could be chemically turned off or on. Switching off M1 doubled the life of a cell, whereas switching off M2 meant that the cells divided forever. A switch back on for M1 and aging returned – it's all rather unsettling, isn't it?

What about our perception of time? Our internal 'watch' is a bundle of neurons the size of a fat ant in the brain called the suprachiasmatic nucleus. What if we turned the clock so it ran backwards, like in the film *Benjamin Button*?

I've discussed at length the importance of exercise and this was echoed in my *4 Keys* book. One of my favourite studies (although many years ago now) was carried out by the American government. They looked at the fitness levels of 75,000 people who died in 1986 – a big study. They considered just five daily activities: dressing, walking, eating, bathing, and wait for it... not f***ing, but toileting. Seat belts on again now: when they looked at those aged between 64 and 74, only 20% were fully functional, 10% dismal, and the rest in between!

I'd like to talk about an even older study (but again a good one), so let's go back in my time machine now to Baltimore in 1958, when 800 people volunteered to have their aging monitored. Here I have summarised just some of the findings. The people aged in tremendously different ways, and their physical performances also varied widely. A few improved their lung, heart, and kidney function with age, and mental function persisted in those mentally stretching their minds. As sixty-year-olds, they could carry out light to moderate exercise as well as twenty-year-olds could. Their cholesterol did not rise after 55. Glucose tolerance became sadly less with age, however, not everyone succumbed to diabetes. Being mildly fat with middle age did not change longevity. Alcohol was metabolised the same, but the effects of drunkenness were so much worse. Their muscles diminished. Sex could be three times a week or a year at any old age, and one partner convinced the other that they should keep doing it – for health reasons!

What excites me most from this old study is the uniqueness to aging. It was not simply a foregone conclusion of decay and boredom, a lack of exercise or sexual vigour, loneliness and pain – in fact, for some, quite the opposite was true.

Now, if you're feeling old, listen up! I talked about the greatest pieces of work being achieved in old age. St. Peter's Dome was designed when he was in his 90's. Picasso, Shaw, Tolstoy, Verdi, and Alex von Humboldt all continued with their vast work into their 80's. Psychologists taught me that creativity is strongest as we age, especially from the age of 60 onwards. Enjoyable, focused, intelligent, creative thinking is anti-aging.

HOMEWORK:
Make something creative from your existence. Go on – it's anti-aging.

Plan for old age with vigour. One of my patients told me last week that she had nothing to live for; she wouldn't eat, walk in her garden, or work in her greenhouse – she simply dwelled in pain. She just wanted to moan and moan and moan. I said that we might as well spend our time constructively, and as she'd clearly made her mind up that her life was over, I suggested we plan her funeral together, starting with the music. That approach seemed to work – she rang up my secretary saying I had frightened her into eating and living!

Going back 50 years in time – when far fewer women had careers, and life was less manic in general – the American public health department gave

7,000 people a simple questionnaire on lifestyle. It was 1965 and the research was headed up by Nadia Belloc and Lester Breslow. Breslow talked the talk and walked the walk, and was committed to pioneering chronic disease prevention and health behaviour intervention.

Breslow's "work in the Human Population Laboratory (Alameda County Study) quantified health risk practice and lifestyle issues such as exercise, diet, sleep, smoking, and alcohol consumption and defined their relationship to mortality. In the report on *Health Needs of the Nation* for Truman in 1952, [Breslow] said, 'we delineated the issue quite clearly. People make choices. You and I can decide each day on positive health behavior or negative [health behavior], though most [behaviors] become ingrained in us as habits. Such decisions are not made nor habits developed in a vacuum, but in a social context in which we live. If people live with smokers, smoking is more likely; if people live with exercisers, they tend to exercise. Social factors, advertising, availability, are all determinants of each individual's choices. As public health workers, we should make it clear that people do have choices, but they exercise them mainly under social influences'" (Stallworth, 'An Interview With Dr. Lester Breslow', 2003).

Breslow was a person who practiced what he preached, and he has learned from his own research, something that is exemplified by his personal interests and hobbies. In the same interview for the *American Journal of Public Health* in 2003, Breslow said, "You should know I am in my 86th year. I walk 2 and a half miles for 45 minutes 5 days a week." Three years later, at age 89, he reported he was still walking 5 times a week. So what else did he do? "I garden, raising vegetables and fruit. You should have seen the figs this morning. Also in season we have oranges, lemons, plums, peppers, tomatoes, beets, etc. I read mainly professional magazines such as the *American Journal of Public Health*, and other medical and public health journals" (Breslow in Stallworth, 2003).

The questions in his questionnaire were simply these, and your homework is to answer them:
- Do you sleep 7 to 8 hours a night?
- Do you eat breakfast every day?

- No eating between meals?
- Normal weight -5% to +12%?
- Do you indulge in regular exercise, active sport, long walks, or gardening?
- Do you have no more than 2 alcoholic drinks a night?
- Not smoking?

It was a simplistic questionnaire not covering specific diets or psychological stress, however, the results that caught my eye were that middle-aged men (45 years of age) could extend their lives by 20 to 33 years by doing 3 to 6 of these habits, whereas females, on the other hand, could only add 7 years to their lives, and only if they did at least 6 of the 7 habits. At over 64 years of age, if either sexes had a strict diet and supplementation of vitamins (this info was gathered in their data), they didn't get any further benefit in years of healthy longevity by changing their habits. They were already living healthy lives. So, in conclusion, if you were a middle-aged man and you persisted in healthy living, you could add 30 healthy years onto your life. If you took excellent vitamins, that would be the best medicine of all.

I have talked at length in this book about healthy eating, and I would just like to emphasise that at the turn of the century, man would eat only a couple of pounds of sugar in a year – now we do that in a week. Primitive man would consume 6 pounds of veggies, fruit, and nuts a day, to match the calories of just 2 pounds of our type of food.

DO YOU HAVE AN ANTI-AGING PERSONALITY?

Within this book I have discussed how exercise is essentially good for you, and the type and amount you should do. Now, let's go back in time again, as this piece of research caught my eye. In 1973, Jewett looked at lots of personality traits in 79 people aged between 87 to 100 years old, to see if he could link health to certain common traits. In summary, here are the traits.

Well, they were happy, with a constant weight (no yoyo dieting). Good grip strength when you shook hands, reasonable muscle tone and skin, physically active, and they drove a car. Good memory, a keen interest in current events, very intelligent, few worries, independent in vocation, their own boss, mostly their professions were medical, architects, farming, nursery, or law. They enjoyed a good life and a good sense of humour. They had suffered losses in both their business and personal lives and bounced back. They saw life as an adventure, saw the beauty in things, and liked living in the present. Satisfied, only religious in the broadest sense – not extreme. Diets were healthy, low in fat and high in protein, and they enjoyed a variety of foods. They rested in bed for 8 hours, slept for 6 to 7 everyday, and were early risers. Alcohol consumption varied and smoking varied. They used medics less in their lifetime than the average old person uses in a week, and most drank coffee.

ARE YOU EXERCISING ENOUGH AS YOU GET OLDER?

Here is a summary from a research institution in America, specialising in exercise in older people. "Essential to staying strong and vital during older adulthood is participation in regular strengthening exercises, which help to prevent osteoporosis and frailty by stimulating the growth of muscle and bone. Feeling physically strong also promotes mental and emotional health. Strength training exercises are easy to learn, and have been proven safe and effective through years of thorough research" (Seguin et al., 2002).

Experts at the Centres for Disease Control and Prevention at Tufts University NEPS (Nutrition, Exercise, Physiology, and Sarcopenia) Research Lab conduct studies aimed at the understanding of nutritional and physical activity that possess anabolic (growth and repair) properties in skeletal muscle and have the potential to prevent or reverse impaired motor performance and/or physical dysfunction in older adults. They recommend exercising more as we age, not less, as our muscle needs more effort to strengthen, so therefore our metabolism improves AND OUR HEALTH. In the west, a rough figure given to me recently was that 40% of us are sedentary, and – seat belts on please – only 20% could be considered 'active'.

HOMEWORK: Get that butt out of the chair!

PREVENTION – WHERE IS IT IN THIS SO-CALLED INTELLIGENT RACE?

In the study 'US adults get failing grade in healthy lifestyle behaviour', Paul D. Loprinzi et al. "from Oregon State University and the University of Mississippi examined how many adults succeed in four general barometers that could help define healthy behavior: a good diet, moderate exercise, a recommended body fat percentage and being a non-smoker. It's the basic health advice, in other words, that doctors often give to millions of patients all over the world. The results are based on a large study group, 4,745 people from the National Health and Nutrition Examination Survey. It also included several measured behaviors, rather than just relying on self-reported information" (Loprinzi et al., 2016).

Seat belts on now, folks: only 2.7 percent of the US adult population achieved all four of the basic behavioural characteristics that researchers say would constitute a 'healthy lifestyle' and help protect against cardiovascular disease.

BEING FAT IS CAUSING A DIABETIC EPIDEMIC

I've talked about lifestyle having a huge impact on health and aging. Being a fatty and eating rubbishly is a poor health choice.

The "majority of new cases of diabetes in older U.S. adults could be prevented by following modestly healthier lifestyles" (Harvard School of Public Health, 2009).

Really?! Do we really need research to tell us this? Researchers headed up by Dariush Mozaffarian et al. have found "that a combination of five [bad] lifestyle factors could account for nine in 10 new cases of type 2 diabetes in men and women aged 65 and older. The lifestyle factors examined included physical activity, diet, smoking habits, alcohol use, and amount of body fat (as determined by body mass index and waist circumference)" (Roache, Harvard Gazette, 2009).

"The findings highlight that diabetes really is a lifestyle disease and is largely preventable, said lead author Dariush Mozaffarian" (Roache, Harvard Gazette, 2009).

DO WE NEED TO LIVE A HEALTHY LIFE WHEN WE ARE YOUNGER?

"Lifestyle choices made in your 20s can impact your heart health in your 40s," (Liu et al., 2012). Maintaining a healthy lifestyle from young adulthood (your 20's) into your 40's is strongly associated with a low risk of cardiovascular disease in middle age, according to a new study. So, it is important to start healthy habits when you're young and fit, because they stick.

DOES YOUR BODY SHAPE DEPEND ON YOUR PARTNER'S?

"Couples' lifestyle choices impact on obesity risk," states a study by Charley Xia et al. (2016). "The lifestyle a person shares with their partner has a greater influence on their chances of becoming obese than their upbringing, research suggests." So ladies, be careful if your man is getting fat.

WHAT ABOUT KIDS' HEALTH AND LIFESTYLE?

"A UCLA School of Nursing study [in 2013] has found that both healthy-weight and obese children who participated in an intensive lifestyle modification program significantly improved their metabolic and cardiovascular health even with little weight loss" (Laura Perry, UCLA Newsroom).

ROBOT MOTHER BUILDS CUBE BABIES THEN WATCHES THEM TAKE FIRST STEPS

In an article in *The Telegraph* (12th August 2015), it was reported that Cambridge University developed a mother bot that elects which baby bot performs the best at taking its first steps, then refines their design. This mimics biological evolution. The mother can evaluate the quality of movement and its survival based on this. For 10 generations, the fittest baby bot informed the design of the next child, with the ability to carry out the task improving through the generations.

Could it be that robots are where human evolution is heading?

ARE WE SPIRITUAL MACHINES?

So many of our thoughts are directed towards our body and its survival, image, mood, sexuality, nutrition, and exercise. If a robot did not have a biological body, how would it mimic human intelligence? As crazy as it sounds, human bodies of the future may be built by robots – they could be complex physical entities built atom by atom via genetic engineering, creating virtual bodies or bodies that are part-biological, part-robot, with many, many nanobots within. It is happening as we speak: nanorobots are mapping out the human brain. We could have enhanced our biological brains with an intimate connection to nonbiological intelligence, with the human body being enhanced through biotechnology (gene enhancement and replacement) and nanotechnology.

One of my northern patients works out in America in a think tank with scientists who are intimately involved in this, including a world leader in this work, Ray Kurzweil. In one of Kurzweil's books, *Are We Spiritual Machines?*, he concludes, "further evolution of our species will be inextricably bound to our ability to enhance our bodies and minds with integrated computer prosthetics" (Kurzweil, 2002).

"As we combine the brain's pattern recognition methods derived from high-resolution brain scans and reverse engineering efforts with the knowledge sharing, speed, and memory accuracy advantages of nonbiological intelligence, the combination will be formidable" (Kurzweil, 2002).

HOMEWORK:
If you now had new robotic circuits in your head – with knowledge about how to nourish and protect your body – you would be programmed to take better care of yourself. How do you feel about this?

If your dying loved one could have their personality downloaded into a computer before they died, so that their intelligence and brain function continued after their biological body had rotted, would you want that?

THE FUTURE OF PHYSIOTHERAPY

I am hopeful that my books, teaching, and radio slots will help to reignite enthusiasm in holistic treatment. My 10,000-strong list of patients experiencing holistic physio is proof to me that it works, and that it prevents unnecessary ill health. As I write this paragraph, on the news the Prime Minister was discussing the new NHS GP rescue package, and the coming together of GPs, physios, and mental health experts to first line specialists, rather than having a patient seeing a doctor with just one day's training under his belt on spinal treatments.

I found a mention in my professional journal that in Suffolk GP practices, this approach is being trialed, and that it resulted in 30% fewer patients on the waiting list for the GP with musculoskeletal problems, and a 40% reduction in hip and knee replacements even before hands-on treatment and specialist technology like MRT was considered.

As I am editing this book, I had a delightful surprise of receiving the 2016 Excellence in Service award from my professional body of physiotherapists that practice Acupuncture. This, in part, was for recognition of my books, articles, teaching, radio, and of course, my clinics. It is wonderful to know that my peers are behind me in promoting a 'wholistic' physiotherapy future.

SUMMARY PARAGRAPH OF ANTI-AGING TIPS

"One of the most important decisions and experiences I have ever made was to change how I treated my body" (Joseph McClendon, 2008).

New brand names appear all the time, not to mention new treatments, new footwear, new sports surfaces, new gels, and new insoles. My aim with this book is to share my experiences in order to give you some insight into where to seek help, and when to embrace your body's wisdom for preventative measures, helping you to protect yourself against ill health. Basically, I wanted it to be a guidebook based on a quarter of a century of studying and honing physical treatments. It is so important that practitioners know that what suits one patient does not suit the next; I find that the dosage of treatment varies so much from one patient to the next. It can either heal them or send their immune system and pain spiralling out of control – it is just dependent on so many factors, hence my reason for writing the *4 Keys* for my patients. Every human is unique, and every human responds to their very own specific catalyst to initiate a self-healing response.

We know that time does not affect the body uniformly; every cell has its own timeline, and age mirrors your unique self. Age is a three-tiered graph: chronological (your age on the planet), biological (your metabolic, dependent on lifestyle), and your psychological (your perceived age).

"We live inside this unbelievable cosmos, inside our unbelievable bodies – everything so perfect, everything so in tune. I got to think God had a hand in it."
- Ray Charles

Here are some hot tips for anti-aging.

HOMEWORK:
Please read them!

Anti-aging means being present in the moment. Like a young child focused on playing with a toy, they are not thinking about the fact it was better yesterday or that it might be worse tomorrow.

Listen to your body's wisdom. Is it whispering 'no', or 'yes, amazing, go for it! This is so good'? Exercise every day to your own body's tune, although the latter can get you into another kind of trouble!

Listen to your inner guidance, your true north, your intuition. This strengthens as we age. Listen less to marketing whims and other's opinions about how you should lead your life. Instead, internalise your own approval and pleasure at things you create, and measure their worth in your own eyes.

Be mindful that fear, anger, and past hurts will trigger unhelpful emotions. Watch like an observer within and intelligently temper these feelings.

Be wise when making choices about what you like and don't like in your life, and make them mostly healthy choices: landscapes you love, food that is fresh, friends who make you laugh…

Be gentle when judging situations in the media or in relationships with which you have little knowledge. Toxic opinions pollute your cells.

Grow your inner voice like plants in your greenhouse – with patience and care. Toxic thoughts will diminish your creative genius that flows through your body. Truth and love – and leading a purposeful, healthy life – are the greatest gifts you can give your body. Take your own medicine every day.

Purposely create a life that is well wishing, intelligent, purposeful, loving, caring, self-accepting, and non-judgmental, and your body will thank you for it in the later years. Speaking of which, the later years are there to complete the cycle, knitting together the mind, body, and soul to achieve a purposeful, happier, healthier old age. I will talk of the soul's journey in my final volume of the Human Garage.

It is my sincerest wish for you that you live your life as actively and as healthily as you can, for as long as you can. As you lead this healthier life, I also ask you to pass this knowledge on to help others do the same. I want you – regardless of who you were when you started this book – to enjoy a new you, one that is healthier, happier, more toned, more active, and younger looking. I also want to let you know that whatever was wrong with you when you started reading chapter one – too tired, too fat, too unhealthy, too unfit – that it *is* possible to step up. Listen to your body's wisdom; it knows what it needs you to do in order to stay fit. You need to put into place tangible, measurable changes, a lifestyle that has a healthy home-cooking kitchen, a pretty garden with home-grown veggies, and a regular fitness regime.

I am providing you with the resources and the tools to achieve a better life for you and your loved ones; all you have to do is live the dream.

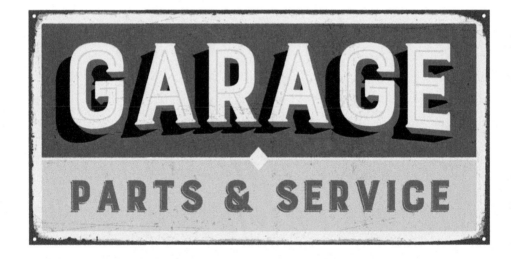

Appendix 1

"It is lovely to meet an old person whose face is deeply lined, a face that has been deeply inhabited, to look in the eyes and find light there."

– *John O'Donohue*

PHYSIOTHERAPY SYMPTOM SORTER

I have rewritten this symptom sorter from an earlier version I wrote for my website: www.painreliefclinic.co.uk.

This information is provided for guidance only and cannot be used as a diagnosis of your condition. It is designed to help you get some clarity about your problem, so you can discuss it further with an expert and obtain an accurate diagnosis.

I will be going through the body starting with the neck, then the shoulder, elbow and hands, thoracic and lumbar spine, pelvis and sacroiliac, hip, knee, and ankle, and finally, the feet.

NECK PROBLEMS

If you answer yes to any of the following you need to see your doctor or physio:

- ☐ Are your hands clumsy?
- ☐ Do you find walking increasingly difficult, or do your legs feel clumsy and stiff?
- ☐ Do you find it difficult to empty your bladder?
- ☐ Do you find you tend to drop things or have difficulty holding things?
- ☐ Does the ground not feel solid when you are walking?

If so, you may be diagnosed with cervical myelopathy.

CERVICAL MYELOPATHY

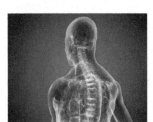

Inflamed neck

Cervical myelopathy occurs when there is pressure on or damage to the spinal cord itself. Cervical spondylosis is a common cause of this condition, as the wear and tear to the vertebra can narrow the canal through which the spinal cord runs.

A prolapse of a cervical disc can also cause myelopathy if the disc prolapse is into the central canal of the vertebra. Although it is very rare for either a tumour or infection to be the cause, a medical opinion and MRI is very important to have. As the nerve fibres run from the brain to the extremities, there can be many symptoms of cervical myelopathy, including:

- ☐ Difficulty with walking, legs feeling clumsy and stiff.
- ☐ Clumsy hands, dropping objects.
- ☐ Difficulty with easily emptying your bladder.

Diagnosis for this is by MRI and neuro consultant, and for treatment options, see a neurologist for advice.

CERVICAL RADICULOPATHY

Do you have pain and numbness in your arms and/or hands?

If symptoms of pain, pins and needles, numbness, and weakness can be felt anywhere from your shoulder to your fingers, you may be told you have cervical radiculopathy (nerve pain down the arm). This provisional diagnosis can be given by a spinal specialist physiotherapist or your chosen physical therapist such as a chiropractor or osteopath.

Radiculopathy is the irritation of the nerve roots at the spinal cord, sufficient enough to cause pain, pins and needles, or weakness across the shoulder and down the arm to the fingers. Radiculopathy can be caused by wear and tear, disc herniation, muscle spasm, or osteophyte growth.

It usually gradually resolves over a few weeks, and the treatment that I would give would be spinal specialist physiotherapy, including modalities such as Acupuncture, Gunn IMS dry needling, laser, soft tissue work, gentle facet joint mobilisations, postural advice, and gentle exercise to progressively strengthen the muscles. The GP can also offer meds to help you through the worst of the pain.

If your symptoms don't improve, your therapist will refer you back to your GP. In more severe cases, where your hands feel clumsy, you have problems with walking, or problems with bladder function start occurring, this may be due to pressure from a worn vertebrae or disc damaging the spinal cord, which is cervical myelopathy. A spinal surgeon will check this out with the aid of MRI scans.

Book to see your GP urgently if:
- The pain gets much worse.
- There is a worsening (numbness), weakness, or you have persistent pins and needles in part of an arm or hand.
- You develop any problems with walking or with passing urine. These symptoms suggest that cervical myelopathy may be developing as a complication of the cervical radiculopathy.
- You develop dizziness or blackouts when turning your head or bending your neck. This can suggest that the vertebral artery – which supplies the brain – is being nipped by the degenerative changes in the spine. This gets more common as we age.

Both cervical radiculopathy and myelopathy can develop from spondylosis (disc wear and tear).

CERVICAL SPONDYLOSIS

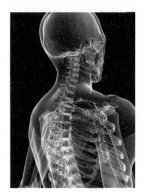

The neck (cervical spine) has seven vertebrae. The top two allow the neck to pivot sideways, and the next five are barrel-shaped, linking to each other at tiny bevelled (facet) joints and cushioned by discs. These discs are tough fibrous structures with a gel-like middle.

Do you have recent stiffness in your neck with mild pain spreading out to your upper back and shoulders?

If so, you may have osteoarthritis and/or cervical spondylosis.

OSTEOARTHRITIS

Osteoarthritis (OA) – the most common type of arthritis – is wear and tear in the smooth cartilage that protects the bones in joints, eventually leading to bone erosion, bone spurs, and unsightly bony end thickening. The joint juice – the synovial fluid – swells and becomes inflamed and sticky, and the attacked bone haemorrhages precious calcium. By the time we are 50 years old, 8 out of 10 of us have OA, and by 60, this goes up to 9 out of 10. Left untreated, OA can have a massive negative impact on quality of life and will eventually need surgery.

Provisional diagnosis is by a physical assessment with a physiotherapist, a GP with specialist interests in arthritis, an osteopath, chiropractor, rheumatologist, or orthopaedic surgeon. Then, you will need confirmation with bloods and X-ray, or MRI.

Personally, my favourite treatment modalities that I use include: physiotherapy-prescribed exercises, electro-acupuncture to give some immediate pain relief with TENS, ultrasound, laser and pulsed shortwave, Gunn IMS assessment for any neuropathic pain overtures, and in less severe cases, shockwave for joint stiffness.

As preventative treatment to help slow the degeneration and further reduce inflammation, we can also use MRT/MBST (magnetic resonance treatment). In order to firefight the pain, we can use GP prescribed medicines, then a long-term nutritional assessment from a nutritional expert with advice on food and supplements.

DO YOU SUFFER FROM HEADACHES?

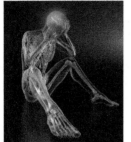

If you have a headache that has lasted more than 48 hours, please contact your GP. Provisional diagnosis will be done by your GP or a headache specialist physiotherapist, with the diagnosis being made by a neurologist and brain MRI.

If you constantly suffer with headaches, you may have one of the following conditions:

CLUSTER HEADACHE

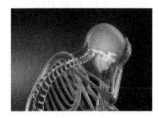

A cluster headache is a less common type of recurrent headache than a migraine, and does not have all the migraine symptoms. The pain in this type of headache is shorter and less severe, and you may also have a watery or bloodshot eye. The symptoms of cluster headaches are characterised by unilateral (one sided) pain, although for some people the side can vary from time to time. The pain is usually centred over one eye, one temple, or the forehead, though it can spread to a larger area, making diagnosis harder. The pain is said to be worse than giving birth.

During a bout of cluster headaches, the pain is often experienced at a similar time each day, often starting at night and waking people up one to two hours after they have gone to sleep. The pain usually reaches its full intensity within 5 to 10 minutes and then continues at this agonising level for between 30 and 60 minutes. For some people, the pain can last for 15 minutes, whereas for others, it has been known to last for up to three hours. It then stops, usually fairly abruptly.

I recently talked with a sufferer, and he explained to me that he was one of the 80% of people with head pain lasting for 4 to 12 weeks a year, often at the same time and often in the spring or autumn. It usually disappeared for several months (and sometimes years) but it would then come back again. This is known as an episodic cluster headache, and the reason for this seasonal timing is not completely known, although it is one of the key aspects of diagnosis and may involve the hypothalamus. The remaining 20% of people do not have these pain free intervals and are said to have 'chronic cluster headaches'.

Provisional diagnosis is often done by your GP or physiotherapist. As physio and painkillers are ineffective, oxygen is one of the safest ways to treat a cluster headache. You need to breathe the oxygen in at a rate of between 7 and 12 litres per minute, and the treatment usually starts to work within 15 to 20 minutes. For some people, the attack is delayed rather than stopping altogether.

MIGRAINE

The most common kind of intense head pain is a migraine, and these can last anywhere from between 4 and 48 hours. It is often felt through a throbbing sensation, and it affects just one side of the head. You can experience vomiting and sensitivity to light and smells, but at its worst your vision is affected with flashing lights and blindness, as well as speech problems and a tingling in the face or fingertips. I remember getting migraines in my 30's when I was running an outpatient department with crazy long waiting lists. I'd had a recent whiplash injury, and my vision used to go suddenly hazy – not fun when you're driving on a motorway.

About one fifth of people with migraines who seek advice believe that cheese, chocolate, and alcohol can trigger the attacks, so food allergy testing can help. My favourite treatment options are Chinese Acupuncture, Gunn IMS dry needling, mobilisations to the neck, nutritionist advice, and for the ladies, a hormone check-up. NLP (neurolinguistics programming) can also help where stress is involved. GP prescribed medicine may be needed too.

TENSION HEADACHE

This is a more common, fairly harmless headache, usually occurring when tired and stressed. It lasts up to six hours and gives pain on both sides of the head, with no other symptoms. Tension headaches are much more common than the cluster headache, thank goodness.

For tension headaches, the provisional diagnosis is done by your GP, and treatment can include: Chinese medicine, hydration, Acupuncture, Gunn IMS, mobilisations to the neck, nutritionist advice, NLP, relaxing massage, Indian head massage, stress counselling, and reiki.

GP prescribed meds should be used only as a last resort. If headaches occur, the cause needs to be found and addressed.

TRIGEMINAL NEURALGIA

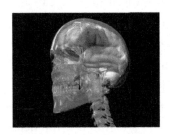

The trigeminal nerve supplies the lower jaw and teeth and can give short, sharp pains like a hot poker when irritated. The *trigeminal nerve* is the fifth cranial nerve and its function is to send pain messages to the brain. When the nerve malfunctions, pain messages are sent at inappropriate times and the pains can be of great severity. It can be triggered by chewing, speaking, or even by the wind.

This condition is more common in older people, probably because the arteries supplying the back of the brain where this nerve enters become stretched and may touch the nerve. It is an extremely severe facial pain that tends to come and go unpredictably in sudden shock-like attacks, and whilst treating the area, even light touch is described as being stabbing, shooting, excruciating, or burning. It usually only lasts for a few seconds, but there can be many bursts of pain in quick succession. It is not easy to treat, and I know; I recently eased – not cured – this condition in a delightful gypsy lady who was losing the battle with this unpleasant condition.

Treatment options that may help the symptoms include: Chinese medicine, electro-acupuncture, TENS, Gunn IMS, NLP, relaxing massage, and GP prescribed medicines. As normal painkillers such as Paracetamol are not effective in treating trigeminal neuralgia, you will normally be prescribed an alternative medication, such as an anticonvulsant (usually used to treat epilepsy) to help control your pain.

These medications were not originally designed to treat pain, but they can help relieve nerve pain by slowing down electrical impulses in the nerves and reducing their ability to transmit pain.

Microvascular decompression (MVD) is an operation that can help relieve trigeminal neuralgia pain without intentionally damaging the trigeminal nerve. Instead, the procedure involves relieving the pressure placed on the nerve by blood vessels that are either touching the nerve or wrapped around it. An alternative way to relieve the pain by damaging the trigeminal nerve that doesn't involve inserting anything through the skin is through stereotactic radiosurgery. This is a fairly new treatment that uses a concentrated beam of radiation to deliberately damage the trigeminal nerve where it enters the brainstem.

WHIPLASH

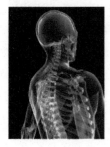

Whiplash is a relatively common injury that occurs to a person's neck following a sudden acceleration-deceleration force, most commonly from motor vehicle accidents. The term 'whiplash injury' describes damage to the vertebrae and soft tissues, while the term 'whiplash associated disorder' describes a more severe and chronic condition.

Fortunately, whiplash is typically not a life-threatening injury, but it can lead to a prolonged period of partial disability. My neck ached for many weeks after a car took out my father's car one dark, wet night in Lincolnshire – I was a sleeping passenger.

While most people involved in minor motor vehicle accidents recover quickly without any chronic symptoms, some continue to experience symptoms for years after the injury. If you fall into this category, Gunn IMS pain clinics may well be the answer.

So what causes whiplash?

Whiplash is most commonly caused by a stationary car being impacted by another from behind, without notice. It is commonly thought that the rear impact causes the head and neck to be forced into hyperextension, and especially the lower part of the neck, as the seat pushes the trunk forward – and therefore the unrestrained head and neck fall backwards. After a short delay, the head and neck then recover and are thrown into a hyper-flexed position.

More recent studies (investigating the condition using high-speed cameras and crash dummies), have shown that after the rear impact, the lower cervical vertebrae forcibly hyperextend, while the upper cervical vertebrae are hyper-flexed. This leads to an abnormal S-shape motion in the cervical spine, and causes damage to the soft tissues between the cervical vertebrae.

My favourite treatment options for acute (recent) whiplash include: physiotherapy, massage, facet joint mobilisations, ultrasound, pulsed shortwave, laser, and gentle Acupuncture. If non-resolving or chronic (long-term), try Gunn IMS, postural and exercise advice, stronger massage, and a counselling healing approach.

TORTICOLLIS (WRY NECK)

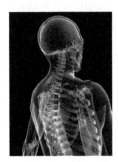

With this, the top of the head generally tilts to one side while the chin tilts to the other side.

Torticollis may be:
- Inherited: Due to specific changes in your genes.
- Acquired: It develops as a result of damage to the nervous system or muscles.

If there is no known cause, it is called idiopathic torticollis. Torticollis may develop in childhood or adulthood.

Provisional diagnosis is done by a physiotherapy assessment.

TEMPORARY TORTICOLLIS

This type of wry neck usually disappears after one or two days, and it can be due to:
- Swollen lymph nodes.
- An ear infection.
- A cold.
- An injury to your head and neck that causes swelling.

Congenital torticollis (present at birth) may occur if the foetal blood supply or muscle development was injured or if the foetus' head is in the wrong position while growing in the womb.

FIXED TORTICOLLIS

Fixed torticollis is also called acute torticollis or permanent torticollis, and it usually occurs due to a problem with the muscular or bony structure.

MUSCULAR TORTICOLLIS

This is the most common type of fixed torticollis, and it results from scarring or tight muscles on one side of the neck.

KLIPPEL-FEIL SYNDROME

This is a rare, congenital form of wry neck, and it occurs when the bones in your baby's neck form incorrectly, notably due to two neck vertebrae being fused together. Children born with this condition may have difficulty with hearing and vision.

CERVICAL DYSTONIA

This rare disorder is sometimes referred to as spasmodic torticollis, as it causes the neck muscles to contract in spasms. If you have cervical dystonia, your head twists or turns painfully to one side, and it may also tilt forward or backward. Cervical dystonia sometimes goes away even without treatment. However, there is a risk of recurrence.

My favourite treatment options for mild cases of wry neck include: physiotherapy, gentle manual traction, mobilisations, Acupuncture, massage, and warmth. If severe, however, it may need a neurologist referral for injections, strong meds, or even surgery. A very useful test is an electromyogram (EMG), which measures electrical activity in your muscles. It can also determine which muscles are affected.

Imaging tests such as X-rays and MRI scans can also be used to find structural problems that might be causing your symptoms.

Your doctor may recommend surgery, such as:
- Fusing abnormal vertebrae.
- Lengthening neck muscles.
- Cutting nerves or muscles.
- Deep brain stimulation to interrupt nerve signals, which is used only in the most severe cases of cervical dystonia

Medications can also be helpful, and they can include:
- Muscle relaxants.
- Medications used to treat the tremors of Parkinson's disease.
- Botulinum toxin injections, repeated every few months.
- Pain medications.

OSTEOARTHRITIS AND FACET JOINT LOCK

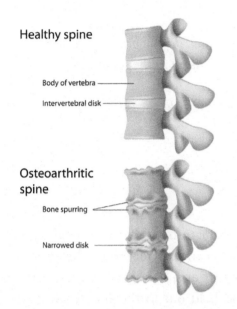

Healthy spine

Body of vertebra

Intervertebral disk

Osteoarthritic spine

Bone spurring

Narrowed disk

Facet joints in the neck (cervical) and lower back (lumbar) can become locked due to muscles going into spasm or a fold occurring in the joint meniscus. This can be caused by a movement or injury that has either happened recently or some time before, and movement will be restricted depending on the position the joint was locked in. To gain a range of motion, other joints near the lock will tend to be excessively moved and so pain will ensue near the lock or sometimes on the opposite side. If a facet joint in the neck is locked, it can cause symptoms in the neck and into the arms, and a lumbar facet joint lock can cause sciatica symptoms. A lack of core stability muscle control is a prime cause of lumbar facet joint lock.

Provisional diagnosis is by physiotherapy assessment, and treatment options to reduce the pain, inflammation, stiffness, and weakness include: physiotherapy, chiropractic or osteopathic mobilisations, manipulation, core stability, specific spinal rehabilitation exercises, posture advice, laser, Acupuncture, Gunn IMS dry needling, shockwave, pulsed shortwave, massage, nutrition, and counselling. MRT can be used as a preventative treatment to slow the deterioration.

SHOULDER PROBLEMS

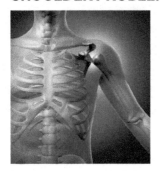

After an acute trauma, do you have severe pain with a 'popping-out' sensation in the shoulder?

If so, you may have a dislocated shoulder.

DISLOCATED SHOULDER

Shoulder dislocation is a very common traumatic injury that can occur across a wide range of sports. In 95% of cases it is an anterior (front) dislocation, where the head of the humerus (the upper arm bone) is forced forwards when the arm is turned outwards, and held out to the side (abducted). Posterior dislocation only accounts for 3% of cases.

With a bankart lesion, the shoulder joint is particularly prone to dislocations due to its high mobility, and lack of stability. Dislocation can cause a labral tear – the labrum is a cup-shaped ring of cartilage, deepening the glenoid fossa into which the arm bone sits. There can be a lot of damage to soft tissue after dislocation.

Provisional diagnosis is by your physio, GP, and X-ray, and follow up treatment should include a time for immediate rest with a sling, then progressive physiotherapy mobilisations. Also, try soft tissue treatment for bruising with electrotherapy modalities and massage.

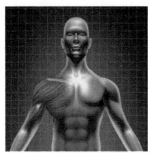

PECTORALIS MAJOR INFLAMMATION

The pectoralis major muscle is a large, powerful muscle at the front of the chest. We need this muscle to rotate the arm inwards, to pull a horizontal arm across the body, to pull the arm from above the head down, and to pull the arm from the side upwards. The weakest spot is where it inserts into the humerus. In weight training, the bench press is the most common reason for injury.

Provisional diagnosis is by a physiotherapy assessment, and treatment can include: initially, ice, and relative rest of the muscle. See a sports therapist or physiotherapist for massage, ultrasound, laser, and a rehab prescribed programme.

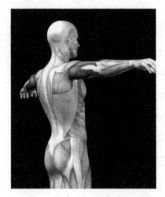

Do you have pain at the front of your shoulder? Does it hurt to lift a straight arm out in front of you?

If so, you may have one of the following conditions:

BICEPS LONG HEAD TENDINITIS

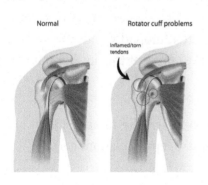

The biceps muscle splits into two tendons at the shoulder. The long tendon runs over the top of the humerus (arm bone), and the head attaches to the top of the shoulder blade. A rupture of this tendon is rare in young athletes, but common in older ones. Inflammation of this tendon is a fairly common complaint, especially with swimmers, rowers, throwers, golfers, and weight lifters.

Provisional diagnosis is by physiotherapy assessment and ultrasound scan, and if tendonitis is confirmed, the treatment of choice can include: initially, relative rest, massage, sports therapy, stretching and strengthening exercises, and a full rehabilitation programme. Electrotherapy – such as pulsed shortwave or MRT – can help reduce inflammation faster.

If the patient is older or a partial tear is also seen on the scan, an orthopaedic opinion may well be needed. If the tendon goes on to tear, the surgeon will need to be consulted in case a repair operation is needed. Furthermore, if pins and needles (or numbness and weakness) are present, a full assessment of the cervical and peripheral nerves is needed.

ROTATOR CUFF INJURY

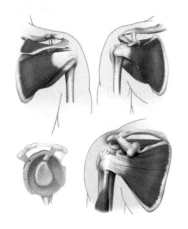

Rotator cuff tendinitis describes the inflammatory response of one or more of the four rotator cuff tendons, due to impingement or overuse, and leading to more and more micro-trauma that can then lead to a tendon rupture.

The inflamed thickening of the tendons often causes the rotator cuff tendons to become trapped under the acromion – like a carpet stuck under a door – causing sub-acromial impingement. Failure to heal then leads to further damage, resulting in a tendinopathy. Early treatment of tendinitis, therefore, is necessary in order to prevent the development of more chronic and serious conditions.

Treatment can include: postural exercises to lessen the impingement and local electrotherapy, such as laser, ultrasound, deep oscillation, or MRT.

Do you have pain when lifting your arm sideways? Does it get worse against resistance?

If so, you may suffer from the following:

SUPRASPINATUS TENDINITIS

Contraction of the supraspinatus (SS) muscle leads to abduction (lifting up sideways) of the arm at the shoulder joint. It works so hard during the first 15 degrees of its arc, and beyond 15 degrees the deltoid muscle supports the abducting of the arm, helping out strongly. When you get inflammation of this tendon, it leads to supraspinatus tendinitis. You will get shoulder pain with movement from the inflammation, and pain at night, as well as weakness in the shoulder and arm. There is also the possibility of tenderness and swelling in the upper front part of the shoulder, and in some severe cases, a difficulty to raise the arm to shoulder level – a painful arc from 60 to 120 degrees.

I learnt some useful diagnostic shoulder tests from two hunky shoulder surgeons, Roger Hackney and Vinod Kathuria, and the tests have rather strange names: Neer's impingement, Hawkins-Kennedy, and the Empty Can Test, the latter of which indicates a problem with SS.

TREATMENTS FOR ROTATOR CUFF TENDINITIS

NSAIDs (non-steroidal anti-inflammatory drugs) are often prescribed for the management of acute inflammation, providing you have a strong stomach. Ice packs, gels, and creams – either NSAID or herbal – can help reduce pain and inflammation and should be applied to the painful area for 15 minutes at a time, at regular intervals throughout the day. Electrotherapy – as in ultrasound, pulsed shortwave, deep oscillation, and laser – all help, as do gentle shoulder mobilisations, massage, and postural exercises. Sport specific rehab exercises guide you back to full fitness.

The provisional diagnosis is by physiotherapy assessment, and a diagnosis of the degree of damage is carried out via an ultrasound scan.

THE INTERPLAY OF SHOULDER MUSCLES

The supraspinatus is just one of four rotator cuff muscles, its partners in crime being infraspinatus, subscapularis, and teres minor. The infraspinatus is a thick triangular muscle, which occupies the chief part of the infraspinatous fossa (a sculptured dent in the back of the shoulder blade). As one of the four muscles of the rotator cuff, the main function of the infraspinatus is to externally rotate the humerus (back hand in tennis) and stabilise the shoulder joint.

The subscapularis is a large triangular muscle that fills the subscapular fossa (the front of the shoulder blade) and inserts into the lesser tubercle (bony knob) of the humerus, as well as the front of the capsule of the shoulder joint. The orthopaedic assessment will include specific tests to move the shoulder into specific positions in order to detect pain, indicating a tear. The name of these tests are the Gerber lift off, the bear hug, and the belly press! There is no singular imaging device or technique available for a satisfying and complete subscapularis examination, but the combination of MRI and ultrasound scans work well, ultimately seeing it in surgery.

The rotator cuff muscles are a group of muscles that work together to provide the glenohumeral (shoulder) joint with dynamic stability, helping to control the joint during rotation. The scapula (shoulder blade) plays an important role in shoulder impingement syndrome. It is a wide, flat bone lying on the posterior thoracic wall that provides an attachment for three different groups of muscles – and it looks like the *Star Trek Enterprise*.

The subscapularis, infraspinatus, teres minor, and supraspinatus intrinsic muscles attach to the surface of the scapula and rotate the glenohumeral joint, along with humeral abduction (sideways). The extrinsic muscles include the biceps, triceps, and deltoid muscles, and these attach to the nobbly bits of bone called the coracoid process, the supraglenoid tubercle of the scapula, the infraglenoid tubercle of the scapula, and the spine of the scapula. It's as if these muscles all have their own coat hook, like in kid's changing rooms, and these muscles are responsible for several actions of the shoulder joint.

THE SPORTY SHOULDER

The third group of muscles with funny names are mainly responsible for both the stabilisation and rotation of the shoulder blade. They are the trapezius, serratus anterior, levator scapulae, and rhomboid muscles, and they attach to the medial, superior (upper), and inferior (under) borders of the scapula. Each of these muscles has their own role in shoulder function, and must be in balance with each other in order to avoid shoulder problems, like the tension on kite strings. Abnormal scapular (shoulder blade) function is called scapular dyskinesis.

The arm bone must be slid down and turned to avoid jamming up; the shoulder blade, during a throwing or serving, has to elevate the acromion process (the spoon-shaped bit overhanging the humerus head). If the scapula fails to properly lift the acromion, impingement may occur during the cocking and acceleration phase of an overhead activity. I see this a lot with my patients and describe it like the rubber stopper wedged under my door, stopping it from closing.

The two muscles most commonly inhibited/being lazy during this first part of an overhead motion are the serratus anterior and the lower trapezius. These two muscles act as a force couple within the glenohumeral (shoulder) joint to properly elevate the acromion process. If a muscle imbalance exists, shoulder impingement may occur, and this can usually be diagnosed by history and physical exam. During a physical exam, I twist or elevate the patient's arm to test for reproducible pain (using the Neer sign and Hawkins-Kennedy test). These tests help localise the problem to the rotator cuff, however, the Neer sign may also be seen with subacromial bursitis, which is when the bursal sac gets inflamed and swollen, like a wet, thickened carpet jamming in the door.

You can inject lidocaine and a corticosteroid into the bursa – I used to in hospital and I still do in my current clinic – and while it can be a quick fix, it is a very unpleasant injection to receive. If there is an immediate improved range of motion and a decrease in pain, this is considered a positive 'impingement test'. It not only supports the diagnosis for impingement syndrome, but it is also therapeutic, and other treatments include electrotherapy, postural exercise, and dry needling.

Plain X-rays of the shoulder can be used to detect joint problems, including acromioclavicular arthritis, osteoarthritis, and calcification. However, ultrasonography, arthrography, and MRI must be used in order to detect any rotator cuff muscle pathology/problems. MRI is the best imaging test prior to arthroscopic surgery. Impingement syndrome is usually treated conservatively, but sometimes it is treated with arthroscopic surgery or open surgery. I have seen a lot of these operations, and they can be done with a local anaesthetic.

Non-surgical treatment includes rest from painful hobbies, as well as physical therapy and electrotherapy treatments to maintain a pain free range of movement, improving posture and gaining a gradual pain free strengthening of the shoulder muscles. As discussed before, in order to improve overall pain and function, treatment can also include: joint mobilisation, Acupuncture, soft tissue therapy, therapeutic taping, rotator cuff strengthening, and rehab education regarding the cause and mechanism of the condition. TENS, deep oscillations, NSAIDs, and ice packs may also be used for pain relief. If nothing is helping and you do not have a muscle tear, then injections of corticosteroid and local anaesthetic may be used for persistent impingement syndrome. The total number of injections is generally limited to three, due to possible side effects from the corticosteroid.

I have watched Mr Hackney do this operation on several occasions, and also, on occasion, Mr Kathuria as well. A number of surgical interventions are available – depending on the nature of the pathology and the age of the patient – and surgery may be done arthroscopically (through a scope) or as open surgery. The impinging structures in the subacromial space may be widened by resection of the distal clavicle (the collar bone) and the excision of osteophytes (bony spikes) on the under-surface of the acromioclavicular joint. Damaged rotator cuff muscles can be surgically repaired, and this may be the only way a shoulder can function again. My mother had this surgery, and while she had a lengthy recovery, she also had excellent results.

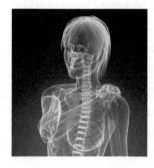 Muscles attach to bone by tendons, and the inflammation of these tendons is called shoulder tendinitis, a type of tendinopathy. Tendinitis (also tendonitis) means the inflammation of a tendon, and the term tendinitis should be reserved for tendon injuries that involve acute injuries with inflammation.

Chronic tendinitis, chronic tendinopathy, or chronic tendon injury all refer to damage to a tendon at a cellular level (the suffix 'osis' means chronic degeneration without inflammation). Damage is caused by microtears in the tendon, and an increase in tendon repair cells. This may lead to reduced tensile strength. I remember Mr Hackney correcting me about tennis elbow – he said it is degeneration, not inflammation. He was referring to degenerative changes in the collagenous matrix, hypercellularity, hypervascularity, and a lack of inflammatory cells. The term tendonITIS (inflamed) is different to tendinOSIS (meaning wear and tear).

Corticosteroids are drugs that reduce inflammation, and they are injected along with a small amount of a numbing (haha) drug called lidocaine. They can make a tendon very weak; I used to fear a 'twang' sound after my injection as if one of my guitar strings were going, so I never carried out more than two jabs in any one tendon. Research shows that tendons are weaker following corticosteroid injections and far more likely to rupture.

By definition, anything that ends in 'itis' means 'inflammation of'. Tendinitis is still a very common diagnosis, though research increasingly documents what is thought to be tendinitis and usually turns out to be tendinosis. Prof Gunn would say that the tendons get damaged due to an increased pull from muscle contractures, and that these muscle contractures present due to supersensitive nerves innervating them.

Tendinitis of the rotator cuff usually occurs over time, and it can be the result of poor posture, keeping the shoulder in one position – such as when on the computer – and not moving it over a period of time. You could be sleeping on the shoulder every night or having your arm bent up over your head. Or you could be doing a lot of activities that require extending the arm over the head at 90 degrees and above. Rotator cuff tendinitis can be developed from cleaning windows, painting ceilings, and manual jobs, as well as playing sports that require extending the arm over the head. This is why the condition may also be referred to as swimmer's, pitcher's, or tennis shoulder.

Often, we don't know why rotator cuff tendinitis occurs, but mostly, over time you are able to regain the full function of the shoulder without any pain. It can affect one or more muscles in the shoulder, and without treatment, it can become a chronic problem.

Diagnosis is by physiotherapy assessment, MRI, and ultrasound scan, and to reiterate, treatment can include: rest from painful activities, ice, sports therapy/physiotherapy, ultrasound, laser, massage, and progressive exercises for posture and muscle imbalance.

CACLIFIED TENDONITIS

This is a form of tendinitis that is characterised by deposits of hydroxyapatite (a crystalline calcium phosphate) in any tendon of the body, but most commonly in the tendons of the rotator cuff (shoulder), causing pain and inflammation. The condition is related to and may cause adhesive capsulitis (frozen shoulder), and three main theories have emerged in an attempt to explain the mechanisms involved in tendon calcification.

The first theory is the theory of reactive calcification and involves an active cellular process, usually followed by spontaneous resorption by phagocytosing multinucleated cells (cell eating), showing a typical osteoclast (bone cell munching) phenotype. The second theory suggests that calcium deposits are formed by a process resembling endochondral ossification (making bone), and the mechanism involves regional hypoxia (low oxygen), which transforms tenocytes (tendon cells) into chondrocytes (cartilage cells). The third theory involves ectopic bone formation from metaplasia of mesenchymal stem cells (cells not as yet assigned to be anything) – which are normally present in tendon tissue – into osteogenic (bone) cells.

As no single theory is satisfactory to explain all cases, calcific tendinopathy is currently believed to be multifactorial – G.O.K. (God only knows!). I'd like to add a quick mention here of extracorporeal (sound waves) shockwave therapy, as after a four day conference in Nice I was sick of hearing about how amazing it was! I have to admit that the highlight was escaping for a trip to Monte Carlo. However, it is excellent for calcific tendinitis, though it is not useful in other types of tendinitis, as it is aggressive and will cause more inflammation.

IMPINGEMENT SYNDROME OF THE SHOULDER CAN BE CAUSED BY OSTEOARTHRITIS

The symptoms of impingement syndrome include pain, weakness, and a loss of movement at the affected shoulder. The pain is often worsened by shoulder overhead movement, and it may occur at night, especially if the patient is lying on the affected shoulder. The onset of the pain may be insidious if it is due to a gradual process such as an osteoarthritic spur, and other symptoms can include a grinding or popping sensation during movement of the shoulder. I often hear crunching in shoulders with OA wear and tear.

When the arm is raised, the subacromial space (the gap between the anterior edge of the acromion and the head of the humerus) narrows, through which the supraspinatus muscle tendon passes. Anything that causes further narrowing impinges the inflamed tendon, resulting in impingement syndrome. This can be caused by bony structures such as subacromial osteoarthritic spurs (bony projections from the acromion, the spoon-shaped part of the shoulder blade where the humerus pushes up against), and also osteoarthritic spurs on the acromioclavicular joint. Thickening or calcification of the coracoacromial ligament will worsen the impingement.

It is useful to get an X-ray to see how arthritic the shoulder is.

ROTATOR CUFF TEAR – HAVE YOU HAD A FALL RECENTLY?

The pathology of tears is common between 40 and 70 years of age, though many patients that have full-thickness tears don't have symptoms, accounting for nearly 40% of rotator cuff injuries. In comparison, patients over the age of 60 with partial and full-thickness tears account for 60% of rotator cuff tears. The supraspinatus is the most commonly injured, and repetitive microtraumas, subacromial impingement, tendon degeneration, and hypo-vascularity (reduced circulation) can lead to a weak, torn muscle, unable to resist shearing forces. Surgery may be needed. My mother had two tendons sewn together last year following two falls. It was a long, slow recovery, but her arm is amazing now.

ROTATOR CUFF ARTHROSCOPIC SURGERY

The rotator cuff requires adequate time to heal by means of conservative (no surgery) treatment or surgical intervention. This slow rehab can last anything from four months to one year, depending on the treatment. Initially, the aim of the treatment is to decrease pain and inflammation by reducing activity and resting the limb. Once the healing process has begun, the focus of physical therapy then changes to increasing pain free strength and range of motion, until full power and movement is attained. Pain relief is essential as it can be a very painful rehabilitation. Deep oscillations, TENS, massage, and electrotherapy are all useful.

CONSERVATIVE REHABILITATION FOR SUPRASPINATUS TEAR

If the tear of the supraspinatus muscle is small, healing without surgical intervention may take between four and nine months, and range of motion (ROM) and pain free exercises are important.

The cycle of rehab is as follows: regain ROM – regain strength – increase range – increase strength. The type of strengthening exercises used during rehab should progress initially from isometric (no movement, just resisted statically), followed by concentric (resistance through movement), and lastly, eccentric (working the muscle whilst it is lengthening). The exercises are integrated into the treatment to provide a return to full functional activities.

Initial Three Weeks: Patient typically in a sling, doing very little in the way of exercise:
- Isometric strengthening.
- Shoulder shrugs.
- Pendulum activities.

Four Weeks:
- Supine (lie on your back) exercises, consisting of abduction (lift out sideways) and external rotation to protect the injured tendon.

Six Weeks:
- Anti-gravity strengthening.
- Progress exercises to full range of movement (ROM) with resistance.

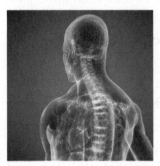

Do you have pain down your arm or in your shoulder? When you move your neck, does this pain change?

If so, you may have one of the following conditions: cervical radiculopathy or spondylosis and osteoarthritis (see neck section).

TRICEPS INFLAMMATION

If you try to push yourself off your chair, does it hurt in your upper arm?

This can happen when you push something far too heavy and get arm pain in your upper arm. The elbow also gets tender and stiff.

The triceps muscles are located at the back of the upper arm, and they act to straighten the elbow and resist the bending of the elbow. Typical actions that can overload the triceps – and in severe cases rupture the tendon – include pushing an excessively heavy object or breaking a fall on your hands.

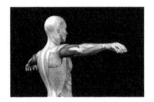

Treatment can include: RICE (rest, ice, compression, and elevation) for two days, ultrasound, laser, sports therapy, and physiotherapy rehab programmes.

ADHESIVE CAPSULITIS (ALSO KNOWN AS FROZEN SHOULDER)

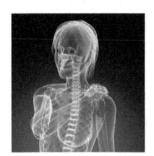

This is a painful and disabling disorder of unclear cause in which the shoulder capsule – the connective tissue surrounding the shoulder joint – is inflamed and stiff, greatly restricting motion and causing chronic pain. Pain is unpleasant, constant, worse at night, and irritated by cold weather. Sudden movements or bumps can provoke even more pain and cramps. It is thought to be caused by injury or trauma to the area and may include an autoimmune and hormonal component.

Treatment may be painful and longwinded, and it can consist of: physical therapy, Gunn IMS with cervical (neck) treatment, shockwave, manipulation, medication, massage therapy, or surgery, as a last resort. A surgeon may also perform manipulation under anaesthesia, which breaks up the adhesions and scar tissue in the joint to help restore some range of motion. Pain and inflammation can be controlled with TENS, Acupuncture, a stiff drink, or analgesics and NSAIDs.

People who suffer from adhesive capsulitis usually experience severe pain and sleep loss for a long time due to pain that gets worse when lying still in restricted positions. It can also lead to depression, can add to problems in the neck and back, and can cause irritability and weight loss due to long-term lack of deep sleep. You may also have extreme difficulty concentrating, working, dressing, or doing housework.

It usually resolves over time even without surgery, and most people will regain about 90% of their shoulder motion. One sign of a frozen shoulder is that the joint becomes so tight and stiff that it is nearly impossible to raise the arm. The movement that is most severely inhibited is the external rotation of the shoulder, and the stiffness and pain can worsen at night, with the pain being dull or aching.

Your physical therapist, osteopath, or chiropractor may suspect a frozen shoulder if a physical examination reveals limited shoulder movement. Frozen shoulder can be diagnosed if limits to the active range of motion (the range of motion from the active use of muscles) are the same or almost the same as the limits to the passive range of motion (the range of motion from a person manipulating the arm and shoulder).

An arthrogram or an MRI scan may confirm the diagnosis, though in practice this is rarely required.

The normal course of a frozen shoulder without treatment has been described as having three stages:
- **Stage One**: The 'freezing' or painful stage. This may last from six weeks to nine months, with a slow onset of worsening pain as the shoulder gets stiffer.
- **Stage Two:** The 'frozen'/sticky/adhesive stage. This is marked by a slow improvement in pain, but the stiffness remains. This lasts from four to nine months.
- **Stage Three:** The 'thawing' or recovery, when shoulder motion slowly returns towards normal and pain is not so much of a problem. This generally lasts from five to 26 months.

Adhesive capsulitis is primarily a clinical diagnosis, though imaging may be used to exclude other causes. Arthrography is usually regarded as the gold standard for imaging diagnosis, though ultrasound and MRI may help in diagnosis by assessing the thickening of the coracohumeral ligament. Another ultrasound finding can be that of 'hypoechoic' material (more blood vessels), surrounding the long head of the biceps tendon at the rotator end. In very painful cases, local injection can help.

Osteopaths, chiropractors, and physiotherapists may suggest treatments such as shockwave, massage therapy, daily extensive stretching, and Gunn IMS dry needling. If these treatments are unsuccessful, however, more invasive painful techniques will be needed. These could include: manipulation under general anaesthesia to break up the adhesions, distension arthrography, and surgery (athroscopy) to cut the adhesions (capsular release).

ELBOW PROBLEMS

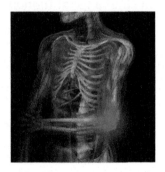

Do you have an extremely painful, swollen elbow that you cannot move, or some deformity?

If so, you may have a dislocated elbow.

DISLOCATED ELBOW

A dislocated elbow occurs usually as a result of a fall or a direct blow, and often involves fractures of the ulna radius and humerus. The most common reason involves falling onto an outstretched hand, with the arm away from the body, and the elbow being forcibly flexed on contact (and usually also with a twisting movement). This results in a posterior dislocation that accounts for up to 90% of all elbow dislocations. In a posterior dislocation, the ulna or the radius (or both) moves backwards and ligament damage will occur. If relocation is not instant, a medic will reduce it and check out the nerves and blood vessels.

Diagnosis is by medical emergency, physiotherapy assessment, and X-ray, and treatment can include: a reduction of the dislocation, sling immobilisation for one to three weeks, and painkillers. Later on you can add gentle mobility exercises, then once movement is back, strengthening, ultrasound, and pulsed shortwave to help the ligament damage.

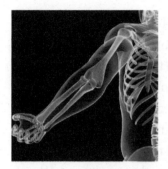

Are normal daily activities painful? Is your elbow becoming stiff, swollen, and losing its range of movement? Is it hard to completely straighten your arm, then is it hard to bend?

If so, you may have osteoarthritis of the elbow (see definition of osteoarthritis).

Do you have elbow pain and a boggy feeling, with a red localised swelling? Do you have limited movement, and pain at rest or upon exertion?

If so, you may have one of the following conditions:

OLECRANON BURSITIS

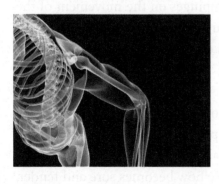

Student's elbow – or olecranon bursitis – is the inflammation/swelling of the bursa that protects the bone at the back of the elbow. Traumatic or repetitive impacts to this area can result in pain and a large swelling at the back of the joint. The bursa is a sack of fluid that helps to prevent friction between bones and the soft tissue over the top of the elbow. Inflammation or bleeding into a bursa can cause it to become very sore, and this can happen by being hit by someone (or a ball, for instance), or a repetitive action.

Treatment can include: RICE (rest, ice, compression, and elevation), phys-iotherapy, sports therapy, and wearing a sling. Advice includes not leaning on the elbow, wearing an elbow guard if playing cricket or contact sports, and initially immobilising the arm. You may need a sac of fluid called a bursa syringed out (aspirated) and a corticosteroid injection.

TENNIS ELBOW

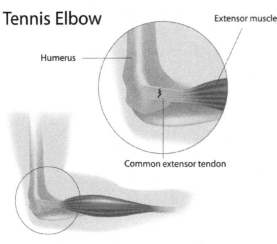

Tennis Elbow

Extensor muscle

Humerus

Common extensor tendon

Right arm, lateral (outside) side

Tendinosis of the com-mon extensor tendon (tennis elbow) is a com-mon cause of elbow pain for adults. Symptoms can include an ache/pain and stiffness to the local area of the tendon at the el-bow, or, when severe, a burning that surrounds the whole joint around the affected tendon. The pain is usually worse dur-ing and after activity, and the next day it will be stiffer as swelling impinges on the movement of the tendon. Repetitive typing, sport, or stressful situations in life can tie in with the onset of the pain. Swelling in a region of micro-damage or partial tear may be detected visually or by touch.

Tennis elbow tendinosis is due to tendon overuse and the failed healing of the tendon. In addition, the extensor carpi radialis brevis muscle (which extends the elbow) plays a key role. Tennis elbow or lateral epicondylitis is a condition in which the outer part of the elbow becomes sore and tender, and the forearm muscles and tendons become damaged from overuse – repeating the same strenuous motions. This leads to pain and tenderness on the outside of the elbow.

Any activity (including tennis) that involves the repetitive use of the extensor muscles of the forearm can cause acute or chronic tendonitis of the insertion of these muscles at the lateral epicondyle of the elbow. The condition is common in carpenters and labourers who swing a hammer/tool with their forearm.

GOLFER'S ELBOW

Golfer's elbow – or medial epicondylitis – is tendinosis of the medial epicondyle of the elbow, and is in some ways similar to tennis elbow. The anterior forearm contains several muscles that are involved with flexing the digits of the hand, as well as flexing and pronating the wrist. The tendons of these muscles come together in a common tendinous sheath, which originates from the medial epicondyle of the humerus at the elbow joint. In response to minor injury – or simply for no obvious reason – this point of insertion becomes inflamed.

Before anaesthetics and steroids are used, physiotherapy treatment after rest, ice, compression, and elevation (RICE) will typically be used. This will help to decrease inflammation, and rest will help the overuse injury. The patient can use an elbow brace or splint for compression, the splint being made in 30-45 degrees of the elbow bend. A simple daytime elbow brace may also be a useful alternative.

Exercise prescription is for muscle/tendon reconditioning, starting with stretching and the gradual strengthening of the flexor-pronator muscles. Strengthening will slowly begin with isometrics (static contractions) and will then progress to eccentric exercises (working into stretching with loading), helping to get a range of motion back to where it once was. Simple analgesic medication has a place in the beginning, as do oral anti-inflammatory meds (NSAIDs) – these will help to control pain due to inflammation. A more invasive treatment is the injection, which causes an initial exacerbation of symptoms lasting from 24 to 48 hours.

Here are the treatments in summary: physiotherapy, brace, deep tissue massage, Gunn IMS dry needling, ultrasound, shockwave, laser, deep oscillations, Acupuncture, posture, exercises with stretches, pulsed shortwave, and MRT.

INJURED TENDONS/TENDINOSIS AND MEDICAL TREATMENTS

An injured tendon is very slow to heal; partial tears heal by the rapid healing response of type-III collagen, which is weaker than normal tendon. Recurrence of the injury in the damaged region of the tendon is common. Rehabilitation, rest, and a gradual return to the activity is sensible.

There is evidence to suggest that tendinosis is not an inflammatory disorder. Therefore, anti-inflammatory drugs are not an effective treatment, and inflammation is not the cause of this type of tendon dysfunction. Initial recovery is said to be within two to three months, with full recovery usually within three to six months. Most people (80%) will fully recover within 12 months, depending on treatment effectiveness. If therapy doesn't work, you can then move onto surgery, consisting of the excision of the abnormal tissue. The time required to recover fully from surgery is about four to six months. Delaying exercise until after the initial inflammatory stage of repair could promote tissue repair and remodelling.

AUTOLOGOUS TENOCYTE INJECTION

Dr Cameron, a delightful Scottish doctor, explained this procedure to me: this is when your own blood is injected back into you. For example, a tenocyte injection could be used for the treatment of severe, chronic, resistant tennis elbow (lateral epicondylitis). A needle biopsy could be taken from the patellar (knee cap) tendon, and the extracted tendon cells expanded by in vitro culture. The tenocytes could then be injected into the injured tendinopathy site – the origin of the extensor carpi radialis brevis (extensor) tendon – under the guidance of an ultrasound. After this little-known treatment, it has been stated that patients showed improved clinical function and structural repair at the origin of the common extensor tendon.

SOFT TISSUE MOBILIZATION

Augmented Soft Tissue Mobilization (ASTM) is a form of manual therapy that has been shown in studies on rats to speed the healing of tendons by increasing fibroblast activity (cells that rebuild connective tissue).

ECCENTRIC LOADING

This simply involves eccentric loading exercises involving the lengthening of muscular contractions.

INFLATABLE BRACE

The use of an inflatable brace (AirHeel) was shown to be as effective as eccentric loading in the treatment of chronic Achilles tendinopathy. Both modalities produced significant reduction in pain scores, but their combination was no more effective than either treatment alone.

SHOCKWAVE THERAPY

I use this. Research agrees that shockwave therapy (SWT) is effective in treating calcific tendinosis. In rat subjects, SWT increased the levels of healing hormones and proteins leading to increased cell proliferation and tissue regeneration in tendons.

TENDON BIOENGINEERING

The future of non-surgical care for tendinosis is bioengineering, as ligament reconstruction is possible using mesenchymal stem cells and a silk scaffold. These stem cells are capable of seeding the repair of damaged tendons, and autologous tenocyte implantation is currently being tested for tendinosis.

INJECTIONS OF MICRO RNA (GENE EXPRESSION REGULATORS)

Scientists have found that miR-29a – a single <u>microRNA</u> – through its interaction with a protein (interleukin 33) plays a key role in regulating the production of collagens in tendon disease. A loss of miR-29a from human tendons increases <u>collagen type-3</u> production, a key feature of tendon disease. The replacement of miR-29a in the damaged tendon cells in the lab then restores collagen production to pre-injury levels. A trial will put injections of microRNA – small molecules that help regulate gene expression – into the tendon in order to decrease the production of type 3 collagen and switch to type-1.

ALLOGENEIC ADIPOSE-DERIVED MESENCHYMAL STEM CELLS

In November 2013, researchers at the Seoul National University Hospital looked at allogeneic adipose-derived mesenchymal stem cells (ALLO-ASC) for the treatment of at least six-month-old tennis elbow tendon injuries. Adipose-derived mesenchymal stem cells were given to the patients by an ultrasonography-guided injection.

ELASTOGRAPHY ULTRASOUND TO ESTIMATE TENDON STIFFNESS

Researchers have tried to analyse the effect of treatment on tendons, and tendon tissue strain and its mechanical properties can be looked at by using elastography (an acoustical imaging technique that measures strain distributions in tissues from stress or compression). Strain is inversely related to stiffness, so under stress, tissue that displays less strain is assumed to be stiffer than tissue that exhibits more strain. Elastography, therefore, is an indirect method to estimate tissue stiffness. Acoustoelastography is another ultrasound technique, one that relates ultrasonic wave amplitude changes to the mechanical properties of a tendon.

LIGAMENT LAXITY, HYPERMOBILITY

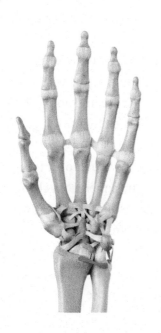

Ligamentous laxity is a cause of chronic body pain characterised by loose ligaments, and when this condition affects joints in the entire body, it is called 'generalised joint hypermobility'. I see a lot of this in some parts of the body but rarely in all the joints, which occurs in 5% of cases and may be genetic. Loose ligaments can appear in a variety of ways and at varying levels of severity.

TENDON AND LIGAMENT

Someone with ligamentous laxity has loose ligaments. Unlike other diseases, the diagnosis does not require the presence of loose tendons, muscles or blood vessels, hyperlax skin, or other connective tissue problems.

With inheritable connective tissue disorders associated with joint hypermobility (such as Marfan syndrome and Ehlers-Danlos syndrome types I-III, VII, and XI), the joint laxity (where the joint is not stabilised enough by the ligaments) is usually apparent as kids. I remember treating a family with this disorder following a car crash – it's OK, you can take your seat belts off, it was a happy ending: they all recovered completely.

Referred pain is created by ligamentous laxity around a joint, but is felt at some distance from the injury. These painful points that refer pain elsewhere are called trigger points, and they respond well to therapy. Excessive joint movement also creates many 'protective actions' by adjacent tissues, and muscles will contract in spasm in an attempt to pull the joint back to the correct location or stabilise it. When this occurs in the back, you need strong muscles, otherwise orthopaedic surgeons will often try to reduce vertebral instability by fusing the vertebrae with bone and/or metal fixation.

Lax ligaments do not support joints as well as healthy ones, and your joint proprioception will be poor, making you prone to injury as well as postural overcompensation for the weakness using other parts of the body. With good exercises you may improve over time and lose some of your hyperlaxity.

Right, it's time to get your seat belts on again now: individuals over the age of 40 with very lax joints have recurrent joint problems and suffer from chronic pain. Back patients with spinal ligament laxity may also suffer from early osteoarthritis and disc degeneration. Also, they may find themselves with disorders involving nerve compression, chondromalacia patellae (inflammation behind the kneecap), excessive anterior mandibular (jaw bone) movement, mitral valve (in the heart), prolapse, uterine prolapse (womb), and varicose veins.

HANDS

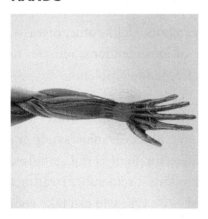

WRIST IMPINGEMENT/ IMPACTION SYNDROMES

This is pain in the wrist due to the pinching of structures within the wrist joint, usually during a traumatic end of range wrist movement (e.g. a fall onto an outstretched hand), and typically with the wrist in extension (stretched back) and in combination with weight bearing forces through the affected wrist (such as during gymnastics). Symptoms may increase upon firmly touching the affected region of the wrist, and on certain wrist movements (e.g. wrist extension). The painful wrist will be sore to the touch with restricted wrist joint mobility and often swelling.

Treatment can include: physiotherapy, home advice regarding supporting the bandage cooling, and RICE.

DE QUERVAIN'S TENOSYNOVITIS

Symptoms include pain and tenderness on the thumb side of the wrist, where the tendons pass through a narrow tunnel and attach to the base of the thumb. Crepitus or a creaking sensation may be felt when moving the wrist.

OVERSTRETCHED THUMB OR FINGERS

A thumb sprain occurs when the thumb is bent out of its normal range of movement, usually backwards. Damage occurs to the ligaments supporting the joint at the bottom of the thumb, and symptoms include pain in the web of the thumb when it is moved, and swelling over the metacarpophalangeal joint (at the base of the thumb). You may also have laxity and instability in the joint.

Treatment can include: RICE, strapping, thumb support, physiotherapy with gentle exercises, and laser.

OVERSTRETCHED FINGERS

Have you really overstretched your fingers and do they really throb?

This is the tearing of the connective tissue and/or the ligaments holding the bones of the finger together, typically after excessive stretching of the joint in one direction. It is associated with pain upon firmly touching the joint, restricted joint mobility, and often swelling.

Treatment can include: strapping, relative rest, and physiotherapy with home exercises.

Does your little finger tingle?

'Handlebar palsy' is the name given to a condition suffered by cyclists, and symptoms at rest and when moving the wrist can include: numbness, tingling, and weakness over the outside of the hand, little finger, and the outer half of the ring finger. In cyclists, this may mean checking the bike set-up, such as the height of the saddle and the handlebars, and the wrist position when riding. Correcting these problems will usually stop the symptoms.

Do your thumb and fingers get stiff after rest?

OSTEOARTHRITIS

With osteoarthritis, your wrist, thumb, and fingers get stiff in the morning and after rest. The joints thicken, and cysts form on your finger joints due to calcific spurs – these are called Bouchard's nodes. These unsightly lumps appear on your fingers. Treatment can include: physiotherapy, home exercises such as playing the piano, laser, deep oscillation, shockwave, and MRT.

Thumb Arthritis

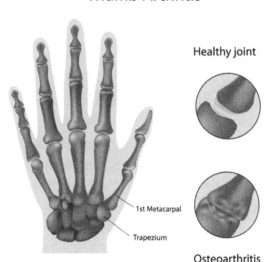

Healthy joint

1st Metacarpal

Trapezium

Osteoarthritis

Do you have a swollen wrist?

If so, this can be made worse by the bursa, a small sack of fluid that lubricates where tendons move in your joints. If the bursa is subjected to repeated trauma or friction then it can become inflamed and swollen, causing pain in the wrist.

HAMATE FRACTURE

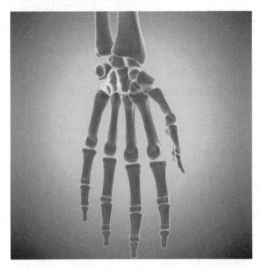

This is when you injure your hand with a recoil – such as an old-fashioned car engine start – or fall, and it hurts in your palm. It can happen when hitting the ground during a golf swing, swinging a tennis racket or baseball bat, playing volleyball, or due to a fall onto an outstretched hand. The break is in one of the wrist bones located on the thumb side of the wrist called a scaphoid. Swelling, tenderness on touching the thumb side of the wrist bone, and a markedly reduced wrist function are also present. Laser can help, as well as MRT to speed up the healing.

COLLES FRACTURE

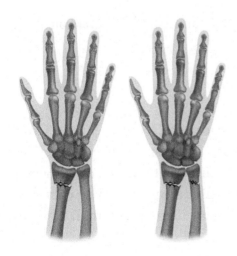

Colles Fracture

This break is in the radius bone near the wrist, and it is usually due to a fall onto an outstretched hand. Severe pain, that is usually located on the thumb side of the wrist, may radiate into the thumb, hand, or forearm. As well as swelling, there is tenderness on palpating the affected region of the wrist, a markedly reduced wrist function, and sometimes, bone deformity. It will need a cast before any therapy can begin.

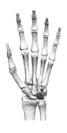

This is a break in one of the small wrist bones – the lunate – which is located in the middle of your wrist. Following a fall onto an outstretched hand, severe wrist pain from the time of the injury settles to an ache and can radiate into the hand or forearm. There is swelling and tenderness upon firmly touching it and the severe ache is on the thumb side.

BOXER'S FRACTURE

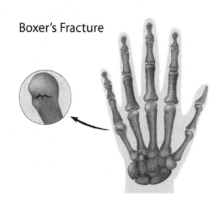

Boxer's Fracture

This is when you punch the wall in frustration, your hand swells up, and it's difficult to move your fingers. It is likely that you have broken the knuckle, called the 'metacarpal bones' of the hand. This is usually due to a punch, hence why it's called boxer's fracture, but basically this is a direct blow to the back of your hand or a fall onto an outstretched hand. This can result in a severe pain in the hand and can radiate into the wrist or fingers. It will swell and be sore to touch, giving you poor hand function, and sometimes a bony deformity.

Treatment can include: strapping, RICE, and gentle progression finger exercises once the bones have healed.

PHALANGE FRACTURE

Your husband slams the end of your finger in a car door and you feel an intense pain – this could be a break in one of the small bones of the finger called the phalanges. This mostly occurs due to a traumatic direct blow to the finger such as during contact sports. This can result in severe pain in the affected finger, swelling, tenderness, a markedly reduced finger function, and sometimes bony deformity.

FLEXOR TENDON INJURY (JERSEY FINGER)

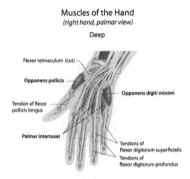

Muscles of the Hand
(right hand, palmar view)

Deep

Flexor retinaculum (cut)

Opponens pollicis

Opponens digiti minimi

Tendon of flexor
pollicis longus

Palmar interossei

Tendons of
flexor digitorum superficialis

Tendons of
flexor digitorum profundus

This is a tear in one of the flexor tendons in your finger. You will have pain in the fingertip and an inability to bend the finger. Tenderness on the pad of the finger will be present, along with swelling and bruising, which will develop later.

TRIGGER FINGER

Does your finger suddenly jam up for no reason?

This a form of tenosynovitis, meaning that your finger becomes bent in towards the palm of your hand. Tenosynovitis is an inflammatory condition of the sheath that surrounds a tendon. The inflamed and thickened tendon cannot slide through the tunnel, therefore, the finger gets stuck in a bent position and clicks or locks. If you have a repetitive job, rheumatoid arthritis, or diabetes, you are more at risk. MRI is needed for a clear diagnosis, and treatment may well include surgery, but if not severe, RICE, physiotherapy, laser, and splinting may help.

TRIGGER THUMB

Does your thumb lock?

'Trigger thumb' is a form of tenosynovitis that occurs in the flexor tendon of the thumb – the thickening of the tendon causes it to get stuck and hold the thumb in a flexed position. Treatment is often surgery, however, RICE, physio exercises, laser, and splinting may ease mild cases.

ULNAR NERVE IRRITATION IN THE THUMB

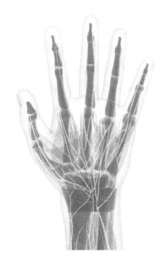

Have you been rubbing your thumb and getting a tingling sensation?

'Bowler's thumb' is an overuse injury resulting from compression or repeated friction on the inside of the thumb, causing pressure on the ulnar nerve. You get thumb pain with numbness, and tingling in the end of the thumb.

FINGER TENDON INJURY

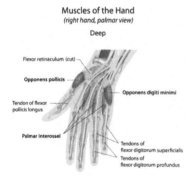

Muscles of the Hand
(right hand, palmar view)
Deep

Flexor retinaculum (cut)
Opponens pollicis
Tendon of flexor pollicis longus
Palmar interossei
Opponens digiti minimi
Tendons of flexor digitorum superficialis
Tendons of flexor digitorum profundus

If you catch your finger on a dry ski slope mat – like my father did – it can cause a tearing of the connective tissue surrounding one of the finger joints with separation of the bones, meaning that the joint surfaces are no longer next to each other, and the finger is deformed. This injury occurs as a result of a traumatic impact to the finger – most often with ball sports, horse riding, or skiing – and causes severe pain in the finger. At the time you get a feeling of the finger 'popping out', leaving a deformity of the finger joint, and sometimes pins and needles or numbness remains due to tendon nerve irritation.

A boutonniere deformity – or 'button hole' deformity – is an injury to a tendon in one of the fingers, right down to the mid bone, resulting in a deformed shape. This usually occurs after an impact to a bent finger, forcefully bending it and rupturing the extensor tendon. Treatment may include: surgery or a splint, then intensive physiotherapy.

FINGER LIGAMENT INJURY

This is when you bend your finger back too far and it really hurts; the volar plate is a very thick ligament which joins two bones in the finger, and a volar plate injury occurs when the finger is bent back the wrong way too far, spraining or tearing the ligament. Treatment is initially RICE and strapping, then gentle stretches.

FASCIAL THICKENING IN PALM

'Dupuytren's contracture' is a condition that affects the hand and fingers, causing the fingers to bend in towards the palm of the hand. Massage and stretching helps, but sadly surgery is often needed in order to regain finger range.

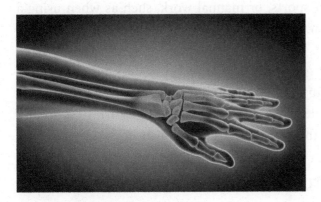

WRIST SPRAIN

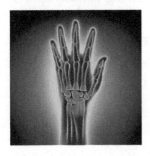

A wrist sprain is an injury to any of the ligaments that join bone to bone in the wrist. Sudden pain in the wrist (with swelling) will often occur after a traumatic impact or a twisting of the wrist, and sprains can vary from very mild to very bad. Repetitive sprains may develop into tendonitis or tendinopathy, inflammation, then the degeneration of the tendons. Pain in the wrist continues with joint stiffness in the morning, local swelling, and tenderness over the tendon.

WRIST LIGAMENT DISRUPTION

This is the tearing of connective tissue and/or ligaments of the joint located between the ends of the forearm bones just before the wrist (distal radioulnar joint), typically as a result of a fall onto an outstretched hand, with twisting. The wrist is painful and swollen, and when touching the joint, wrist joint mobility is less (particularly with regards to the rotation of the wrist).

TFCC TEAR

TFCC (triangular fibrocartilage complex) occurs when there is damage to cartilage tissue located on the little finger side of the wrist joint, usually due to excessive compression forces with twisting or side bending forces through the wrist – such as a fall onto an outstretched hand. Or it can occur during gymnastics, racket sports, or manual work, such as when using a hammer. Pain is located on the little finger side of the wrist and can radiate into the forearm or hand. There is tenderness on touching the wrist, as well as swelling, reduced grip strength, and often a clicking or catching sensation. It is not easy to diagnose, but a scan can help. Both a sports physiotherapist and consultant need to advise on your return to sport and treatment. Depending on the level of severity, it may need surgery.

FINGER TENDON RUPTURES

This is the complete tearing of one or more finger tendons, following a traumatic incident such as an impact to the finger during contact sports. Pain and swelling in the finger may radiate into the hand, there may be a significant weakness of the affected finger, and a deformity of the finger that cannot be straightened. Pain increases on touching the affected tendon, and treatment can include: splinting, laser, ultrasound, and gentle progressive rehab.

CARPAL TUNNEL

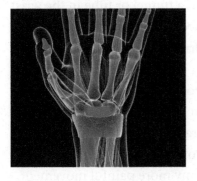

Are your fingers getting weaker, and do they tingle and bother you at night?

Carpal tunnel is a dull ache in the wrist and forearm that may radiate into the hand and fingers. The pain is worse at night, and weakness in the fingers and hand may occur, as well as a tingling or burning sensation. This can be caused by trauma, aging, or repetitive stress, and diabetics are more at risk. Symptoms are caused by the compression of the median nerve in the wrist as it passes through a narrow channel in the wrist called the carpal tunnel, which also houses the flexor digitorum superficialis and flexor pollicis longus tendons of the forearm.

Treatment can include: Gunn IMS dry needling for the neck at C5/6, Acupuncture, physiotherapy postural exercises, RICE, and splinting. Initially, mobility and gentle stretching exercises should be done to restore the full pain free range of motion at the joint. Later, static (no movement) strengthening exercises can begin, and finally, normal strength can be restored through dynamic/moving exercises with resistance bands/ dumbbells. Investigations may also be performed to confirm the diagnosis including MRI scan, ultrasound imaging, electromyography, or a nerve conduction study.

DE QUERVERAIN'S

This is tenderness on the thumb side of the wrist where the tendons pass through a narrow tunnel and attach to the base of the thumb. Crepitus – a creaking sensation – may be felt when moving the wrist. Finkelstein's test is used to help diagnose De Quervain's tenosynovitis: here, the thumb is placed in the palm of the hand and the wrist moved sideways towards the little pinky finger side to stretch the tendons. If pain is felt, the test is positive.

The tendons of the abductor pollicis brevis (thumb) and extensor pollicis longus muscles (also the thumb) pass through a tunnel or tube in the wrist and attach at the base of the thumb. This tube or sheath surrounding the tendons can become inflamed, preventing normal movement of the tendon and also creating pain. It is the inflammation of the sheath that surrounds the tendon as opposed to the actual tendon itself. Tennis, squash, or badminton – as well as canoeing, ten pin bowling, and golf – can cause this, and treatment can include: rest, ice, ultrasound, and a stretching and strengthening program. Rest is important to allow healing, and often, a wrist splint can ensure rest and help prevent any more painful movement.

THORACIC SPINE

Do you feel pain in the upper and mid back? Does your spine curve outwards a lot in this area, and then back in a lot below?

If so, you may have Scheuermann's disease.

This is a 'hunchbacked' condition, affecting children normally of teenage years. It is believed to be caused by genetic failings in the blood supply to growing cartilage, and bone cells die off in the spinal vertebrae where they should be growing, leaving a very curved, over thoracic spine. This leads to back ache.

Treatment, especially during teens, would be specialised physiotherapy exercises and pain-relieving electrotherapy.

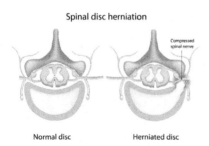

Spinal disc herniation

Compressed spinal nerve

Normal disc   Herniated disc

Do you feel pain in your mid back, that can feel like a band going all around to the front of your chest?

Have you experienced arm or leg weakness or numbness, pins and needles, or bladder/ bowel changes?

THORACIC DISC HERNIATION

Discs can be damaged by trauma or repetitive overloading – such as heavy lifting – and will degenerate with age but get less troublesome. In some conditions the fibrous ring will tear, allowing the soft inner contents to rupture through (herniate). This process is known as 'disc herniation' and is most common in the two lowest discs in the lumbar spine.

Disc herniation can cause the compression of the exiting nerves or the nerve root and can result in symptoms such as local pain, pain in the torso and/or limbs, pins and needles, loss of strength, and loss of motor control. In some cases, loss of bladder or bowels can also occur.

Diagnosis is by physiotherapy assessment, MRI, and orthopaedic consultation, and treatment can include: MBST, GunnIMS, Acupuncture, and exercise with physiotherapy. Severe cases may need surgery.

KYPHOSIS POSTURAL SCOLIOSIS

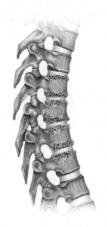

Scoliosis can occur from birth, or it can develop slowly in childhood, with the child often not realising that anything is amiss as often there is no pain. In the majority of cases children do not need treatment as the condition self corrects, though a brace can help to prevent the condition from worsening.

For adults the condition is usually painful, with the pain local to the curvature in the spine and sometimes into the legs, along with numbness and weakness. Other symptoms can include loss of bladder and bowel control, and treatment is usually conservative, with surgery only considered in severe cases. Scoliosis occurs in around 70% of adults over 65.

Diagnosis is by physiotherapy assessment, X-ray, and orthopaedic opinion, and treatment can include: physiotherapy, mobilisations, Theraflex, Acupuncture, Gunn IMS dry needling, strengthening and stretching, and deep tissue <u>massage</u>. For one-sided sports, at the end of the game, practice using your other arm.

Do you have pain when moving the spine, twisting, and side bending? Does deep breathing or coughing increase that pain?

If so, you may have costovertebral joint ligament sprains.

COSTOVERTEBRAL JOINT LIGAMENT SPRAINS

The costovertebral joints are located in the upper (thoracic) spine and occur where each rib meets the spinal vertebrae on both sides of the spine. Any activity, through trauma, certain movements, or repetitive activity – which overloads the joint – can cause injury to one or more of the costovertebral joints. Pain may be felt immediately, or on the following morning, combined with stiffness. The pain will be felt at the spine, or it may travel around the chest and into the arm, and will be made worse by deep breathing, coughing, sneezing, or by bending and twisting.

In most cases the condition will heal in about six weeks, provided that aggravating activities are avoided and that the physiotherapy regime is followed. Diagnosis is by physiotherapy assessment, and treatment can include: initially RICE then physiotherapy to prescribe mobility exercises, Acupuncture, ultrasound, pulsed shortwave, mobilisations and manipulations, and postural advice. You may also see a sports therapist for some soft tissue therapy.
On a sudden movement, did you feel a tearing in your upper back?

If so, you may have intervertebral ligament sprains.

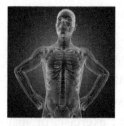

INTERVERTEBRAL LIGAMENT SPRAINS

Ligaments are made of strong fibrous material that is positioned to strengthen and stabilise a joint. They are prone to damage when overloaded, due to, say, a trauma – such as a car accident – or from more everyday activities such as lifting while bending or twisting. Pain will be felt and may be aggravated by deep breathing, coughing, or sneezing. In most cases the ligaments will heal within four weeks, helped by avoiding aggravating activities.

Diagnosis is by physiotherapy assessment, and treatment options include: RICE, sports massage, shockwave, and physiotherapy to prescribe stretching and mobilising exercises.

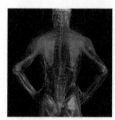

Are your neck muscles and the muscles between your shoulder blades always tight?

If so, you may have chronically tight muscle contractures.

CHRONICALLY TIGHT MUSCLE CONTRACTURES

Diagnosis is by physiotherapy/physical therapy assessment, and treatment can include: posture improvement (especially with the heat), stretching routines, regular sports massage, and strengthening exercises. If persistent or non-resolving, try Gunn IMS and shockwave therapy.

Have you ever had pain suddenly occur in your back with movement, for example, when bending to tie up your laces? Is the pain localised to one spot in your back and does it not radiate out anywhere?

If so, you may have mechanical back pain.

MECHANICAL BACK PAIN

Mechanical back pain is a general category that includes pain from the spinal vertebrae, joints, or soft tissues, but the source of the pain is ill-defined as usually there are no definable causes found from physical examinations or MRI scans. It can occur due to poor posture, lack of exercise, or just aging. Pain does not travel down the limbs – it remains localised – and treatment can include: manipulation, posture and exercise advice, massage, and Acupuncture.

FACET JOINT BLOCK

(Please see description in the neck section). This responds well to specific manipulations, and if straight forward, can be adjusted in just one session – the clunk is very satisfying.

DISC BULGE

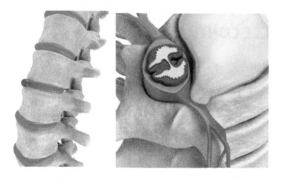

Also referred to as a slipped disc or prolapsed disc, this is when the soft disc cushion between the spinal vertebrae suffers constant loading from daily activity. Often such activities will overload the disc and cause a bulge in the side, but without the fibrous ring rupturing (becoming herniated). This is much like the bulge in a car tyre, caused by hitting a curb.

DISC PROLAPSE

A disc may bulge into the central spinal column or sideways into the exiting nerves and can, if excessive, create compression on the nerves, sufficient enough to cause local or distal pain in the limbs, numbness and weakness, and loss of motor function.

Diagnosis is by physiotherapy assessment, X-ray, and MRI, and treatment can include: Gunn IMS, electro-acupuncture, MBST, laser, and core stability rehab and exercises. If severe, surgery may be needed.

LUMBAR MUSCLE STRAINS AND LIGAMENT SPRAINS

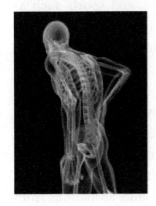 The lower back (lumbar) is in use for most daily activities, and is supported by strong muscles and ligaments to enable it to perform these tasks while still maintaining control. It is therefore more susceptible to injury from incorrect, excessive loading or repetitive loading; injury can occur to the muscles and connecting tendons (strain), or the ligaments (sprain), and the symptoms can be very similar. Typical symptoms include low back and buttock pain, which is aggravated by activity and which reduces with rest.

Lower back strains and sprains most often occur with heavy lifting – particularly when lifting and twisting – but they can also occur with sudden movement or trauma, such as during a car accident. Aggravating factors are poor core stability, obesity, and smoking, and treatment can include: Gunn IMS, physiotherapy, mobilisations, manipulation, core stability rehab and exercises, Acupuncture, shockwave, and massage.

LUMBAR SPONDYLOLYSIS

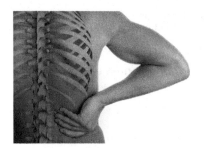

Spondylolysis is a stress fracture in a specific area of the vertebrae called the pars interarticularis, and it most often occurs at the bottom of the lumbar spine at L5. The fracture leads to a separation of the nearby facet joints.

Spondylolysis appears to have a hereditary link of having thinner bone structure at the pars interarticularis, which makes the probability of fracture higher. Activities where the back is repeatedly impacted while overextended (hyperextended) are prone to causing spondylolysis, and sports such as fast bowling, cricket, tennis, and gymnastics have a higher probability of repeatedly causing this condition. The problem is more common in young males, with the peak being at 16 years old.

Spondylolysis is the most common cause of spondylolisthesis, and if left untreated, spondylolysis can cause spinal stenosis, radiculopathy, and compression of the spinal cord in the lumbar region (cauda equina syndrome). Treatment can include: initially, a brace if severe, then laser, extensive core stability, one on one physiotherapy, and abstaining from aggravating activities. In severe cases, surgery may be needed.

SPONDYLOLISTHESIS

This can be either forward (anterior) or rearward (posterior) displacement of the vertebral column, and the first signs are a tightening back and hamstrings, which will lead to postural changes, the buttocks muscles (gluts) weakening, and a waddling walk. The back aches along with sciatica, causing shooting pains down the leg, from the buttock to the foot. Further symptoms can include tingling and numbness with a slipping sensation, and pain on sitting to standing. Inflammation and pain will increase with activity. If the slippage is less than 50%, the symptoms can be mild with some sciatic pain on increased activity.

The source of the pain is believed to be from tension in the centre of the inferior disc, and the nerve tunnel narrowing (foraminal stenosis) at the level of the slip. Biomechanical studies to explain the pain are found wanting. The lack of restraint on movement from the inferior facet joints adds to the stress on the disc, and slips over 50% represent only 10% of cases. Symptoms are progressive and painful, and you may also suffer from biomechanical issues, gait problems, tight hamstrings, and neurological changes (reflexes and numbness).

Posterior-only fusions tend to have more progression of their spondylolisthesis, following surgery and more pain, and degenerative changes can cause a narrowing of the spinal cord. Symptoms are the same as with spinal stenosis, neurogenic claudication, or radiculopathy, with or without back pain.

Neurogenic claudication is thought to result from central canal narrowing that is exacerbated by the listhesis (forward slip). The classic symptoms of neurogenic claudication include bilateral, posterior leg pain, which worsens with increased activity and is relieved by sitting or forward bending.

Spondylolisthesis runs in families, showing a possible genetic link. There are five types:
- Isthmic
- Degenerative
- Dysplastic
- Traumatic
- Pathologic

ISTHMIC

Isthmic spondylolisthesis (also called spondylolytic spondylolisthesis as it results from spondylolysis) is the most common form of spondylolisthesis and is a common condition. The spondylolytic defect is usually acquired between the ages of six and 16 years, and the slip often occurs shortly thereafter. Once the slip has occurred, it rarely continues to progress.

DEGENERATIVE

Degenerative spondylolisthesis is a disease of the older patients that develops as a result of facet joints getting arthritic and losing their nice chiselled shape, allowing a slip. 30 to 60% of women over 65 with osteoporosis have this problem, and these slips can go unnoticed unless there are problems with stenosis (symptoms of neurogenic claudication). This may require surgery.

DYSPLASTIC

Dysplastic spondylolisthesis is rare, and to get this you are born with damaged facet joints at the lumbar sacral junction.

TRAUMATIC

Traumatic spondylolisthesis is very rare, though it can happen in sporting accidents and may be associated with acute fracture of the inferior facets or pars interarticularis. It is currently thought that the pars interarticularis defect develops from small stress fractures that fail to heal and therefore form a chronic nonunion. There have been reports that the defect is more common among athletes who participate in sports with repeated hyperextension, such as fast bowling in cricket, gymnastics, and ballet. It is treated in the same manner as with other spinal fractures.

PATHOLOGIC

Pathologic spondylolisthesis is the last type and is also very rare. This type can occur following damage to the posterior elements from cancer secondaries or metabolic bone disease.

Treatment for these conditions can include: drugs, physiotherapy, Acupuncture, biomechanical analysis, core stability rehab, and stretches to tighten hip flexors and lumbar paraspinal muscles. If severe, seek an orthopaedic opinion, and possibly surgery.

Do you have a dull ache in the lumbar spine, both buttocks, and thighs, but not below the knees? Do you also have a dull ache after sleeping?

If so, you may have one of the following conditions: facet joint osteoarthritis or mechanical back pain (explained in the thoracic section).

Do you have any of following: burning pain, tingling, pins and needles, numbness, weakness, or coldness? Does the pain follow a line down your leg?

If so, you may have one of the following conditions:

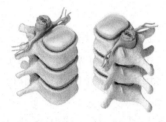

IRRITATED SPINAL NERVES EXITING SPINAL CORD

A nerve can be compressed by a muscle contracture, disc bulge, herniation, or osteophyte growth. The pain travels down into the muscles and tissue relating to the level in the lumbar spine where it is trapped – L1, L2, etc. It can also cause digestive changes and relate to neck issues, and the pain can also track down into the groin. Problems at the lumbar 2 and 3 disc level could be mistaken for groin and hip problems, and you can feel numbness in your upper leg in the front of your thigh.

L4/5 can give you pain caused by numbness in your ankle, and if the compression is chronic, you can see hair loss in the specific skin area (dermatome).

L5/S1 can give big toe pain, and this pain will travel down the back of the leg all the way into the foot. The hamstrings at the back of the thigh can be shortened or in spasm, with the calf muscles being more at risk from injury, and the plantar fascia in the sole of the foot getting tight. Numbness can be felt, or a tingling in the toes and outer aspect of the foot. Pins and needles, numbness, and pain can also occur if a peripheral nerve is affected.

A combination of problems with bladder or bowel, saddle anaesthesia (numbness around the anus), plus weakness in one or both legs, is a rare condition, resulting from a disc pressing on the spinal cord. MRI is very useful in helping to diagnose severe unrelenting pain or repeating episodes. However, bulging discs are very common and only cause a problem if the nerve is trapped.

SCIATICA

If you have sciatica, the most important treatment you can have is to get skilled and early hands-on therapy with Acupuncture – that way, you are more likely to prevent further episodes. Here is what you need to do to help the healing process during your treatment:

- Keep gently active whilst the disc is healing, and avoid activities that stir it up.
- Avoid sitting for long periods of time.
- Swap a chair for a fit ball for some of the time, and a slightly reclined, correctly aligned chair at other times.
- Drink more fluids and set new, small step goals each day.
- Get treatment and discuss this with your therapist/doctor.
- If looking at a new mattress, remember that there is no evidence to say a firm one is better. Get your back fixed before making an expensive mistake. Invest in a good mattress suitable for your weight and age. If you fear your bed is too firm, get a topper.
- If the pain is severe, see your GP for medication.
- If all else fails, a neurosurgeon may need to operate.

Diagnosis is by a pain specialist and physiotherapy assessment, and treatment can include: Gunn IMS, MBST, electro-acupuncture, physiotherapy and manipulation, laser, ultrasound, core stability, and massage.
Do you keep having spinal fractures?

If so, you may have osteoporosis.

OSTEOPOROSIS

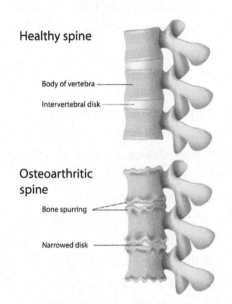

Healthy spine

Body of vertebra

Intervertebral disk

Osteoarthritic spine

Bone spurring

Narrowed disk

Osteoporosis is a silent disease of bone thinning that many people suffer from with no awareness whatsoever until the bones start breaking or crumbling. The pain associated with this condition can be severe and can effectively destroy any quality of life. One in three women and one in twelve men over 50 suffer from osteoporosis. In the UK alone there are three million individuals with osteoporosis, and these suffer from 230,000 breaks a year.

When you get a spinal fracture the pain is band-like, chronic, and over the years it gives you a hunched posture, also known as a dowager's hump. MBST can be used to stimulate the growth of new bone, and this causes the bones to regenerate, becoming thicker and stronger and giving significant pain relief.

Treatment can include: MBST, nutritionist advice, exercise prescription, pain relief treatment such as laser with acupuncture, and meds.

Have you felt a snapping sensation when you bring your knee towards and away from your waist, sometimes with a popping noise and pain, and does the pain reduce with rest?

If so, you may be suffering from snapping hip.

SNAPPING HIP

Snapping hip syndrome is more common in athletes due to repeated strenuous movements of the hip, and it is mainly caused by a tendon catching on a bony prominence and then releasing, much like when you pluck a guitar string.

There are three main causes of snapping hip syndrome:
- The greater trochanter is the bony protrusion you can feel on the side at the top of your leg near the hip joint. The iliotibial band (ITB) is a strong and broad tendon that passes over this area and down to the knee on the outside of the leg. The snapping of the ITB across the greater trochanter is the primary cause of snapping hip.
- The most important muscle for bringing the thigh forward (hip flexor) is the iliopsoas major muscle, which runs from the lower spine inside the torso and then across the front of the hip joint. It can snap across the pelvis, and this condition is also known as 'dancer's hip'.
- Although not so common, the cartilage in the hip joint can sometimes tear, causing noise as the hip moves.

Diagnosis is by physiotherapy assessment, ultrasound scan, MRI, or biomechanical assessment, and treatment can include: physiotherapy, strengthening and stretching rehab, shockwave, corticosteroid injection, and if non-resolving, surgery.

Do you get brief, sudden pain down the front of your thigh, or sudden twinges with your leg giving way, meaning you are unable to walk for a while?

It can just be increasing knee stiffness and pain, but you may have the following:

LOOSE BODY

The top of the shin bone (tibia) has a coating of cartilage, as well as two meniscal cups for the long thigh bone (femur) to move in. The menisci have a number of important roles in the function on the knee, such as spreading the load across the top of the shin bone (tibia), plus helping to both absorb shocks and stabilise the knee.

The lateral meniscus is less prone to tearing than the medial meniscus, and this tends to occur with twisting while weight bearing, which is common in many sports. Aggravating factors include aging, as much of the body's connective tissue becomes more rigid and less elastic with age, and typical symptoms include significant pain if the knee is rotated or if a sudden load increase occurs, as in jumping.

The menisci have poor blood supply and often will not heal. In cases where conservative treatment does not work, surgery is indicated with either repair or removal of the torn tissue. Recovery times will vary widely depending on the grade of the injury, and could be up to several months.

Diagnosis is by physiotherapy assessment and MRI, and treatment can include: RICE, physiotherapy, gentle specific rehab, knee brace, TENS, laser, ultrasound, sports massage, mobilisations, and if deemed necessary, a surgeon referral.

Do you get pain in the buttocks, for no apparent reason? Does walking make it worse?

If so, you may have one of the following conditions:

GLUTEAL BURSITIS

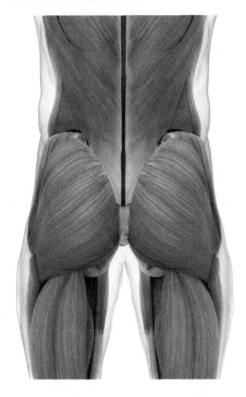

Gluteal bursitis causes pain on the side of the hip, making it uncomfortable to cross your legs or walk up the stairs. Pain from gluteal bursitis can be worse in the morning, and sitting a lot can irritate the condition further.

Diagnosis is by physiotherapy assessment, X-rays to rule out osteoarthritis, and MRI, and treatment can include: ultrasound, pulsed shortwave, massage, ice, physiotherapy, and corticosteroid injection.

The vertebrae in the spine are connected to each other via the disc and two facet joints, one on each side, and the facet joints have cartilage and synovial fluid to lubricate them, allowing for low friction movement. Osteoarthritis in the facet joints can lead to cartilage loss, inflammation in the synovial fluid, bone on bone contact, and bony spurs, all of which can contribute to the pain and stiffness typically felt. Symptoms tend to be worse after inactivity and then improve as activity is underway, as the movement helps lubricate the joint. Activity throughout the day tends to bring the pain back.

OSTEOARTHRITIS

Osteoarthritis (OA), the most common type of arthritis, is wear and tear in the smooth cartilage that protects the bones in joints, eventually leading to bone erosion, bone spurs, and unsightly bony end thickening. The joint juice – the synovial fluid – swells and becomes inflamed and sticky, and the attacked bone haemorrhages precious calcium. By the time we are 50 years old, 8 out of 10 of us have OA, and by 60, 9 out of 10. Left untreated, OA can have a massive negative impact on quality of life and will eventually need surgery.

Diagnosis is by physiotherapy assessment and X-ray, and treatment options include: physiotherapy, MBST, rehab, and shockwave.

RADICULOPATHY

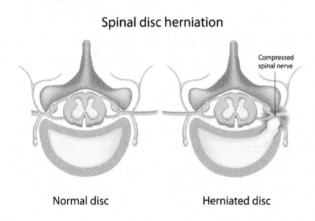

Spinal disc herniation

Compressed spinal nerve

Normal disc   Herniated disc

This describes a nerve problem, but one where the problem lies at the root, close to the spine. Neuropathy is also a nerve problem in which the nerves are not functioning correctly, with typical symptoms including pain, pins and needles, numbness, and muscle weakness. Neuropathic problems can occur as a result of interference with the nerves not at the nerve root, whereas radiculopathy is specifically caused at the nerve root. Thus radiculopathy is one type of neuropathy.

HIP PROBLEMS AND SACRAL ILIAC

Do you get pain slowly developing in the front of your upper thigh for no apparent reason, which has maybe been going on for years? Is it painful if someone tries to push your legs together or twist your leg outwards?

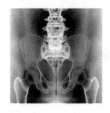

If so, you may have iliopsoas bursitis.

ILIOPSOAS BURSITIS

The Iliopsoas consists of three muscles that lie deep in the body, connecting the lower spine and pelvis to the thigh bone (femur). The Iliopsoas act to flex the hip. The Iliopsoas bursa is the largest in the body and eases friction of the soft tissue over the top of the hip capsule. Iliopsoas bursitis usually occurs with tendinitis of the psoas tendon, and symptoms can include pain that spreads deep into the groin, the front of the hip, down the front of the thigh to the knee, and into the lower back and buttock. These symptoms can sometimes be confused with hip osteoarthritis or rheumatoid arthritis, and the condition can link with snapping hip, trochanteric bursitis, torn hip labrum, lumbar spine and lumbosacral problems, groin injuries, and more.

Diagnosis is by physiotherapy assessment, X-ray, and MRI, and treatment can include: specialised sports physiotherapy, pulsed shortwave, deep tissue massage, Acupuncture, specific rehab strengthening of the hip, pelvis, abdominal muscles and back, stretching out the opposing muscles to take the load off the iliopsoas and stabilise the pelvis, NSAIDs, and corticosteroid injection.

The iliopsoas muscles attach between the lower back and pelvis and into the femur. They move the knee towards the chest and are very active in kicking, hurdling, and running. When the iliopsoas muscles are put under stretch, the fibres are in tension – too much and they fail. The level of iliopsoas strain is graded, and most tend to be grade II:
- Grade I: Small number of fibres torn, some pain, full function.
- Grade II: Significant fibres torn, major loss of function.
- Grade III: All muscle fibres torn/ruptured with major function.

RHEUMATOID ARTHRITIS OF THE HIP

Hip RA can cause symptoms such as severe pain, stiffness, and swelling, and with RA's hip pain, you may have discomfort and stiffness in the thigh and groin very similar to osteoarthritis. However, other symptoms of RA include fatigue, loss of appetite, pain, swelling, and stiffness in other joints, and these can come on gradually or suddenly. Inflammatory, seronegative arthritis occurs when the body's immune system becomes overactive and attacks healthy tissues. It can affect several joints throughout the body at the same time, as well as many organs, such as the skin, eyes, and heart.

There are three types of inflammatory arthritis that most often cause symptoms in the hip joint:
- Rheumatoid arthritis.
- Ankylosing spondylitis.
- Systemic lupus erythematosus.

Although there is no cure for inflammatory arthritis, there have been many advances in treatments to ease the symptoms, particularly with new medications. Early diagnosis and treatment can help patients maintain mobility and function by preventing severe damage to the joint.

RHEUMATOID ARTHRITIS

In rheumatoid arthritis, the synovium thickens, swells, and produces chemical substances that attack and destroy the articular cartilage covering the bone. Rheumatoid arthritis often involves the same joint on both sides of the body, so both hips may be affected.

ANKYLOSING SPONDYLITIS

Ankylosing spondylitis is a chronic inflammation of the spine that most often causes lower back pain and stiffness. It may also affect other joints, including the hips.

SYSTEMIC LUPUS ERYTHEMATOSUS

Systemic lupus erythematosus can cause inflammation in any part of the body, and most often affects the joints, skin, and the nervous system. The disease is most prevalent in young adult women, who have a higher incidence of osteonecrosis (death) of the hip, a disease that causes bone cells to die, weakens the bone structure, and leads to disabling arthritis.

Blood tests may reveal whether a rheumatoid factor – or any other antibody indicative of inflammatory arthritis – is present.

NON-SURGICAL TREATMENT

Most people find that some combination of the following treatment methods works best.

NON-STEROIDAL ANTI-INFLAMMATORY DRUGS (NSAIDS)

Drugs such as Naproxen and Ibuprofen may relieve pain and help reduce inflammation. NSAIDs are available in both over-the-counter and prescription forms.

CORTICOSTEROIDS

Medications such as Prednisone are potent anti-inflammatories. They can be taken by mouth, by injection, or as creams.

DISEASE-MODIFYING ANTIRHEUMATIC DRUGS (DMARDS)

These drugs act on the immune system to help slow down the progression of disease. Methotrexate and Sulfasalazine are commonly prescribed DMARDs.

PHYSICAL THERAPY

Specific exercises help increase the range of motion in your hip and strengthen the muscles that support the joint. Acupuncture, laser, and massage can ease the pain, and in addition, regular, moderate exercise may decrease stiffness and improve endurance. Swimming is a preferred exercise for people with ankylosing spondylitis because spinal motion may be limited.

ASSISTIVE DEVICES

This can include using a cane, a walker, a long-handled shoehorn, or a reacher.

SURGICAL TREATMENT FOR RA HIP

If non-surgical treatments do not sufficiently relieve your pain, your doctor may recommend surgery, and the type of surgery performed depends on several factors, including: your age, the hip damage, disease, and severity. The most common surgical procedures performed for inflammatory arthritis of the hip include total hip replacement and synovectomy (the removal of the synovium/lining).

TOTAL HIP REPLACEMENT

The surgeon will remove the damaged cartilage and bone, and then position new metal or plastic joint surfaces in order to restore the function of your hip. Total hip replacement is often recommended for patients with rheumatoid arthritis or ankylosing spondylitis to relieve the pain and improve their range of motion.

Do you have a severe stabbing pain in your hip, upper buttock, front of the thigh, your knee, and sometimes down to your ankle?

If so, you may have radiculopathy (see the spine section).

Do you have a dull pain in your lower back, one or both buttocks, and possibly your groin, radiating sometimes to your feet? Is it uncomfortable to put one cheek on a chair?

If so, you may have sacroiliac joint dysfunction.

SACROILIAC JOINT DYSFUNCTION

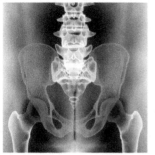

The sacroiliac joint is a very strong joint that lies at the junction between the sacrum of the spine and the pelvis – it is almost immobile and is key to load transference. Sacroiliac joint dysfunction can be due to leg length discrepancy, injury, or pregnancy.

Finding out if the sacroiliac joint is inflamed is not easy, as it can hardly move, and it is difficult to palpate or manipulate. X-rays and MRI scans can read as normal, and both the hip and lower back can refer pain here.

Diagnosis is by physiotherapy assessment or biomechanical assessment, and treatment can include: mobilisations, physiotherapy, exercises, Acupuncture, orthotics, and corticosteroid injection.

Do you have groin pain? Does lifting a straight leg, doing sit-ups, or coughing make it worse?

If so, you may have a hernia.

HERNIA

A hernia is a protrusion through a weakened wall, and there are many types of hernia affecting the stomach, abdominal organs and tissue, and groin. The most common are abdominal hernias, where adipose tissue or abdominal organs can push through, whereas hiatal are when the stomach protrudes, and inguinal hernias can be found in the groin. Men may experience a dragging feeling, or pain and swelling in the testicles. Spinal discs can also become herniated.

Hernia symptoms can include a vague pain with a palpable lump, and strangulated hernias can cause vomiting, fever, and severe pain. There

362

are numerous causes of hernias, some of which require surgery, though this varies greatly according to the size and location of the hernia, and the techniques involved. If the procedure is done with keyhole surgery, the recovery time is much faster. Muscle reinforcement techniques used with synthetic mesh are called tension free repairs, and results from the use of synthetic mesh show a lower reoccurrence of herniation and a faster recovery, though there are higher recorded levels of chronic pain, infection, and rejection. Conservative recovery can sometimes be successful with weight loss, gentle muscle toning, and avoiding strenuous activities.

Diagnosis is by your GP or sports physiotherapy exam and a CT scan, and the treatment can include weight loss, gentle rehab and exercises, and surgery.

Do you have hip pain and a reduced range of movement, plus clicking on movement? Is it difficult to flex or rotate the joint?

Do you have a locking, clicking, or catching sensation in your hip joint, plus pain in your hip/groin with stiffness in your hip joint?

If so, you may have a hip labral tear.

HIP LABRAL TEAR

A hip labral tear can happen without any symptoms, and only MRI – ideally using a dye – can diagnose this. It basically involves the ring of cartilage (called the labrum) that follows the outside rim of the socket of your hip joint. The labrum acts like a rubber seal or gasket to help hold the ball at the top of your thighbone securely within your hip socket. Athletes who participate in such sports as ice hockey, soccer, football, golf, and ballet are at a higher risk of developing a hip labral tear. Structural abnormalities of the hip can also lead to a hip labral tear, such as Perthes' hip – a misshapen head of femur that you are born with.

LABRAL TEAR

The hip labrum is a cartilage ring that deepens the hip socket by adding a rim, allowing flexibility and motion. A labral tear has two main causes:
- Degenerative, due to overuse. This can be seen in early osteoarthritis.
- Acute trauma in association with dislocation, and common with sudden twisting actions.

Labral tears are difficult to diagnose as they are similar to hernias, snapping hip syndrome, and bursitis, and although a labrum is torn, this does not necessarily mean that it is the cause of the symptoms. Typical symptoms include groin pain, clicking in the hip, and limited movement of the hip joint.

Arthroscopic techniques – which were developed for hips in the 1990's – awakened an interest in labral tears, and reattachment of labral tears through surgery is now showing good results with athletes.

Provisional diagnosis is by physiotherapy assessment, then MRI with dye to distinguish pathology. If a labral tear is suspected, treatment can include an orthopaedic assessment, rehabilitation, physiotherapy, MRT, and possibly (in rare instances) surgery with a scope. With orthopaedic surgery and post-op physiotherapy rehab, recovery is typically six to 12 weeks.

Do you have *hip pain on walking or running? Does your hip feel tender and warm over the bony bump on the side of your hip? Is it sore to lie on?*

If so, you may have trochanteric bursitis.

TROCHANTERIC BURSITIS

The bursa sits over the outer side of the hip, located where you have a palpable bony prominence, the greater trochanter. Because the bursa lies between fascia and muscles, a **trochanteric bursitis** diagnosis can be unclear, especially as there is no obvious cause for it. Local trauma, osteoarthritis, and hip replacement, however, are candidates. In rare cases the bursa is surgically removed, followed by a six-week recovery period with physiotherapy.

Provisional diagnosis is by physiotherapy assessment, X-ray to rule out bony pathology, and ultrasound to diagnose. Treatment can include: RICE, pulsed shortwave, Acupuncture, physiotherapy, graded exercises, and corticosteroid injection.

Do you have hip pain, which increases on movement or loading? It is difficult to walk and are you stiff after rest or sleep?

Do you experience joint stiffness that occurs as you are getting out of bed, or joint stiffness after you sit for a long time? Do you have any pain, swelling, or tenderness in the hip joint, or a sound or feeling ('crunching') of bone rubbing against bone?

If so, you may have hip osteoarthritis.

HIP OSTEOARTHRITIS

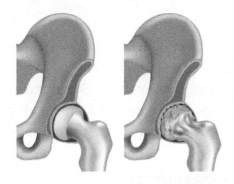

Healthy hip joint   Osteoarthritis

This occurs when inflammation and injury to a joint cause a breaking down of cartilage tissue. In turn, that breakdown causes pain, swelling, and deformity. Cartilage is a firm, elastic coating that covers the ends of bones in healthy joints, made up of water and proteins. The function of cartilage is to reduce friction in the joint and serve as a 'shock absorber', and the shock-absorbing quality of normal cartilage comes from its ability to change shape when compressed. It can do this because of its high water content. Although cartilage may undergo some repair when damaged, the body does not grow new cartilage after it is injured, and its ability to do this declines with age as well.

You're most likely to feel pain deep at the front of your groin, but also at the side and front of your thigh, in your buttock, or down to your knee (this is called radiated pain). If you have severe hip osteoarthritis, you may find that your affected leg seems a little shorter than the other because of the bone on either side of your joint being crunched up due to muscle spasms. Men and women are equally likely to develop hip osteoarthritis, and it can start from your late 40's onwards. You may be at greater risk if you had hip problems at birth (congenital dislocation), or abnormal hip development in childhood, such as Perthes' disease. Physical work and obesity may also increase the risk, but there's often no clear cause.

Your doctor may arrange X-rays or other tests – including <u>blood</u> tests and examination of the fluid in the joints – usually to eliminate other <u>types of arthritis</u>. He or she may also recommend a special type of X-ray where dye is injected into the hip joint (known as an arthrogram), or an MRI or CT scan. Treatment can involve: losing excess weight, <u>exercise</u> prescription, physiotherapy with mobilisation techniques, MRT to help repair the joint, pulsed shortwave, Acupuncture, Gunn IMS assessment for spinal involvement, gait analysis to check footwear, and possibly a stick or Nordic poles to walk with.

Medicines prescribed may include Paracetamol, a non-steroidal anti-inflammatory medicine such as Ibuprofen, or a prescription pain medication. These treatments mostly control pain and inflammation. Surgery may be needed for a resurfacing or total hip replacement if Grade 4. For complementary and alternative therapies, see www.arthritisresearchuk.org.

AVASCULAR NECROSIS OF THE FEMORAL HEAD

Avascular necrosis is a disease in which a lack or interruption of blood supply leads to cellular death within hours (necrosis). One of the more common sites for avascular necrosis is at the head of the thigh bone (femur), resulting from the death of the bone cells which are responsible for breaking down and rebuilding all bones. Avascular necrosis of the femoral head affects the hip joint and will not only damage the bone, but also the articular surfaces of the joint (osteochondritis dissecans).

Avascular necrosis is most common in the middle aged – typically 30 to 50 years old – and the preferred treatment for the hip is resurfacing, as hip replacements do not have sufficient longevity for anyone other than older patients. An alternative is drug therapy to promote bone building. Many proposed causes for avascular necrosis are being investigated, though rheumatoid arthritis and lupus are known ones. Sports trauma can also upset the blood supply and create this problem, for example, in water-skiing. Trauma is caused by extreme dislocation of the hip, where the ball of the hip joint is dislodged from the socket (subluxation).

Symptoms of avascular necrosis of the femoral head include pain in the lateral hip, groin, buttock, or knee, which is made worse by weight bearing. Hip movements are especially sore when the leg is rotated inwards (medial rotation).

Provisional diagnosis is by physiotherapy assessment, MRI, bone scan, and scope, and treatment includes: surgeon opinion, physiotherapy, MBST, nutrition, and hip replacement.

Do you have hip stiffness? Is it worse after rest or sleep?

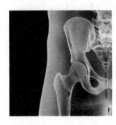

If so, you may have:

TROCHANTERIC BURSITIS

The bursa sits over the outer side of the hip, located where you have a palpable bony prominence, the greater trochanter. Because the bursa lies between fascia and muscle tendons, a trochanteric bursitis diagnosis can be unclear, especially as there is no obvious cause for trochanteric bursitis. Local trauma, osteoarthritis, and hip replacement, however, are candidates.

In rare cases the bursa is surgically removed, followed by a six-week recovery period with physiotherapy.

Provisional diagnosis is by physiotherapy assessment, X-ray to rule out bony pathology, and ultrasound to diagnose. Treatment can include: RICE, pulsed shortwave, Acupuncture, physiotherapy, graded exercises, and corticosteroid injection.

Do you have pain down one or both legs to the foot? Is sitting painful? Do you find it helps to roll one buttock off the seat?

If so, you may have piriformis syndrome.

PIRIFORMIS SYNDROME

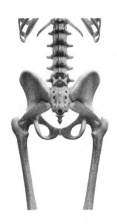

The piriformis muscle sits below the gluteus muscles in the bottom and runs across the sciatic nerve. In about 10% of the population, the sciatic nerve runs through the piriformis, and if the piriformis goes into spasm, it is prone to irritate the sciatic nerve and give typical sciatica symptoms in the affected leg of pain, pins and needles, and tenderness. The piriformis muscle tends to go into spasm due to nerve irritation in the lumbar spine, or problems in the hip joint.

Provisional diagnosis is by physiotherapy assessment, and treatment can include: Gunn IMS, electro-acupuncture, shockwave, and physiotherapy.

Do you have an ache in the front of your thigh and groin, which gets worse with activity? (This is most likely in athletes).

If so, you may have iliopsoas strain.

ILIOPSOAS STRAIN

The iliopsoas (IP) muscles attach between the lower back and the pelvis and into the femur. They move the knee towards the chest and are very active in kicking, hurdling, and running. When the iliopsoas muscles are put under stretch, the fibres are in tension – too much and they fail. The level of iliopsoas strain is graded and most tend to be grade II:

- Grade I: Small number of fibres torn, some pain, full function.
- Grade II: Significant fibres torn, major loss of function.
- Grade III: All muscle fibres torn/ruptured with major function loss.

Diagnosis is by sports physiotherapy assessment, and treatment can include: physiotherapy, specific sports massage and stretching, then rehab to work towards a neutral pelvis.

Do you have pain at the base of your buttocks, which gets worse on sprinting and stretching?

If so, you may have a hamstring strain.

HAMSTRING STRAIN

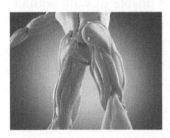 Hamstring strains are common amongst sprinters, long jumpers, and hurdlers, as well as in sports where hard sprinting is required, such as football or hockey, and aging increases the risk. Most of the injuries occur in the biceps femoris muscle, especially during sprinting. Injuries occur just before foot strike. Hamstring tendinitis can occur at either end of the three muscles where the hamstring tendons attach to the bone.

The hamstrings are comprised of three posterior thigh muscles: semimembranosus, semitendinosus, and biceps femoris, and they span the thigh from the ischial tuberosity at the bottom of the pelvis, to attach below the knee. They connect by tendon to the tibia and fibula below the knee and ischial tuberosity. At the top (proximal), the hamstrings attach to the bottom of the pelvis at the ischial tuberosity. The odd man out is the biceps femoris, where only one head attaches to the ischial tuberosity and the other head attaches to the femur. For this reason, the rectus femoris tends to be injured the most frequently. The hamstrings extend the hip and flex the knee, and while they are not active in normal walking or standing, they come into their own in running, jumping, and climbing. Athletes depend on healthy, well-conditioned hamstrings.

There are three grades of strain:
- Grade I: Minor strain with some pain, though the individual may be able to continue sport. Use ice, compression bandage, and massage, and get assessed by a sports physio – you may need to rest from sport for up to three weeks. With grade I, gentle jogging at seven days is fine, and fast sprinting by three weeks.
- Grade II: There is immediate pain which is more severe than the pain of a grade I injury, and it is confirmed by pain upon the stretch and contraction of the muscle. It can be also felt with a 'ping' feeling, like elastic in the muscle. You may be out of your sport from four to six weeks depending on the treatment you receive.
- Grade III: Hamstring strain is a severe injury. There is an immediate burning or stabbing pain and the athlete is unable to walk without pain. The muscle is completely torn and there may be a large lump of muscle tissue above a depression where the tear is. You will need crutches or sticks to walk initially, then when walking any distance, and you may need to take up to three months off the aggravating activity. Three months of sports rehab, massage, and treatment will be needed, and surgery if severe.

After a few days with grade II and III injuries, a large bruise may appear below the injury site, caused by the bleeding within the tissues. Grade III will need intensive icing every two hours for twenty minutes, elevate, rest, and a compression bandage. After about five days, you can start active rehab.

With all grades, as soon as pain permits, it is important to begin a prescribed program of stretching and range-of-motion exercises. Your sports therapist/physiotherapist will help you avoid prolonged inactivity resulting in muscle shrinkage (atrophy) and scar tissue (fibrosis). Excessive scar tissue is incompatible with healthy muscle function, and atrophy and scarring (fibrosis) are best avoided or reduced by prescribed exercise and stretching early in the rehabilitation process. This can be followed by massage and shockwave, then a graded rehab program return to sport encourages the tissue to stay pliable.

Rehab needs to include sprinting, as the hamstrings work hard to decelerate the lower leg as it swings out. It is in this phase – just before the foot hits the floor – that the hamstrings have to remain injury free, as they are maximally activated at maximum length.

As strength returns, resistance exercise is increased and Therabands can be useful. This is closely followed by core work. Fit ball work is great for stability, as both the trunk and pelvis get more stable, and sporting drills can follow the core stability training.

HAMSTRING TENDINITIS

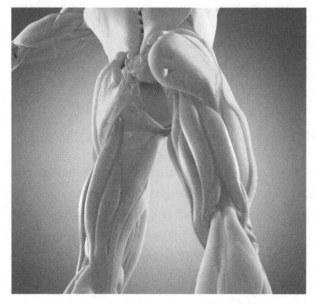

Hamstring tendinitis can occur at either end of the three muscles where the hamstring tendons attach to bone. The hamstrings are comprised of three posterior thigh muscles: semimembranosus, semitendinosus, and biceps femoris, and they span the thigh from the ischial tuberosity at the bottom of the pelvis, to attach below the knee. They connect by tendon to the tibia and fibula below the knee and ischial tuberosity. At the top (proximal), the hamstrings attach to the bottom of the pelvis at the ischial tuberosity. The odd man out is the biceps femoris, where only one head attaches to the ischial tuberosity and the other head attaches to the femur. For this reason, the rectus femoris tends to be injured the most frequently. The hamstrings extend the hip and flex the knee, and while they are not active in normal walking or standing, they come into their own in running, jumping, and climbing. Athletes depend on healthy, well-conditioned hamstrings.

It will hurt to stretch, pull, and sprint, and it can follow an unhealed tear or repetitive overuse. Your sports therapist will advise on RICE, stretching, and strengthening, and advice on a full rehab program is important. Massage and shockwave will also help to reduce scar tissue. Occasionally, hamstring syndrome occurs, where fibrous adhesions irritate the sciatic nerve as it passes above the ischial tuberosity. If shockwave cannot help, surgery may be needed.

Diagnosis is by physiotherapy assessment and ultrasound scan, and treatment can include: RICE, shockwave, and strengthening and stretching with massage.

Do you have pain inside your hip or pelvis, or up to your back? When lifting your knee or stretching your hip, does it gets worse?

If so, you may have ischiogluteal bursitis.

ISCHIOGLUTEAL BURSITIS

The ischiogluteal bursa sits between the ischial tuberosity, at the base of the pelvis, and the hamstring muscles. It mimics hamstring problems – similar to hamstring tendonitis – and may come on after a lot of sprinting. Once a bursa becomes swollen and inflamed, it can make it difficult to move the joint, and a tell tale sign of bursitis is worsening symptoms after massage, and improvement with cooling. A common cause is a fall, and occasionally crystal deposits due to gout or infection.

Provisional diagnosis is by physiotherapy assessment, and for conformation, MRI, and treatment can include: rest from the aggravating activity, physiotherapy, and pulsed shortwave.

Have you had an injury to your upper anterior thigh that hasn't got better?

If so, it could be a quads strain at the attachment onto the pelvis.

QUADS STRAIN (NEAR HIP)

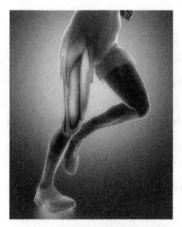 The rectus femoris central tendon inserts at the pelvis in two locations, the direct and the indirect head. The indirect head is deeper, and flattens and rotates before it blends into the rectus femoris muscle at the central tendon. Injuries in this area are thought to occur due to the two parts acting independently, resulting in a shearing at the central tendon. Symptoms can eventually become apparent months after the injury, and recovery time with a comprehensive rehab program can be three to six times longer than a normal quads muscle strain.

Diagnosis is by physiotherapy assessment, with MRI to confirm, and treatment can include: RICE, massage, physiotherapy, shockwave, and prescribed exercise and stretching.

Has the belly of your quads felt tender and weak for a long time, and has it been painful to run and kick?

If so, you may have quadriceps strain.

QUADRICEPS STRAIN

The quads comprise of four muscles: rectus femoris, vastus lateralis, vastus intermedius, and vastus medialis. These muscles cause hip flexion and knee extension, and they arise from the pelvis and femur (thigh bone) and insert via the patella tendon on the tibia (shin bone). Only the rectus femoris attaches above the hip joint into the pelvis, and as a result, is far more vulnerable to injury.

Strains are graded in the usual way: mild, moderate, and complete tear. The usual symptom is immediate pain, and depending on the severity of the strain, swelling and bruising can also occur. The location of the injury can sometimes be felt – a complete tear may feel like a hole.

It is important not to stress the area and to control swelling as quickly as possible. The injury will heal in time – typically in two to six weeks, depending on the severity of the injury. Management of the scar tissue formation is important to regain full capability. In some cases, a strain can occur deep in the rectus femoris muscle, which will require significantly longer rehab.

Diagnosis is by sports physiotherapy assessment, and MRI if severe, and treatment can include: RICE, maintaining exercise by cycling (if not painful), sports massage, ultrasound, laser, and sports specific rehab.

Have you felt a sudden onset of pain – possibly a swelling in your thigh – most likely after a sprint start, rapid change of direction, jumping, or martial arts kick? Have you had traumatic pain to your inner thigh, and if you try to close your legs against resistance, is it too sore?

If so, you may have adductor longus strain, or rider's strain.

ADDUCTOR LONGUS STRAIN

The adductors are located on the inside of the thigh and act to close the legs together. Adductor longus strain is common in football, hockey, tennis, horse riding, and karate, and it tends to happen when the athlete needs to quickly change direction and the adductors are subjected to high forces, such as in a football tackle where an adducting foot is about to kick the ball and meets an opponent's leg. This type of strain is responsible for 62% of groin injuries.

Diagnosis is by physiotherapy assessment and treatment can include: physiotherapy, shockwave, massage, and if acute, ultrasound and pulsed shortwave. Recovery can be lengthy – up to five months.

Have you had a bruising injury some months ago? Do you now feel a bony lump there?

If so, you may have myositis ossificans.

MYOSITIS OSSIFICANS

This is an uncommon condition in which bone is formed inside an injured muscle. Many sports are prone to muscle injury – such as football, rugby, martial arts, and hockey – and these injuries can lead to heavy internal bleeding, evident as bruising and swelling, and can also result in a blood clot, which is an ideal breeding ground for calcification. Left untreated, the calcification can continue to develop and may take over much of the injured site over several months.

The key to prevent myositis ossificans – or the growth of bone by calcification within the injured muscle – is to seek treatment as early as possible after the injury. Once formed, the bone can only be removed surgically and the current guidelines advise waiting up to 12 months to minimise the risk of further bone growth post-surgery. The cause of myositis ossificans is not understood, and there *is* a risk of further bone growth post-surgery.

Diagnosis is by physiotherapy assessment, X-ray to confirm the diagnosis, and checks to confirm it is non-malignant. Treatment can include: drugs to relieve the symptoms, and surgery.

Have you suffered a blow to the front mid high (quads)? Are the muscles swollen and sore?

If so, you may have quadriceps contusion, or 'dead leg'.

DEAD LEG

There are three grades of contusion, and grades I and II are commonly known as 'dead leg':
- Grade I: The thigh will feel tight and mildly uncomfortable on walking or extending the knee.
- Grade II: You will be unable to run or walk quickly, and unable to bend the knee fully.
- Grade III: A muscle tear with severe pain, you will be unable to walk without crutches or contract muscles. You will be out of competition for six to 12 weeks.

The quads comprise of four muscles: rectus femoris, vastus lateralis, vastus intermedius, and vastus medialis. These muscles cause hip flexion and knee extension, and they arise from the pelvis and femur (thigh bone) and insert via the patella tendon on the tibia (shin bone). The quads are easily kicked in contact sports, sometimes leading to a severe bruise or tear (grouped as contusion) that can take weeks or months to heal. A quads contusion can be swollen, sore, and bruised.

A contusion injury results in a crushing force on your muscle tissue, and the body's protective response is to wall-off the area of damage from the unaffected muscle in order to prevent damaging chemicals – released due to the injury – from further damaging more muscle. This results in an overall decrease in the oxygen to the surrounding tissue. This walling-off causes stiffness, creating an internal splint to prevent further injury and slowing down healing. Repeated overuse causes microscopic soft tissue failure, inflammation, and rupture. Healing involves inflammatory cells, macrophages clearing necrotic cells, and muscle cells regeneration.

Treatment can include: physiotherapy, ultrasound, pulsed shortwave, light massage, and gentle prescribed rehab.

Do you have localised pain at the back of your thigh?
Does it hurt to bend your knee against resistance, and does it feel weak?
Do your hamstrings feel tight when you stretch them?
If so, you may have hamstring strain.

HAMSTRING STRAIN

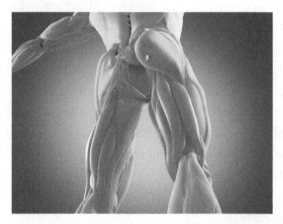

Tight hamstrings, SI joint dysfunction, and lumbar spine radiculopathy all have to be assessed in order to confirm hamstring strain; just because the hamstrings may feel tight, they may not be short and therefore stretching does not always help. The brain feels tightness as a signal that something is wrong; it cannot perceive shortness in length. Therefore, overstretched muscles can feel tight, and the problem could be coming from the lower back, from the pelvis, or from the sciatic nerve. Back problems can cause short hamstrings and vice versa – lots of sitting or driving without core stability can cause this. You need to have a rehab stretching program specific to you and your sporting needs.

Diagnosis is by sports therapist/physiotherapy assessment.

The hamstring muscles run down the back of the thigh, and there are three of them:

Pulled Hamstring

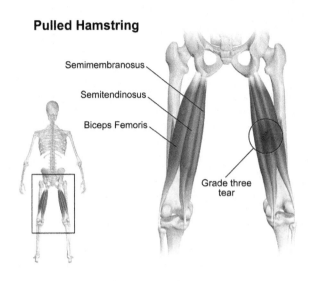

- Semitendinosus
- Semimembranosus
- Biceps femoris

They start at the bottom of the pelvis at a place called the ischial tuberosity, crossing at the knee joint and ending at the lower leg. Hamstring muscle fibres join with the tough, connective fascia of the hamstring tendons attaching to bones. The hamstring muscle group helps you extend your leg straight back, as well as bending your knee.

During a hamstring strain, one or more of these muscles gets overloaded, and the muscles might even start to tear. You're likely to get a hamstring strain during activities that involve a lot of running and jumping, or sudden stopping and starting. The three grades of hamstring injury are:

- Grade I: A mild muscle strain.
- Grade II: A partial muscle tear.
- Grade III: A complete muscle tear.

The length of time it takes to recover from a hamstring strain or tear will depend on how severe the injury is. A minor muscle pull (grade I) may take a few days to heal, whereas it could take weeks or even months to recover from a muscle tear (grade II or III).

Getting a hamstring strain is also more likely if:

- You don't warm up before exercising.
- The muscles in the front of your thigh (the quadriceps) are tight as they pull your pelvis forward and tighten the hamstrings.
- You have weak glutes (bottom muscles). Glutes and hamstrings work

together; if the glutes are weak, the hamstrings can be overloaded and become strained.

Treatment can include the following:

- Avoid putting weight on the leg as best you can. If the pain is severe, you may need crutches until it goes away – ask your doctor or physio if they're needed.
- ICE: Ice your leg to reduce pain and swelling. Do it for 20 minutes every four hours for two to three days, or until the pain is gone. Compress your leg. Use an elastic bandage around the leg to keep down swelling. Elevate your leg on a pillow when you're sitting or lying down.
- Take anti-inflammatory painkillers and painkillers from your pharmacist or GP. Non-steroidal anti-inflammatory drugs (NSAIDs) – like Ibuprofen or Naproxen – will help with pain and swelling. However, these drugs may have side effects, such as an increased risk of bleeding and ulcers. They should only be used short-term, unless your doctor specifically says otherwise.
- Practice stretching and strengthening exercises if your doctor/physical therapist recommends them. Strengthening your hamstrings is one way to protect against hamstring strain.
- Sports massage, shockwave, stretching, and rehab will all help to speed up recovery.

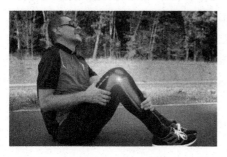

Are you unable to move your knee after a sudden trauma? Is the joint deformed, swollen, and cannot bear weight?

If so, you may have a dislocated knee.

DISLOCATED KNEE

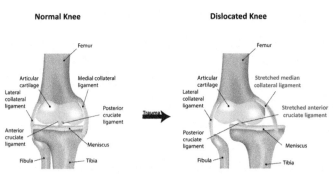

Dislocation of the Knee

Normal Knee

Dislocated Knee

This is a serious injury, and it describes the situation when the thigh bone (femur) loses all contact with the lower leg bones (the tibia and fibula). For this to happen there is usually substantial damage to the tissues around the knee, often including complete tearing of the cruciate ligaments (ACL & PCL), plus damage to the collateral ligaments and menisci, so it has the potential to cause significant damage to important vascular (blood) vessels and nerves. Immediate attention is required as this injury can lead to the loss of the leg.

After repositioning the knee, ongoing surveillance of the nerves and blood vessels may be needed, and due to the level of damage, surgical reconstruction is usually required.

Diagnosis is by physiotherapy assessment, X-ray, and MRI, with urgent medical attention needed. Treatment can include: having the joint repositioned by a medical practitioner, gentle progressive physiotherapy, having your blood vessels and nerves monitored, thorough rehab for mobility, balance, and strength, and possible surgery.

Did you have a blow to the outside of your knee? Is your foot weak when you lift it to walk?

Do you have a tingling/numbness on the outside of your leg?

If so, you may have peroneal nerve injury or radiculopathy (see spinal section).

380

PERONEAL NERVE INJURY

The peroneal nerve branches off from the sciatic nerve and is responsible for innervating the muscles that raise the foot and toes. Damage to the nerve can thus lead to spontaneous foot drop or weakness in lifting the foot. Other symptoms include a tingling or numbness on the outside of the lower leg, and pain down the shin or the top of the foot.

Diagnosis is by EMG tests, orthopaedic surgeon, or a back specialist.

Peroneal nerve injuries have a poor chance of recovery, worsening with time, so it is cimportant to be assessed quickly by a specialist who can determine whether to proceed with surgery or go down a more conservative route – typical conservative options include physiotherapy and orthotics.

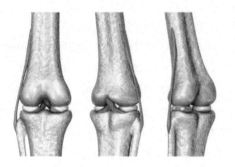

Did you have a sudden onset of localised acute pain on the inner side of your knee, which is painful after a twisting injury and is still mildly painful when touched?

If so, you may have a medial coronary ligament.

MEDIAL CORONARY LIGAMENT

The top of the shin bone (tibia) has a coating of cartilage, with two meniscal cups for the long thigh bone (femur) to move in. The medial meniscus is attached at the medial, lower edge to the tibia by the medial coronary ligament, and the lateral meniscus is attached at the lateral, lower edge to the tibia by the lateral coronary ligament. These ligaments act to stabilise the menisci and help limit knee rotation injury to the coronary ligaments.

Injury is most likely to occur with sudden, sharp direction changes, especially when the foot is planted securely, forcing a rotation of the lower leg (tibia) relative to the thigh (femur). Such injuries are common in football, rugby, tennis, squash, dancing, and martial arts, and aggravating factors include poor biomechanics and laxity in the four major stabilising knee ligaments (ACL, PCL, MCL, and LCL). Injury can be from acute trauma – which normally causes immediate, sharp pain – or chronic overuse, such as from long distance running.

Diagnosis is by physiotherapy assessment and possibly scope, and the medial coronary ligament usually heals conservatively.

Do you have a golf ball-shaped swelling at the back of your knee?

If so, you may have a popliteal cyst.

POPLITEAL CYST

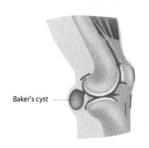

Baker's cyst

This is also known as a baker's cyst. Irritation to the knee can be caused by a number of factors, such as osteoarthritis and rheumatoid arthritis, biomechanical problems, and meniscal tears. Any form of irritation can lead to swelling due to excess synovial fluid production, and if this causes sufficient pressure, it can lead to a cyst forming at the back of the knee. The cyst may or may not cause pain and/or restricted range of knee motion.

Assessment is important in order to differentiate from a tumour or deep vein thrombosis. Diagnosis is by physiotherapy assessment to find the cause – possibly osteoarthritis or a cartilage leak – and treatment can include: RICE (depending on the cause) and occasionally surgery.

Do you have a gradual onset of knee pain on the inner side, plus limited range of movement, especially when it comes to bending? Is the knee stiff on rest?

If so, you may have osteoarthritis, and you are more likely to suffer from this if:

- **You're in your late 40s or older** – your muscles have become weaker, your body is less able to heal itself, and your knee joints have gradually worn out over time.
- **You're a woman** – osteoarthritis is more common and more severe in women.
- **You're overweight** – this increases the chances of osteoarthritis and of it becoming gradually worse.
- **Your parents or siblings have had osteoarthritis.**
- **You've had a knee injury** – for example, a torn meniscus.
- **You've had an operation on your knee** – for example, a meniscectomy (to remove damaged cartilage) or repairs to your cruciate ligaments.
- **You do a repetitive activity or have a hard, physically demanding job,** like a physio.
- **You have another type of joint disease** that has damaged your joints – for example, rheumatoid arthritis or gout.
- See more at: http://www.arthritisresearchuk.org/arthritis.

Main symptoms can include pain (in the knee, or at the end of the day – this usually gets better when you rest), stiffness (especially after rest – this eases as you get moving), crepitus (a creaking, crunching, grinding sensation when you move the joint), hard swellings (caused by osteophytes, calcified bony growths), and soft swellings (caused by extra fluid in the joint). Other symptoms can include: your knee giving way because your muscles have become weak or the joint structure is less stable, your knee not moving as freely or as far as normal, your knees becoming bent and bowed, the muscles around your joint looking thin or wasted, and the joint looking thickened.

It's unusual, but some people have pain in their knee that wakes them up at night. This generally only happens with severe osteoarthritis – Grade III or IV. You'll probably find that your pain will vary, with good days and bad days. This can be due to how active you've been, but sometimes it will just happen for no clear reason.

Some people find that changes in the weather (especially damp weather and low barometric pressure) make their pain and stiffness worse, and this may be because nerve fibres in the capsule of their knee are sensitive to changes in atmospheric pressure.

RHEUMATOID ARTHRITIS

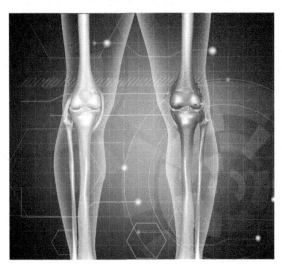

Rheumatoid arthritis is an inflammatory disease that can strike at any age. When arthritis develops following an injury to the knee, it is called post-traumatic arthritis, and this can occur years after a torn meniscus, injury to ligament, or fracture of the knee. Some types of arthritis can also cause fatigue.

Rheumatoid arthritis (RA) is a systemic disease of the immune system, affecting multiple joints in the upper as well as the lower limbs. Knees are one of the most common joints affected by RA, which can occur at any age and which can affect both knees. When RA affects the knee joint, the synovium that lines the ends of the bones thickens and produces an excess of joint juice – it is said to feel like a crisp packet. The immune system supplies inflammatory juices, leading to swelling and damage to the cartilage that normally acts as a cushion within the joint. This then leads to pain and joint erosion.

Symptoms of RA mostly include pain and stiffness of the affected joints, and the pain is more often than not worse in the mornings, a time that is associated with severe stiffness. The joint may become stiff and swollen, making it difficult to bend or straighten the knee, and pain and stiffness is also at its worst after a period of inactivity. The knee may feel weak, it may feel 'locked', or it may 'buckle' as a result of this disease. Due to inflammation, blood tests such as C-reactive protein and erythrocyte sedimentation rate (ESR) may be raised. These are, however, non-specific markers of inflammation as it is not straight forward to diagnose. Rheumatoid factor is a relatively specific test, and there is presence of this indicative factor in nearly 80% of all rheumatoid arthritis sufferers. Presence of rheumatoid factor may NOT be detected in early stages of the disease. In addition, just to really f*** up the diagnosis, around 1 in 20 healthy persons may test positive for rheumatoid factor (RF), hence RF is not absolutely indicative of rheumatoid arthritis.

Several imaging studies such as X-rays, MRI scans, and CT scans may be ordered to look at the extent of joint damage caused by the disease; X-rays typically show a loss of joint space in the affected knee. To ease the symptoms, pain relievers and non-steroidal anti-inflammatory drugs (NSAIDs) are used widely to control the symptoms of rheumatoid arthritis. They are, however, notorious for their side effects due to which they may be used for a short-term basis only. A healthy diet and supplements can also help.

To prevent progression of joint damage, disease-modifying anti-rheumatic drugs (DMARDs) are used. They act by reducing joint swelling and pain, decreasing markers of acute inflammation in the blood, and halting the progressive joint damage. DMARDs include Methotrexate, Sulfasalazine, Leflunomide, Hydroxychloroquine, Gold salts and Cyclosporine. However, everything comes with a price and these are also associated with a varying degree of side effects.

CORTICOSTEROIDS

Corticosteroids are anti-inflammatory agents that may be given as medications or as injections directly into the joint spaces in order to reduce the joint inflammation. I have given these jabs in the past.

BIOLOGICAL AGENTS

A newer approach is to use biological agents such as TNF (tumour necrosis factor), cytokines that kill cells you do not want.

SUPPORTIVE TREATMENT

Supportive treatment includes exercise prescription, physiotherapy, joint protection nutrition, psychological support, and a multitude of alternative medicines.

LIFESTYLE MODIFICATIONS

Lifestyle modifications include losing weight, and changing exercises from running or jumping to swimming or cycling – things that don't carry the risk of damaging the knees. Weight loss can reduce stress on weight bearing joints, such as the knee.

PHYSIOTHERAPY

Physiotherapy is an important part of the treatment of debilitating arthritis, as it helps maintain optimum joint flexibility and strength. Assistive devices – such as a cane, walker, long shoehorn etc. – may help cope with disabilities associated with knee rheumatoid arthritis.

SURGERY

Surgery may be performed to retain joint function or prevent the loss of joint function. Joint replacement therapy may also be chosen, which is vital when joints fail. There are different types of surgery to correct different joint problems, and total or partial knee replacement is often recommended for patients with rheumatoid arthritis.

Do you have inner knee pain after a 'twisting with knee bent' injury, typically with your foot fixed to the ground? Did you feel 'something go' with immediate pain and swelling afterwards?

If so, you may have a medial menisci tear.

MEDIAL MENISCI TEAR

Meniscal Tear

Healthy Knee

Knee with a Torn Meniscus

Healthy Knee: Femur, Articular cartilage, Medial collateral ligament, Lateral collateral ligament, Posterior cruciate ligament, Anterior cruciate ligament, Meniscus, Fibula, Tibia

Knee with a Torn Meniscus: Femur, Articular cartilage, Medial collateral ligament, Lateral collateral ligament, Posterior cruciate ligament, Anterior cruciate ligament, Meniscal tear, Meniscus, Fibula, Tibia

The top of the shin bone (tibia) has a coating of cartilage and then two meniscal cups for the long thigh bone (femur) to move in. The menisci have a number of important roles in the function of the knee, such as spreading the load across the top of the shin bone (tibia), plus helping to both absorb shocks and stabilise the knee.

The menisci are often torn in knee injuries, particularly those involving twisting while the knee is bent, which is common in many sports. Aggravating factors can include aging, as much of the body's connective tissue becomes more rigid and less elastic with age.

The menisci have a poor blood supply and often will not heal. Therefore, in cases where conservative treatment does not work, surgery is indicated with either repair or removal of the torn tissue. The top of the shin bone (tibia) has a coating of cartilage and then two meniscal cups for the long thigh bone (femur) to move in. The menisci have a number of important roles in the function of the knee, such as spreading the load across the top of the shin bone (tibia), plus helping to both absorb shocks and stabilise the knee.

The lateral meniscus is less prone to tearing than the medial meniscus and tends to occur with twisting while weight bearing, which is common in many sports. Aggravating factors can include aging, as much of the body's connective tissue becomes more rigid and less elastic with age. Typical symptoms are significant pain if the knee is rotated, or if a sudden load increase occurs – as in jumping.

Diagnosis is by physiotherapy assessment and MRI, and treatment can include: RICE, physiotherapy, MBST, gentle specific rehab, knee brace, TENS, laser, ultrasound, sports massage, mobilisations, and surgeon referral. Recovery times will vary widely depending on the grade of injury, and may be several months.

SYNOVIAL PLICA

The knee is encased in synovial tissue, and sometimes a fold (**synovial plica**) will remain in the tissue from birth. If the plica is sufficiently large it can become irritated during activity and is then more susceptible to injury from direct trauma or overuse. This type of injury is most common on the medial side of the knee and its symptoms can sometimes be confused with a medial meniscal tear or patellar tendonitis.

In most cases, a **plica** can be treated conservatively, including the use of corticosteroid injections. If the symptoms do not respond, then arthroscopic surgery may be needed.

Diagnosis is by physiotherapy assessment and treatment can include: RICE, physiotherapy, MBST, rehab and exercises, support, sports massage, and TENS. If there is no improvement, MRI and surgeon referral may be needed.

Have you had a blow to the inside of your knee? Is your knee tender and painful on the outer side, most noticeably on the bone just below the knee?

If so, you may have a problem with your collateral ligaments.

COLLATERAL LIGAMENTS

These are found on the sides of your knee. The medial/inner collateral ligament (MCL) connects the femur to the tibia, while the lateral/'outside' collateral ligament (LCL) connects the femur to the thin bone in the lower leg (fibula). The collateral ligaments control the sideways motion of your knee and protect it against sudden movements – the knee joint relies just on these ligaments and the surrounding muscles for stability. Any direct contact to the knee or hard muscle contraction – such as changing direction rapidly while running – can injure a knee ligament. Injuries to the collateral ligaments are usually caused by a force that pushes the knee sideways, and while these are often contact injuries, they're not always.

Medial collateral ligament tears often occur as a result of a direct blow to the outside of the knee, and this pushes the knee inwards (toward the other knee). If there is an MCL injury, the pain is on the inside of the knee; an LCL injury pain is on the outside of the knee. A blow to the outside of the knee does the latter, and you get swelling over the site of the injury. Injury causes instability, and this is when the knee gives way. Injured ligaments are considered 'sprains' and are graded on a severity scale.

- Grade I sprains: The ligament is mildly damaged. It has been slightly stretched, and is still able to keep the knee joint stable.
- Grade II sprains: This stretches the ligament to the point where it becomes loose. It is referred to as a partial tear of the ligament.
- Grade III sprains: This type of sprain is a complete tear of the ligament. The ligament has been split into two pieces, and the knee joint is unstable.

Do you have pain just below the knee? Is it painful to extend the knee, and worse after exercise?

If so, you may have Osgood-Schlatter disease.

OSGOOD-SCHLATTER DISEASE

Anatomy of the Knee Joint

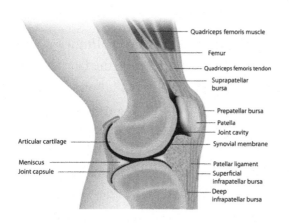

Osgood-Schlatter disease (OSD) – also known as apophysitis of the tibial tubercle, or Lannelongue's disease – is an inflammation of the patellar ligament at the tibial tuberosity. It is characterised by a painful lump just below the knee and is most often seen in young adolescents.

Osgood-Schlatter disease describes the local pain in the tendon under the kneecap (patella), which links the kneecap to the top of the shin bone (tibia). The tendon becomes inflamed and swollen due to repeated tension whilst exercising, and is most common in early teenage boys, particularly those undergoing a strong growth phase. In some cases the tendon becomes calcified.

Osgood-Schlatter disease occurs most often in children who participate in sports that involve running, jumping, and swift changes of direction – such as soccer, basketball, figure skating, and ballet. While Osgood-Schlatter disease is more common in boys, the gender gap is narrowing as more girls become involved with sports. Age ranges differ by sex because girls experience puberty earlier than boys, so the Osgood-Schlatter disease typically occurs in boys aged 13 to 14 and girls aged 11 to 12. The condition usually resolves on its own, once the child's bones stop growing; the discomfort can last from weeks to months and may recur until your child has stopped growing.

Provisional diagnosis is by physiotherapy assessment and X-Ray, and treatment can include: RICE, massage, and a specific rehab program. If severe, casts, patella tendon straps, or braces may be needed.

Do you have pain in the knee on movement? Does the movement feel boggy, and is there swelling?

If so, you may have knee bursitis.

KNEE BURSITIS

A bursa is a sac of synovial fluid that is positioned to cushion joints and help tendons move more freely and with less friction. The overuse of joints and tendons can cause tendinitis and inflammation of the bursa, which is called bursitis. The primary action of the quads is to straighten the leg at the knee, and these four strong muscles all connect to the upper kneecap (patella) through the suprapatellar tendon. Overuse of this tendon – or local trauma – can cause tendinitis and also bursitis of the underlying suprapatellar bursa, plus nearby infrapatellar and prepatellar bursae.

The infrapatellar bursa is located under the tendon connecting the bottom of the kneecap to the shin bone, the infrapatellar tendon. This area is prone to injury from any biomechanical misalignment. Inflammation of the infrapatellar bursa is also known as 'clergyman's knee', as historically, clergymen were prone to this condition due to frequent kneeling. A similar condition occurs with the bursa in front of the kneecap – the prepatellar bursa – known as 'housemaid's knee'. Infrapatellar bursitis can often coincide with infrapatellar tendinitis, or jumper's knee.

Diagnosis is by physiotherapy assessment, and treatment can include: gentle progressive physiotherapy, training of correct lifting techniques, laser, electrotherapy, MBST, and biomechanical assessment. If non-responding, corticosteroid injections may be used.

Do you have pain in the knee with swelling, creaking, and pain on running? Does your knee feel as if it catches and is unstable?

If so, you may have osteochondritis dissecans.

OSTEOCHONDRITIS DISSECANS

In most cases this affects the knee joint, but it can also occur in other body joints. Osteochondritis dissecans describes the separation of a piece of cartilage, plus a small piece of bone from one of the bones in the joint. This is caused by a local weakening in the bone due to insufficient blood supply and mainly occurs following a trauma to the joint. In some cases surgery may be needed to repair the bone, but in many cases the problem will self heal.

Diagnosis is by physiotherapy assessment with orthopaedic opinion, X-ray, and MRI, and treatment can include: RICE, MBST, and physiotherapy. If not healing, surgery may be needed.

Are you tender just above the kneecap, possibly with swelling? Do you get the same pain if someone else bends your knee or if you try to straighten your knee against resistance?

SUPRAPATELLAR TENDON

Overuse of the suprapatellar tendon – or local trauma – can cause tendinitis and also bursitis of the underlying suprapatellar bursa, plus the nearby infrapatellar and prepatellar bursae. This area is prone to injury from any biomechanical misalignment.

Diagnosis is by physiotherapy assessment, and to confirm, MRI, and treatment can include: gentle progressive physiotherapy, MBST, laser, ultrasound, biomechanical assessment, and training of the correct lifting technique.

CHONDROMALACIA PATELLA

This describes the condition where the back of the kneecap (patella) – which is normally covered in cartilage to provide a smooth, low friction contact with the thigh bone (femur) – is damaged, leading to a painful and sometimes noisy contact. It is more common in women and tends to be more prevalent in under 30's.

Chondromalacia patella could be caused by a number of factors:
- Individual knee misalignment problems.
- Overuse.
- Poor tracking due to muscle imbalance or hypermobility.
- Trauma.
- Normal wear and tear from aging.

Diagnosis is by physiotherapy assessment, X-ray, scope, and biomechanical assessment, and treatments can include: physiotherapy, MBST, shockwave, sports massage, muscle strengthening, stretching and balancing, orthotics, possible knee support, or taping. If unresponsive, try scope for plica or surgery.

HYPERMOBILITY

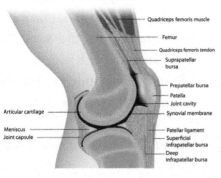

Anatomy of the Knee Joint

This is commonly referred to as being 'double jointed', and it is a condition where joints are allowed to move further than in a normal joint. People who have hypermobility tend to be more prone to sprains and strains, and are generally more accident-prone. The implications of hypermobility include:

- More rapid muscle fatigue as muscles have to compensate for joint laxity.
- More muscle pain than normal.

- Greater prevalence to childhood growing pains.
- Increased joint wear and tear and hence early onset osteoarthritis.
- More easily dislocated joints, especially in the shoulder.
- Prone to lower limb joint pain.
- Increased risk of spinal disc bulge and spondylolisthesis.

Diagnosis is by physiotherapy assessment and/or a rheumatologist, and treatment can include: orthotics, which can help assist lower limb joint pain.

Is it tender just below your kneecap? Is it painful to contract your quads, or after exertion?

If so, you may have infrapatellar tendinitis.

INFRAPATELLAR TENDINITIS

This condition is also known as jumper's knee. The straightening of the knee is achieved primarily through the quads and their attachment to the top of the kneecap (patella) with a very strong tendon. This force is transferred through the kneecap down to the lower leg by the infrapatellar tendon, which connects the lower part of the kneecap to the shin bone (tibia). Tendinitis is a condition where the tendon becomes irritated and inflamed. Infrapatellar tendinitis is most often caused by overuse and is particularly common in sports involving repeated jumping, such as football and netball. This condition can often occur with infrapatellar bursitis.

Diagnosis is by physiotherapy assessment, grading by the severity of pain and swelling, and MRI, and treatment can include: RICE, rest from aggravating activities, gentle progressive physiotherapy, sports rehab, laser, ultrasound, and MBST. If severe, a sports surgeon referral may be needed.

Is there tenderness and possible swelling on the outer side of your knee? Is knee movement restricted, and does it hurt to squat?

Is your knee tender on the inner side around the joint line?

As covered earlier, the inner side of your knee could be tender for a number of reasons, but most likely, it is a sprain to the medial collateral ligament (MCL). This is a common injury in skiing and contact sports, and comes in grades I to III.

- Grade I: Mild sprain.
- Grade II: Partial tear.
- Grade III: Complete rupture and the knee feels unstable.

COLLATERAL AND CRUCIATE LIGAMENT COMBINED INJURY AND MEDIAL MENISCI TEARS

Was there an audible crack at injury? Does the knee feel unstable, and does the pain feel deep in the knee? Is it warm and swollen?

Is swelling pronounced within 24 hours, and does it feel thick rather than fluid? Is it painful at the end range of movement of your knee?

If so, you may have a combined injury.

The knee is stabilised by four major ligaments: not just the collaterals, but also the anterior cruciate ligament (ACL) and posterior cruciate ligaments (PCL). The medial collateral ligament (MCL) connects to the femur (the long thigh bone) and the tibia (the shin bone), its task being to stabilise the inside of the knee (medial) and prevent it from opening up. However, it can be damaged in conjunction with the ACL. The MCL is most often injured when the outside of the knee is struck from the side, and depending on the amount of force, this will overload the MCL to cause anything from a mild sprain to complete rupture. This is a common injury in skiing and contact sports. Often, an MCL injury coincides with an anterior cruciate ligament (ACL) injury or a meniscal tear, and can injure both the medial and lateral coronary ligaments. This type of injury is common to football.

Grade I and II injuries will be painful over the ligament and will result in swelling within one or two days. With a full thickness tear – grade III – the knee will feel unstable and it will be difficult to bend it. Grades I and II will require ceasing the sport for one to four weeks, whereas a grade III tear will need bracing for at least six weeks. Surgery is not often needed.

Diagnosis is by physiotherapy assessment, specific test for grading I to III, MRI if a suspected grade III, and sports surgeon consultation. Treatment can include: RICE, physiotherapy, rest from training, knee brace if grades II or III, sports massage, ultrasound, pulsed shortwave, laser, MBST, and rehab that includes proprioception work for rough ground. Full recovery only comes with rehab.

CRUCIATE LIGAMENTS ACL AND/OR PCL SPRAIN

Torn Anterior Cruciate Ligament (ACL)

Normal Knee

Knee with Torn ACL

To reiterate, the knee is stabilised by four major ligaments, the medial (MCL) and lateral (LCL) collateral ligaments, and the anterior (ACL) and posterior (PCL) cruciate ligaments. The ACL and PCL lie deep within the knee joint, and of these, the ACL is much more prone to injury in sport, typically with a non-contact rapid deceleration whilst running or a twisting fall. This may also coincide with a MCL and medial meniscal injury. If the pain is behind the knee, it is more likely PCL.

PCL injuries are most common when the knee is bent and the shin is forced backwards – this is common in car accidents or in sports when a player lands hard on the knees with the knees fully flexed.

Diagnosis is by physiotherapy assessment, MRI, endoscope, and X-ray, and treatment can include: RICE, stopping the sport, physiotherapy, MBST, brace, rehab and exercises, and possible surgeon referral and prescribed pre-surgery rehab.

LOWER LEG

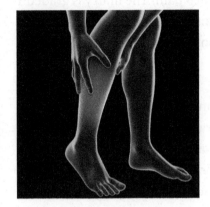

Did you get a sudden severe pain at mid-calf, with pain on walking ever since?

If so, you may have gastrocnemius and soleus strain.

GASTROCNEMIUS AND SOLEUS STRAIN

The calf is made up of two well-known muscles, the gastrocnemius and soleus, and a little known muscle, the plantaris. These muscles all join at the achilles tendon.

The largest muscle – the gastrocnemius – lies above the soleus and attaches above the knee joint, helping to bend the knee, whereas the soleus attaches below the knee and has no effect on the knee. Both muscles act to flex the foot down (plantarflex) through the achilles tendon. Gastrocnemius is the stronger plantar flexor when the knee is straight, with the soleus becoming stronger when the knee is bent. The gastrocnemius is more at risk of straining due to crossing two joints, and most often it is the medial head that is strained. The muscle has a high density of two fast twitch muscles, and in sport its action has been described as being like a whip.

Soleus is considered low risk to injury – mostly slow twitch fibres – and injury tends to be slower and less traumatic than with gastrocnemius, with mild calf tightness. Walking and running can provoke discomfort that can rumble on for weeks. The plantaris also crosses the knee and ankle, it is considered vestigial, and isolated strains are difficult to identify.

A calf strain usually happens at the place where the gastrocnemius muscle joins the tendon, and starts with a sudden sharp pain. The injury is graded 1 to 3. It is possible to strain a combination of muscles, or in isolation. Physical tests – and ultimately, ultrasound scanning or MRI – give diagnostic information.

- Grade I: Twinge pain in lower leg, some aching up to five days, and you can still play sport. Initially, therapists will be careful of strong massage, and your sports injury therapist will give technology and massage as the tissue heals at appropriate stages, before progressing on to rehab in order to strengthen and stretch, helping elongate the scar tissue. Shockwave also aids with scar tissue treatment. Strengthening starts with unloaded isometric, then isotonic and dynamic. It often takes 10 days for the tensile strength to allow this to be pain free, then you will need to do sport specific skill drills, and finally, plyometrics, i.e. hopping and jumping. Complete recovery is the goal before returning to sport. Rare complications do occur, such as myositis ossificans and compartment syndrome. Diagnosis is by physiotherapy assessment to grade and specify muscle rehab.
- Grade II: Pain on walking and initially a sharp pain in the back of the calf, bruising and some swelling, aching for a week, and pain on resisted plantar flexion (pointing toes). Treatment can include massage, electrotherapy, and specific sport physio rehab.
- Grade III: Severe pain, and you are unable to contract the muscle. There is obvious swelling and bruising. If full rupture muscle, the tear is palpable and Sever's test positive. I have seen a handful of these.

Orthopaedic opinion and an ultrasound scan are both needed to confirm diagnosis before treatment, which can include: RICE, heel raises to ease stress on the tendon and bilateral to avoid back issues, and physiotherapy followed by shockwave, rehab massage, and stretches for grades I and II. Sport specific rehab for strengthening and balance work can also help, as well as a biomechanics check. For grade III, an orthopaedic surgical referral is always needed in case of surgery.

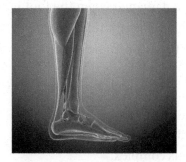

Did you get sudden pain on the outside of the lower leg with or without a blow? Also, does pulling your toes and foot up feel weak?

If so, you may have anterior compartment syndrome.

ANTERIOR COMPARTMENT SYNDROME

The (front) anterior compartment space has a fascial enclosure and osseous enclosure of muscles. Anterior compartment syndrome can affect tibialis anterior, extensor hallucis longus, extensor digitorum longus, and peroneus tertius, and it is potentially much more serious than shin splints. Increased pressure in the compartment can stop venous (blood) flow, which causes more swelling and pressure that can cause tissue death. The process may start with muscle swelling, then you'll start to feel the pain. The skin may look taut and red, and the common fibular nerve may give more pain and numbness.

For a test guideline, remember the 5 P's: Pain, Pallor, Paraesthesia, Pulselessness, Paralysis.

This condition requires urgent medical attention, then later on, physiotherapy and a biomechanical assessment. Treatment can include: RICE, medical attention, biomechanical assessment, ultrasound, pulsed shortwave, massage, and a rehab program including exercising the upper body or cycling.

Do you get foot pain on stopping or starting from running? Do you have swelling and pain on the big toe joint? Does it hurt to pull your big toe up?

If so, you may have a metatarsophalangeal joint injury.

METATARSOPHALANGEAL JOINT INJURY

The big toe joint at the base of the big toe can be damaged when the foot is jammed into the ground – such as when pushing off for running – resulting in forced over straightening (hyperextension) of the joint. Typical symptoms include pain at the base of the toe.

There are 3 grades:
- Grade I: Minor tearing of capsuloligamentous complex.
- Grade II: Partial tear of capsuloligamentous complex.
- Grade III: Complete tear of capsuloligamentous complex and plantar plate torn from the toe bone, the proximal phalanx of the metatarsal head.
- Diagnosis is by physical exam by physio or GP and then X-ray, and treatment can include: physiotherapy, laser, MBST/MRT, pulsed shortwave, Acupuncture, brace, and firm shoes to prevent bending. Non-weight bearing activity for two days, using a stick or crutches. Buddy tape for shoes. Then, strengthening rehab over three to four weeks, allowing the injury to heal before returning to normal sport.

Do you get localised pain on the bone on the outer side of the lower leg (fibula)? Is it worse when weight bearing, especially if you have flat feet?

If so, you may have a fibula stress fracture.

FIBULA STRESS FRACTURE

This happens when either the compressive forces due to repetitive weight bearing, or the stress caused by the contraction of muscles that attach to the fibula, get too much and cause bony damage. Pain will be felt in the outer lower leg, often after running on hard ground or excessively, and in more severe cases, there may be night pain. MBST/MRT and laser can help the repair process, and rehab needs to be graded from non-weight bearing to full impact. Progression goes from cycling and swimming to water running and dynamic proprioceptive work, and finally, plyometrics.

Provisional diagnosis is by physiotherapy assessment, X-ray, biomechanical assessment, CT, and bone scan, and treatment can include: MBST, laser, orthotics, complete rest until the bone is healed, support, massage, and a gradual return to sport.

Do you get pain in an infected area? Is it sore and difficult to move the limb?

If so, you may have osteomyelitis.

OSTEOMYELITIS

This is a bone infection, and you will feel ill in addition to having a local bump over a bone with tenderness. Bacteria (staphylococcus aureus) is the most common cause of osteomyelitis, and increased risk factors include:
- Poor immune system.
- Following hip prosthesis surgery.
- Fracture.
- Alcoholic or drug abuse.

Diagnosis is by GP for scans and bloods, and treatment options include: seeing a medic, drugs, and nutrition.

Do you get pain in the lower third of your shin bone (tibia) after running long distances, and if you press there?

If so, you may have a tibia stress fracture.

TIBIA STRESS FRACTURE

This is an incomplete crack in the shin bone. Several muscles attach to the tibia and when they contract they pull on the bone. If the loading is too excessive or repetitive, this can lead to stress fractures. A tibia stress fracture causes tenderness and pain, which tends to mostly be on the inner shin bone.

Various factors can play a role in the development of a **tibia stress fracture**:
- Training on too hard a surface.
- Poor foot biomechanics.
- Stiff ankle.
- Weak muscles.
- Diet lacking in minerals.
- Too obese to run.

Treatment involves soft tissue work, laser and MBST to fracture sites, Gunn IMS dry needling, guided rehab, and ankle mobs, with a biomechanics overview – especially looking for pronation – and possible orthotics with arch support.

Diagnosis is by physiotherapy assessment, and an X-ray after four weeks to show the bone is healing. Treatment can include: rest, MBST, laser, Gunn IMS, biomechanical assessment, and lower limb non-weight bearing rehab. In most cases, the individual can return to sport in eight to twelve weeks, but if more severe, this could turn into six months.

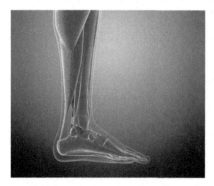

Do you get pain on the back of your heel? Does standing on your tiptoes hurt?

If so, you may have achilles tenosynovitis.

ACHILLES TENOSYNOVITIS

Achilles tenosynovitis and achilles tendinitis usually occur together. Tendons are fibrous structures that attach muscle to bone, covered by sheaths that are lubricated by synovial fluid. Achilles tenosynovitis is also called paratenonitis, which describes the degeneration of the outer sheaf. As the tendon heals, scar tissue forms in the sheaf, attaching itself to the inner part of the tendon and causing tightness, pain, and swelling. The smooth gliding of the tendon is prevented, leading to secondary tearing. Beyond swelling and tightness, it may be possible to feel a lump at the back of the tendon.

There are multiple causes for inflammation:
- Sports activities.
- Competing triathletes.
- Systemic diseases.
- Repetitive movements.
- Poor footwear.
- Inadequate stretching.
- Hard, uneven terrain.
- Previous scar tissue.
- Sudden increase in distance.

Relative rest, cooling, and gels can help, as well as a biomechanical analysis to see if the positioning of the foot or footwear is an issue, local electrotherapy, and sport specific rehab with graded strengthening and balance work. Shockwave will soften the scar tissue, promoting healthy collagen and also promoting blood flow.

Provisional diagnosis is by physiotherapy assessment, ultrasound scan or MRI, and biomechanical assessment, and treatment can include: RICE, massage, physiotherapy, heel raises, orthotics, changing your footwear, shockwave, Gunn IMS, pulsed shortwave, ultrasound, rehab and exercises, and reduced hill running.

Do you get persistent ankle pain with swelling and locking after an ankle sprain or injury?

If so, you may have an osteochondral fracture.

OSTEOCHONDRAL FRACTURE

This is damage to the joint cartilage and underlying bone, and in the ankle this is often caused by trauma, typically from a sports injury where the shin bone is struck on the outside. Persistent ankle sprains can also lead to osteochondral fractures on the inside of the ankle.

Fragments of cartilage and bone are torn from the bone under the shin bone in the ankle (talus). If a fragment of cartilage is still attached to the bone, then conservative treatment of putting the ankle in a cast, plus MBST/MRT will suffice until the fracture is healed. Where fragments are only marginally attached or totally detached, then these are best removed with arthroscopic surgery.

Symptoms of osteochondral fracture include the swelling of the joint, possibly some instability, and a feeling of the joint catching with some grating.

Provisional diagnosis is by physiotherapy assessment and X-ray, and treatment can include: for grades I and II – cycling/swimming, ankle non-weight bearing exercises, laser, MBST/MRT, and a full rehab program for balance and strength. For grades III and IV – scope and surgery to remove the fragment.

Do you get a tingling or numbness in the extremities, stiff muscles or cramps, and a red rash?

If so, you may have hypocalcaemia.

HYPOCALCAEMIA

Calcium regulation is necessary for cell function – including cell membrane integrity – and ionised calcium is needed for nerve conduction, muscle relaxation, contraction, bone mineralisation, and hormones.

Diagnosis is by GP physical exam, and treatment can include: seeing a medic, and then, with their agreement, a nutritionist.

Do you have an ache at the back of the ankle, which is painful on exercise, and worse on stairs or an incline? Is the achilles tender, thickened, and red?

If so, you may have achilles tendinitis.

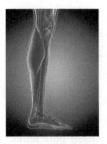

ACHILLES TENDINITIS

Achilles tendinitis is the irritation/inflammation of the large tendon at the back of the ankle. This is an acute condition, rather than the chronic condition called tendinosis. Causes of achilles tendinitis include a lack of flexibility and overpronation, increasing running mileage, more uphill work, poor footwear, and poor biomechanics.

Typically the back of the ankle is very sore after rest, about 4 cm above tendon insertion on the heel bone (calcaneus). Pushing off through the foot will also be difficult. Rehab must allow for adequate rest to stop the tendon getting inflamed. Initially, cycling and swimming is progressed to weight bearing and balance exercises, and then plyometrics.

Diagnosis is by physiotherapy assessment, biomechanical assessment, and MRI scan, and treatment can include: sports rehab exercises, stretches, a training program, MBST, orthotics, physiotherapy, massage, and laser. For the chronic cases, Gunn IMS and shockwave will be needed.

ACHILLES BURSITIS

An increase in running mileage, more uphill work, poor footwear, and poor biomechanics can cause this. Like with achilles tendinitis, the back of the ankle is very sore after rest, about 4 cm above tendon insertion on the heel bone (calcaneus). Pushing off through the foot will also be difficult.

Rehab must allow for adequate rest to stop the tendon getting inflamed. Initially, cycling and swimming is progressed to weight bearing and balance exercises, and then plyometrics.

Diagnosis is by physiotherapy assessment, biomechanical assessment, and MRI scan, and treatment can include: sports rehab exercises, stretches, a training program, MBST, orthotics, physiotherapy, massage, and laser, and for chronic cases, Gunn IMS and shockwave.

Do you have leg pain, but no amount of working your leg muscles or prodding specific places gives a pain?

If so, you may have radiculopathy (see the spinal section).

Do you have pain and swelling over the outside of the ankle, which gets worse with activity?

If so, you may have peroneal tendinitis or a peroneal nerve injury (weakness of foot raise).

PERONEAL TENDINITIS

The two peroneal tendons – the brevis and longus – run outside the lower leg and then behind and underneath the bony prominence on the outside of the ankle (lateral malleolus). A high arch tends to increase the stress through the tendons and thus aggravate the condition.

Peroneal tendinitis tends to be a chronic wear and tear problem resulting from repetitive loading, and in some cases the tendons can become torn. Symptoms of peroneal tendinitis include pain and inflammation on the outside rear of the ankle. This inflammation will cause stiffness, especially after periods of inactivity such as first thing in the morning.

The tendons are activated in direction changes and therefore sports involving rapid changes of direction will aggravate the tendinitis and should be avoided while healing. Biomechanically, a high arch with an inverted ankle (the foot being rotated as if you are trying to look at the bottom of your foot) will predispose you to peroneal problems. A complete tear would be evident with you not being able to move the foot to the side. Occasionally, nearby nerves (sural) are affected and this will cause nerve supersensitivity.

Diagnosis is by physiotherapy assessment, pressing on the peroneal, and a biomechanical assessment for overpronation and excessive eversion. Treatment can include: biomechanical assessment, orthotics with a view to looking at the high arch being a problem, foot plate analysis for pressure around the big toe, rehab with strengthening and stretching the peroneal and calf muscles, and sports.

PERONEAL NERVE INJURY

The peroneal nerve branches off the sciatic nerve and is responsible for innervating the muscles that raise the foot and toes. Damage to the nerve can thus lead to spontaneous foot drop or weakness in lifting the foot. Other symptoms include a tingling or numbness on the outside of the lower leg, and pain down the shin or the top of the foot.

Peroneal nerve injuries have a poor chance of recovery, worsening with time, so it is important to be assessed quickly by a specialist who can determine whether to proceed with surgery or go down a more conservative route – typical conservative options include physiotherapy and orthotics.

Diagnosis is by EMG tests, orthopaedic surgeon, or a back specialist, and treatment can include: Gunn IMS for assessment, physiotherapy, and biomechanical assessment.

Do you have pain over the inside of your lower part of your shin, which gets worse if you bend your foot down? Is there initial pain on training that can be worse the next morning?

If so, you may have shin splints.

SHIN SPLINTS

These are caused by exercise, and the pain comes on after long distance running, or sports that involve sudden turns and stops. The dull pain – which can be felt along the shin bone (tibia) – gets worse without rest. Take the pain as a warning to do activities that put less force through the tibia, then try ice, relative rest, and swimming or cycling while healing – over a couple of weeks. Once the pain is gone, make sure to run on softer ground.

It is not clear what causes microtrauma to the membrane between the bones or small fractures to the periosteum, but to reduce risk, wear good running shoes and orthotics if needed, especially if flat-footed. Run on softer ground, watch your weight, and stretch the achilles tendon before activity. A sports physio will advise you on warming up correctly, and rehab will be needed with a progressive return to your sport.

Provisional diagnosis is by physiotherapy assessment, X-ray, and biomechanical assessment, and treatment can include: orthotics, better trainers, changing your training program and using a softer surface, laser, MBST, mobilising the ankle, nutrition, and weight control. A sports therapist will take you through a graded rehab program.

Do you have unpleasant sensations in your legs, which cease on movement, and worsen in evenings?

If so, you may have restless legs syndrome.

RESTLESS LEGS SYNDROME

This affects the nervous system, and you can experience an overwhelming need to move your legs, as well as a creeping, crawling feeling in the legs. Low dopamine levels can affect this. Restless legs syndrome is occasionally linked to anaemia, kidney failure, or Parkinson's, and it affects around one in ten people.

Diagnosis is by nutritionist, and a Gunn IMS specialist to check for lumbar spondylosis link. Treatment can include: massage, stretching, Gunn IMS, Acupuncture, reducing caffeine and alcohol, increasing your iron intake, increasing your exercise, and dopamine aiding your nutrition.

Have you had a bruising injury some months ago and do you now feel a bony lump there?

If so, you may have myositis ossificans.

MYOSITIS OSSIFICANS

This is an uncommon condition in which bone is formed inside an injured muscle. Many sports are prone to muscle injury – such as football, rugby, martial arts, and hockey – and these injuries can lead to heavy internal bleeding, evident as bruising and swelling, and can also result in a blood clot, which is an ideal breeding ground for calcification. Left untreated, the calcification can continue to develop and may take over much of the injured site over several months.

The key to prevent myositis ossificans – or the growth of bone by calcification within the injured muscle – is to seek treatment as early as possible after the injury. Once formed, the bone can only be removed surgically and the current guidelines advise waiting up to 12 months to minimise the risk of further bone growth post-surgery. The cause of myositis ossificans is not understood, and there *is* a risk of further bone growth post-surgery.

Diagnosis is by physiotherapy assessment, X-ray to confirm the diagnosis, and checks to confirm it is non-malignant. Treatment can include: drugs to relieve the symptoms, and surgery.

If you try to flex your foot up against resistance, does it hurt?

If so, you may have a tibialis anterior strain.

TIBIALIS ANTERIOR STRAIN

The tibialis anterior muscle runs down the outside of the shin, and when it gets sore, you feel pain at the front of the ankle. Its purpose is to lift your foot up and out. With tibialis anterior strain, the tendon can feel creaky and sore and the toes hurt to move up and down. This strain occurs when running on hard ground and is especially vulnerable with racket sports.

Provisional diagnosis is by physiotherapy assessment, and treatment can include: RICE, orthotics, shockwave, ultrasound, laser, physiotherapy, sports strengthening rehab, and proprioceptive exercise.

If you try to rotate your foot in – as if looking at the sole of your foot – against resistance, does it cause pain on the inside of your foot, but does flexing your foot up against resistance not hurt?

If so, you may have tibialis posterior tendinopathy.

TIBIALIS POSTERIOR TENDINOPATHY

The tibialis posterior originates from the back of both calf bones – the tibia and fibula – then travels down the inner side of the leg, with the tendon running behind the inner bony prominence of the ankle (medial malleolus) to attach into the foot bones. It acts to flex the foot down and rotate inwards, as when you're trying to look at the bottom of your foot. It is also an important muscle for maintaining the arch of the foot.

A problem with tibialis posterior tendinopathy can occur either with a sudden force or repeated overuse, the latter being the more common. Symptoms of tibialis posterior tendinopathy include pain in the inner lower leg and ankle, which is made worse when running over uneven ground. Sore to touch, it can be stiff in the morning, and this can go on for weeks.

Degeneration of the tendon causes pain on the inside of the foot, and the pain is made worse if someone else tries to lift the outside of the foot (passive eversion) or if you try to press the inside of your foot down against resistance (resisted inversion). Some noise may be apparent when the tendon is activated (crepitus). In severe cases of tibialis posterior tendinopathy, the tendon can become detached and pull some of the underlying bone away (partial avulsion).

Sports prone to tibialis posterior tendinopathy include:
- Speed skaters, as they have prolonged stretching and eversion of the feet.
- Runners who develop by training around bends.

If you have flat feet or you are not fit with good balance reactions, you will be more at risk of experiencing this injury.

Diagnosis is by physiotherapy assessment, MRI or ultrasound scan to confirm, and biomechanical assessment, and treatment can include: looking at your posture, orthotics to correct overpronation, physiotherapy, shockwave, laser, prescriptive proprioceptive strengthening, and rehab sports therapy to change your running program to avoid running around bends. It can take months to achieve full recovery, depending on how chronic the condition is.

FEET

Are you a dancer? Is it tender on the sole of your foot? (Dancers tend to repeatedly impact load the sole of the foot, making this area tender.)

If so, you may have metatarsalgia.

METATARSALGIA

The metatarsals are the five long bones in the midfoot which connect the toes to the group of bones at the ankle. The metatarsals meet the toe bone (phalanges) at the ball of the foot, and metatarsalgia is pain in this area. Symptoms may also include pins and needles, numbness in the toes, and a burning or sharp pain.

There are many potential causes of metatarsalgia including being overweight, wearing tight and/or high heeled shoes, any sport which causes high impact loading, and thinning of the fat pad on the bottom of the foot, which is typical with aging and the foot structure itself. Both flat and excessively arched feet can aggravate the condition, and related conditions which could contribute include osteoarthritis, gout, Morton's neuroma, and diabetes.

Provisional diagnosis is by physiotherapy assessment, X-ray, ultrasound scan, bloods, and biomechanical assessment, and treatment options include: physiotherapy and exercises, orthotics, Acupuncture, toe mobilisations, stretches and graded exercises, and wearing padded, spacious shoes.

Are your toes stiff? Can you only pull your toes up by 45 degrees or less? Do you get pain on walking?

If so, you may have osteoarthritis of the toes.

OSTEOARTHRITIS OF THE TOES

Osteoarthritis is a condition where the cartilage that coats the end of the bones at joints to provide a smooth motion is worn away, eventually leaving bone on bone contact. The symptoms of osteoarthritis include pain and stiffness, worsening as the condition develops.

Treatment options are <u>MBST</u> plus physiotherapy and exercise.

Does your ankle click or have loss of movement? Is one ankle stiffer, has less movement than the other, and is noisy? Comparing the two ankles, is one joint stiffer with more loss of movement when you flex your foot down? Does it clunk and creak when moving? Does it feel blocked with a 'hard end' feel?

If so, you may have osteoarthritic changes.

OSTEOARTHRITIC CHANGES

The ankle joint is subject to considerable loading from normal daily activities, something that is much higher with impact loading such as with running or jumping. The ankle area has a lot of bones and joints, and this combined with the loading makes it vulnerable to both wear and tear and injury. It is no surprise that the ankle is the most injured joint in the body and therefore vulnerable to osteoarthritis. Additional contributing factors include poor foot mechanics such as flat feet (overpronated) or high arched feet (supinated).

Provisional diagnosis of this condition is by physiotherapy assessment plus X-ray, and treatment options include: MBST/MRT plus physiotherapy, rehab, and Acupuncture.

Do you get severe pain under the heel when you first stand? If you have been sitting or lying – especially first thing in the morning – do you get severe pain under the heel, but if you wiggle your ankle it is not painful?

If so, you may have plantar fasciitis.

PLANTAR FASCIITIS

This condition is also known as 'policeman's foot'. The fascia is a strong tendon that connects the heel bone (calcaneus) to the toes and acts as a shock absorber, supporting the arch in the underside of the foot. Pain is most often felt where the fascia connects to the underside of the heel bone, and this can be due to being overweight from inactivity, excessive heel strike loading as in running, or having excessively tight calf muscles. The pain and tightness will most likely be felt first thing in the morning or after periods of inactivity.

Plantar fasciitis responds well to shockwave therapy on the fascia combined with calf stretching if necessary. For chronic tendon problems, MBST can help calm the condition. If the feet are incorrectly aligned, then orthotics will help resolve the underlying cause.

Provisional diagnosis is by physiotherapy assessment plus biomechanical assessment, and treatment options include: ice, stretching, night splint, taping, massage, orthotics, shockwave, and physiotherapy. Then you can consider MBST/MRT.

Do you have a blood blister, bruising, and possible tenderness?

If so, you may have a haematoma.

HAEMATOMA

A haematoma is swelling caused by the accumulation of clotted blood, and if the haematoma compresses a local nerve it can cause pain. These are quite common in contact sports, and such injuries can occur either inside or outside a muscle. Muscle strains will typically restrict the range of movement, but those outside of muscles can be more persistent and more restrictive.

Treatment options include: RICE, physiotherapy, and electrotherapy, and if resolved, you may need aspiration.

Have you had a recent trauma to a toe by kicking something hard or dropping something heavy on it? Do you now get foot and/or toe pain, which is worse on standing? Are you unable to move your foot in the full range of motion?

If so, you may have broken toes.

BROKEN TOES

Broken toes are fairly common injuries, but in most cases do not require treatment and will self heal in around four to six weeks. If the toe is misaligned it may need to be reset, which your GP can do under anaesthetic.

If the big toe is broken, it may need to be put in a cast. If you have walked a lot or play a lot of contact sport, you can get a stress fracture in your toes.

Laser or MRT accelerates the healing process and you have to ease up on the aggravating activities. Treatment can include: stiff shoes, laser, and strapping.

Does it hurt if someone else flexes your ankle by pulling your foot down, but you can stand on your toes and it does not hurt? Is the back of your heel tender?

If so, you may have posterior impingement syndrome.

POSTERIOR IMPINGEMENT SYNDROME

This condition is also known as 'dancer's heel', as it is very common with ballet dancers. Pain is felt at the back of the ankle – at the base of the thin bone running down the outside of the calf (fibula) – and is aggravated if the foot is pointed downwards (plantar flexion). The pain is due to tissue inflammation in this area, caused by the trapping, or impingement, of tissue as the foot is flexed. Usually standing on tiptoe will elicit the pain.

Rest and ice are advisable to reduce any swelling, and it's possible that a cast may be needed for four weeks. In some cases, a corticosteroid injection is advised to control inflammation.

Provisional diagnosis is by physiotherapy assessment plus biomechanical assessment with dancing shoes, and treatment can include: rest, ice, physiotherapy, orthotics, cast, and corticosteroid injection.

Do you have swelling over the outside of your ankle and does it hurt when you do a combination of flexing your foot down and turning the sole inwards, as if to look at the sole of your foot?

If so, you may have ligament strain or tear.

415

LIGAMENT STRAIN OR TEAR

The ankle is a hinge joint between the leg and the foot, allowing up and down movement. The bones of the leg (tibia and fibula) form a slot, and the talus bone of the foot fits between them. The talus connects to the tibia and fibula by strong bands of tissue called ligaments, and each ligament is made of many fibres of collagen, which is extremely strong.

The ligament on the inside of the ankle (the deltoid ligament) has two layers; the deepest one is the most important. This ligament is mainly torn in association with severe fractures of the ankle bones, and sporting injuries of this ligament are rare. The ligament on the outside of the ankle (lateral ligament) is made up of three separate bands: one at the front (anterior talo-fibular ligament), one in the middle (calcaneo-fibular ligament) and one at the back (posterior talo-fibular ligament). The front and middle bands are the ligaments that are injured in a sprain.

The tibia and fibula form a joint between themselves just above the ankle, and this also has strong ligaments, one at the front and one at the back (tibio-fibular ligaments). The ligament at the front is involved in 10-20% of ankle sprains, and this injury is important, as it takes a long time to heal, although it usually heals without the need for surgical treatment.

How do the ankle ligaments get injured?

Most ankle ligament injuries are caused when the foot twists inwards. All of the body's weight is then placed on the lateral ankle ligaments. The anterior and middle fibres of the ankle tear/sprain the ankle. Occasionally small pieces of bone may be torn off with the ligaments.

In a few cases I have seen a twisting force on the ankle cause other damage: the bones around the ankle may have fractured, a piece of the cartilage lining the ankle may be chipped off, ligaments connecting other bones in the foot may be torn, or the tendons around the ankle may be damaged. X-rays (conducted later on) show these bony injuries.

Although a couple of days' rest is useful – as well as a stick – it is best to start taking some weight on the injured ankle reasonably soon after injury, usually within 2-3 days. Also, start to exercise and stretch the injured ankle as soon as possible after the injury, taking advice from experts.

Normally a sprained ankle will recover within 6-8 weeks, although it may tend to swell for a few months longer. Treatment can include: physiotherapy, strapping, a gradual return to activities with rehab prescription, and electrotherapy.

Do you get pain on walking at the big toe? Can you not lift the big toe beyond 45 degrees? (The big toe – or hallux – should normally lift well beyond 45)

If so, you may have osteoarthritis of the first MTP joint.

OSTEOARTHRITIS OF FIRST MTP JOINT

This is osteoarthritis in the joint at the base of the big toe. The metatarsals are the long bones in the midfoot that join the ankle bones to the toe bones – the phalangeals at the MTP joint. The big toe is the first toe.

The restriction of the toe joint is carried out when not weight bearing. A similar test when weight bearing is called the Windlass test, which looks at the ease of the toe to be lifted up and also tests for flat feet. Bunions (hallux valgus) deformity at the base of the big toe may be associated with OA, but not necessarily.

Provisional diagnosis is by physiotherapy assessment and X-ray, and treatment can include: physiotherapy with MBST/MRT, and shockwave.

So, this concludes our whistle stop tour through the notebook of a physio – hopefully you've learnt something about muscle and nerve problems, and hopefully you can use this guide in the future if you start experiencing any pain or discomfort.

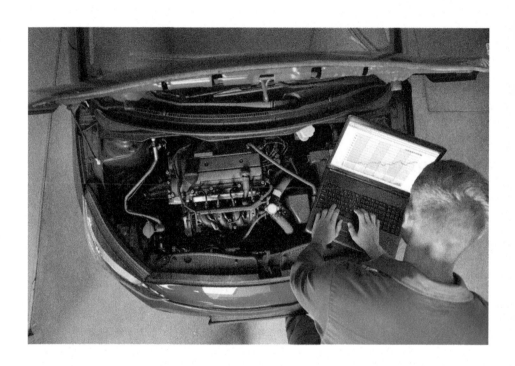

Appendix 2

"Do not deprive me of my age. I have earned it."

– *May Sarton*

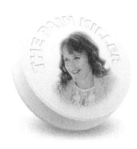

Your Greatest Wealth Is Your Health

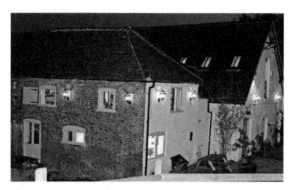

Cromwell House, Wolseley Bridge Clinic

The midlands holistic physiotherapy clinic is in a refurbished Grade II listed building, called Cromwell House, as it is thought that Oliver Cromwell stayed here before the battle at Hopton Heath, near Stafford.

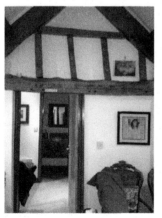

Clinic waiting room

Upon arrival, it feels like stepping into your home rather than a clinic. The energy is conducive to healing as it is surrounded by an Area of Outstanding Natural Beauty, on the edge of Cannock Chase in Staffordshire.

MRT WILLEY BARN Wolseley Bridge

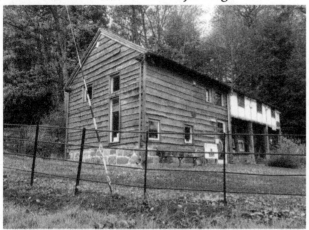

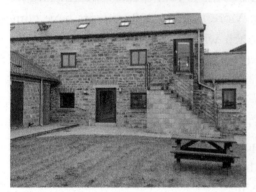

Harrogate, Spa Bottom Farm

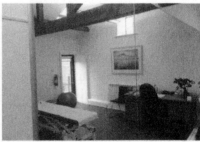

My new venture, Spa Bottom Farm, is near to my darling little nephews, who are both under five at the time of writing this book. Strangely enough, Cromwell was busy around here too, destroying the place and burning witches. There will be more about this in my Soul volume.

The midlands clinic was set up to educate and help patients and practitioners in many aspects of musculoskeletal health, aimed not just at firefighting their symptoms but informing people of them too.

I want for you all to see your body as your temple – not just a vehicle – and one that is built on pillars of health. Each pillar represents a different aspect and each needs to be strong for you to have a long and healthy life. Your temple is only as strong as the weakest pillar. This is what inspired me to present and write *The 4 Keys to Health*, as by the time I got around to publishing my book, everyone was talking about 'pillars' of everything, so keys it was.

So, when you come to our clinics and we look at you – that's myself and my team – we want every aspect of you to be as robust as it can be, whether it be mindset, diet and nutrition, exercise and fitness, or lifestyle and stress. Your ability to heal from an injury and your speed of recovery depends on all of these factors. This project has been ongoing, and it originally evolved in my home practice. It is the foundation for my presentations on pain around the world, my Z factor shows, and my book on the 4 keys to health.

We believe that a long, healthy, pain free life is your greatest wealth, and we will strive to help you achieve this. More than 10,000 patients have gone through this kind of therapy approach with me, and are now no longer immobile and needing pain meds; they are testament to this approach of preventative medicine.

Instead of just treating your injury or pain, we would like to prevent your problem from reoccurring, and to achieve this we need you to embrace the preventative approach of optimum health, which can:

- Move you towards a pain free life.
- Regain your physical fitness.
- Help you live a longer and healthier life.
- Reignite your passion for life.
- Make you feel more energetic and vital.
- Give you more resistance to illness and disease.

WHAT IS OPTIMUM HEALTH?

The achievement of optimum health can be likened to the Parthenon; for the building to have optimum strength, each of the stone pillars must be strong and well built, otherwise the building will crumble and fall.

Optimum Health Parthenon

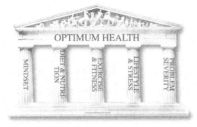

Picture optimum health as that building; every one of your health pillars needs to be strong or your health will come crashing down. For optimum health you need to learn the power of your own mind to control and drive your subconscious thoughts, and you also need to understand that your body is a complex biological machine made up of billions of cells. These tiny cells crave good nutrition and oxygen to grow and flourish. Therefore, adding regular exercise is vital to maintain good blood flow, muscle tone, and strong bones, as well as helping to keep you trim and combat the stress that goes with our modern lifestyle.

HOW DO WE GET YOU THERE?

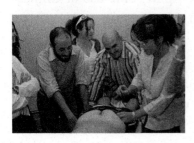

Once we fully understand the severity of your problem and your starting point, we will make a specific treatment plan to get you to your goals, using the appropriate skills and technologies. Whether or not you come to one of my holistic physiotherapy clinics or similar clinics, or one of my presentations, you will soon have my life's work at your fingertips with my Human Garage series of books.

CHINESE MEDICINE

Chinese Medicine and Acupuncture offers a gentle approach to putting your body back in balance. As a holistic approach, it is particularly good at treating conditions where there is an internal imbalance, such as period pain, pregnancy, menopause, IBS, and worry and anxiety.

Chinese Medicine and Acupuncture has been proven to:
- Rebalance your body.
- Reduce pain.
- Increase flexibility.

Chinese Medicine is a complete medical system with a history going back thousands of years. The basis of the treatment starts with questioning, observation, and pulse and tongue diagnosis, to work out in which way your body is out of balance – something that is called Syndrome Differentiation. It also treats local pain problems with 'Ah shi' (which literally translates as 'that's it') point needling. Treatment is a combination of herbal medicine, Acupuncture, diet, massage, and exercise. The effect of generating chi or 'vital energy' can be experienced through Tai Chi or Qigong.

Most people have heard of Acupuncture, though this is normally western Acupuncture, which combines needling to local areas of pain or spasm, 'Ah shi' points – sometimes called trigger points – plus some use of Chinese Acupuncture points, but without reference to the principles and theory of Syndrome Differentiation.

Acupuncture is a treatment that has been and continues to be debated heavily by western medical practitioners. The views are widespread – some GP Practices and NHS hospitals openly use Acupuncture while others don't. One year, NICE (government guidelines) gives Acupuncture a gold standard for treating, for example, back pain, while another year it vanishes again.

Perhaps a broader and more logical perspective can be seen in China, the birthplace of Acupuncture. China is rapidly developing, and as a result, it is reforming its approach to medical care. The approach that China is taking is to evaluate the effectiveness of traditional Chinese medicine in comparison to western techniques, selecting the most effective in clinical trials. China teaches both western and eastern medical courses, though in many cases China continues to use traditional Chinese medicine as the preferred treatment option.

ELECTROACUPUNCTURE

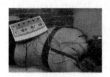

Electroacupuncture

- Chronic spinal neuropathic pain relief.
- Acute and post-operative pain relief.
- Acute back pain relief.
- Osteoarthritic pain and sports injuries.

Electro acupuncture is often likened to TENS, but it is more effective in the treatment of chronic pain, and therefore it is often used by physiotherapists for the treatment of chronic pain. Also, benefits continue after treatment and improve with repeated treatments. TENS, on the other hand, is only effective while the treatment is active, but is beneficial for acute and post-op pain relief. It is also helpful for reducing pain during a course of IMS treatment.

TENS

Transcutaneous electrical nerve stimulation (TENS) is a method of pain relief involving the use of a mild electrical current produced by the device to stimulate the nerves for therapeutic purposes. TENS, by definition, covers the complete range of transcutaneously applied currents used for nerve excitation.

A TENS machine is a small, battery-operated device that has leads connected to 4 sticky pads called electrodes. TENS is applied at high frequency (>50 Hz), with an intensity below motor contraction (sensory intensity), or low frequency (<10 Hz), with an intensity that produces motor contraction. The physiotherapist will demonstrate how to use all the settings and where to place the pads.

The development of the modern TENS unit is generally credited to C. Norman Shealy, and a few studies have shown objective evidence that TENS may modulate or suppress pain signals. One showed that electric stimulation of A-beta sensory fibers reliably suppressed the A-delta fiber (touch). Two other studies used functional magnetic resonance imaging (fMRI) to look at brain activity: one showed that high-frequency TENS decreased pain with carpal tunnel syndrome, the other showed that low-frequency TENS decreased shoulder impingement pain and modulated pain-induced activation in the brain. A head-mounted TENS device called Cefaly was approved in 2014, for the prevention of migraines. The Cefaly device was found effective in preventing migraine attacks in a randomised sham-controlled trial. This was the first TENS device which the FDA approved for pain prevention, as opposed to pain suppression.

LASER ACUPUNCTURE

Laser Acupuncture
- Reduce pain and swelling.
- Promote tissue healing.
- Promote bone healing.

Therapeutic laser – sometimes called cold lasers – use pure light to speed cell repair. A physiotherapist will often use a therapeutic laser as part of their treatment as it is effective in reducing pain and swelling. Different wavelengths can be used to treat skin conditions, muscle and tendinopathy, and bone healing.

It is unclear how LLLT (low level laser therapy) might work. However, photochemical reactions are well known in biological research; it may be that the light applied in low level laser therapy might react with the respiratory enzyme cytochrome c oxidase, which is involved in the electron transport chain in mitochondria.

The research is not terribly positive – while anecdotal evidence is strong, Cochrane reviews, sadly, are not. I was trained how to use laser by Prof Gunn and Omega Lasers, and I find it very useful in combination with needling.

A 2008 Cochrane Library review concluded that LLLT has insufficient evidence for treatment of nonspecific low back pain, a finding echoed in a 2010 review of chronic low back pain. A 2015 review found benefits in nonspecific chronic low back pain. Another 2015 review found benefits in shoulder tendinopathy. A 2014 Cochrane review found tentative evidence that it may help in frozen shoulders.

MANUAL MANIPULATION

Joint manipulation is a passive movement made to a patient's joint by a therapist, and it is aimed at producing a therapeutic effect at a synovial joint (a fibrous joint capsule filled with synovial fluid). The degree of force and the angle of application to free up a joint is taught by different professional bodies. Physiotherapy has Cyriax, Maitland, McKenzie, and Nags and Snags schools of training. Chiropractors and Osteopaths have their own too.

THERAFLEX ROBOTIC SPINAL MANIPULATION

At least 60% of the UK population suffer from back problems. There are many causes for back pain, and one of those causes is a spine which becomes inflexible. In simple terms, there are 17 vertebral bones from the bottom of the neck to the base of the spine, and if we imagine that each of these should allow an element of rotation and flexibility, then if any of these joints become seized, it begins to cause problems in overall flexibility, resulting in pain.

Physiotherapy is an effective treatment for improving spinal flexibility, however, a physiotherapist's ability to manipulate spinal vertebrae is limited by the force they can apply with their hands. Theraflex robotic spinal manipulation provides the physiotherapist with a powerful technology to manipulate the whole spine with ease.

HOW DOES THERAFLEX SPINAL MANIPULATION WORK?

Theraflex has three modes of operation, each of which can be minutely adjusted for force and speed, thus matching the patient requirements exactly.

MUSCLE RELAXATION

On this setting, the device rapidly taps on the muscles either side of the spine. By running this up and down the spine, the physiotherapist is able to stimulate muscle relaxation along the whole length of the spine, quickly and effectively. Most patients find this setting extremely comfortable and relaxing.

REFLEX STIMULATION

The second stage of treatment involves stimulation of the spinal reflexes. This is achieved by a gentle tapping over the full length of the spine, triggering the spinal reflexes to create further relaxation in preparation for spinal manipulation.

VERTEBRAL MANIPULATION

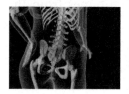 In the final stage of Theraflex treatment, the physiotherapist is able to manipulate each neighbouring vertebrae to move independently of each other, reducing the friction between them. In practice, the treatment mobilises the facet joints between each pair of neighbouring vertebrae. The net result of this treatment is to regain the flexibility in the full length of the spine, as originally intended. To achieve this, several treatments may be required, as each treatment progressively improves flexibility.

WHAT DOES THERAFLEX TREAT?

Theraflex is able to treat a number of conditions, the most common being general stiffness of the spine, but we have also successfully treated:

- Mild Scoliosis, a mild side flexion in the spine.
- Mild Kyphosis, hump back posture.

It also helps with the symptoms of:
- Osteoarthritis.
- Sciatica.
- Spinal Disc Pain.

THERAFLEX AS PREVENTATIVE TREATMENT

As a maintenance treatment, Theraflex helps keep the spine supple and prevents many of the pain problems associated with a stiff spine. This treatment has helped golfers improve their handicap by enhancing the smoothness of their golf swing thanks to increased spinal flexibility.

PULSED SHORTWAVE

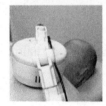

Pulsed Shortwave Close Up

- Increase range of movement of joints.
- Reduction of pain and inflammation for acute and chronic conditions.
- Increase blood flow.

Pulsed shortwave uses high frequency electromagnetic waves to produce thermal and non-thermal effects in deeps tissues. An advantage of pulsed shortwave over ultrasound is that a much larger, deeper area can be treated and the heating effect will last longer (if necessary), giving the practitioner more time to work on the treated area.

A damaged cell that is inflamed has a reduced cell membrane potential, meaning that the cell can't function correctly. This causes an ionic imbalance, and cellular osmotic pressures go awry. PSWD (pulsed shortwave diathermy) is said to restore normal cell membrane transport and ionic balance. The theory is not fully understood, but it is believed that it's to do with ionic transport and sodium/potassium pumped by the pulsed energy (Sanseverion, 1980). Energy is absorbed in the membrane (Luben and Cleary, 1996), and via signal transduction, it stimulates intracellular effects.

RADIAL SHOCKWAVE

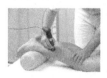 *Shockwave treatment of Achilles Tendinitis*

Radial shockwave has been extensively used in mainland Europe for many years, but as it has only recently been introduced to the UK, it is not commonly available here. It has, however, recently gained NICE approval. Extensive research around the world is pushing the boundaries of radial shockwave forward at a rapid pace and many new applications are being developed all the time.

The hubby and I have travelled to Europe for education on shockwave use, and have had training from an orthopaedic consultant who runs a major shockwave clinic in Luxembourg.

Shockwave is particularly effective in the treatment of:
- Plantar fasciitis/policeman's foot.
- Tendon calcification.
- Adhesive capsulitis/frozen shoulder.
- Achilles tendonitis.
- Reducing lumbar spasm.
- Piriformis syndrome.
- Tennis elbow.
- Iliotibial band syndrome.
- Improving osteoarthritic joint mobility.

SHOCKWAVE TREATMENT OF EPICONDYLITIS / TENNIS ELBOW

Many patients who have come to us with osteoarthritic joints have felt immediate improvement in joint flexibility. For those who choose not to undergo joint replacement surgery, shockwave offers a maintenance alternative, and ultimate relief from the condition of osteoarthritis; preliminary treatment with shockwave (to loosen the joint), followed by MBST (to regrow the cartilage), is the best solution in preventative care to slow down osteoarthritis.

There is so much supporting research out there. We attended a shockwave seminar in Southern France a few years back and listened to three days of research presentations from around the world, often at seven minutes a presentation. There was so much information to share!

For example, Ogden et al. (Shockwave Therapy for Chronic Proximal Plantar Fasciitis: A Meta-Analysis, 2014) presented at the 4th annual meeting of the International Society for Musculoskeletal shockwave Therapy, Berlin, Germany, in May 2001.

Pleiner et al., 2004, states that in a randomised controlled trial, extracorporeal shockwave treatment is effective in treating calcific tendonitis of the shoulder.

ULTRASOUND THERAPY

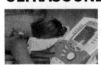

Ultrasound

- Reduces fibrous scar tissue.
- Speeds soft tissue injury healing.
- Increases local blood flow.
- Increases collagen production in tendons and ligaments.

Ultrasound in physiotherapy uses high frequency sound waves to accelerate the treatment of an inflammatory condition. The depth of penetration is controlled through the frequency.

INTERFERENTIAL THERAPY

- Reduce Swelling.
- Reduce muscle spasm.
- Treat acute joint pain.

Interferential therapy is most often used to treat conditions where there is muscle spasm, swelling, or joint pain, resulting from an acute injury. It works on the same pain gate theory as TENS and, like TENS, involves the use of stick-on pads around the area to be treated.

DEEP OSCILLATION-ELECTROSTATIC

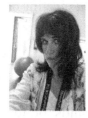 I love this – the technology can be used through your hands. It's so much fun.

DEEP OSCILLATION

I was introduced to this again recently at an AACP conference in 2016. Just after this event, bronchitis hit me again and I was amazed at the effect of this technology on my lungs; I could breathe afterwards and slept much better.

It is easy to use and cost effective, the results including pain relief, anti-inflammatory effects, the reduction of oedema, the acceleration of wound healing, and it is anti-fibrotic and can be used straight after an injury.

I came across three good pieces of research on this, though there are a lot more out there: Jahr et al., 2008, Aliyev, 2009, and Aliyev, 2012.

TREATING SPORTS INJURIES AND BACK PAIN WITH DEEP OSCILLATION

Press Release

Nicky Snazell, Consultant Physiotherapist, adds DEEP OSCILLA-TION® to her high-tech Pain Relief Clinics

Julie Soroczyn, M.D. of PhysioPod® UK Ltd. Consultant Physio and health celebrity Nicky Snazell

"DEEP OSCILLATION® was initially implemented in the UK for the management and treatment of Lymphoedema and Lipoedema but it is now used increasingly within the elite sporting world and in private physiotherapy clinics. It was at the AACP Conference in May 2016 that Nicky Snazell first learned of DEEP OSCILLATION® therapy.

So what is DEEP OSCILLATION®?

DEEP OSCILLATION® is an internationally patented, proven technology based on the effects of creating an electrostatic field in the tissue of the patient. Easy application is from clinician to patient/client via vinyl gloved hands; utilizing all normal massage movements or via circular movements over the tissue with a handheld applicator but without pressure, protecting the clinician's hands. The special structure of DEEP OSCILLATION® allows the creation of biologically effective oscillations in the treated tissue using electrostatic attraction and friction. In contrast to other therapies, these pleasant oscillations have a gentle and deep-acting effect on all tissue components to an 8 cm depth (through skin, connective tissue, subcutaneous fat, muscles, blood, and lymph vessels).

Because of the non-invasive, non-traumatic, gentle nature of this therapy, very early possibilities of application are possible following injury and from Day One post-operatively. Chronic conditions can also be worked upon with effective results.

It is clinically proven to significantly reduce pain, anti-inflammatory, swelling and bruising, resulting in a dynamic wound healing with less resultant scar tissue. Stubborn fibrosis and scar tissue are also effectively broken down. Sensitivity, range of motion, and function are regained with a quicker return to normal activities than with conventional therapies alone.

It is also FDA Approved. Normal massage contraindications apply plus pregnancy and pacemaker."

DYNAMIC SCANNING

As you walk across the GaitScan plate, 4096 sensors are set to scan the plantar surface of the foot in motion. The GaitScan system records timing sequences during gait, and captures the relative pressure for each of ten distinct anatomical landmarks. The result is the detection of imbalances and other indicators of common lower limb pathologies.

PRESSURE MAPPING

GaitScan gives you the ability to view a patient's foot (plantar) pressure distribution in both 2D and 3D. The synchronised mode allows for a direct right and left foot comparison, and displays the centre of pressure – or 'gait line' of the foot – throughout the gait cycle. Detailed images allow for the easy identification of high-pressure areas and existing biomechanical inefficiencies. It can be an early predictor of osteoarthritis in the lower limb, and can help to avoid injuries by prescribing orthotics where clearly a biomechanical abnormality needs addressing.

DIETARY PAIN RELIEF

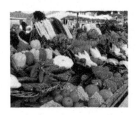

When presented with a medical issue, it is easy to overlook diet and nutrition as a potential cause of the problem. It is a sad fact that our health in the UK is not as good as it could be – you only have to look at

the rapidly increasing obesity evident on our streets every day. Through simple changes to your diet, however, it is possible to:
- Minimise your risk of heart disease, diabetes, and arthritis.
- Live a longer and healthier life.
- Maximise your life every day.

Cases of heart disease, stroke, and diabetes are all increasing, and there is a very clear relationship between this and the proliferation of sugar-loaded and highly processed food that is becoming ever more popular. Such a rapid change in health cannot have occurred by evolution. After all, we have been on this planet for hundreds of thousands of years, and we are seeing rapid change over the last 30 to 40 years.

No food manufacturer is going to tell you that their products are bad for your health, even if they know they are. Ultimately, you are what you eat, and only you are responsible for that.

The facts are that many of the UK's health problems are preventable; the proof is that other countries with healthier diets have fewer health problems than we do. For example, recent data shows that the UK is the 6th WORST country for breast cancer and that women are 50% more likely to die than in Spain. So, we could be 50% better if we do and eat what they do and eat.

How many older people do you know who are having a really hard time with poor health or pain, with it getting worse every day? A common phrase to describe this is we 'live short and die long'. Do you want that to be you? It doesn't have to be that way. It's your choice. You just need to get your mind-set focused on prevention – why wait until it's happened and then hope that surgery or drugs will save you? We can help guide you towards better diet and health.

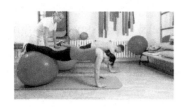

Exercise class

REHABILITATION CLINIC

EXERCISE CLASS

At the clinic we will ensure that you are safe and ready to start exercising, and then we will tailor a program to your needs. This program must contain specific stretches and exercises – prescribed only to you. Never, ever use someone else's prescription, as it may make you worse. You need both a balanced body, and good core strength to minimise damaging, abnormal stress. Studies have shown a 67% improvement when the rehab program has been prescribed by a physiotherapist.

We can help you develop a highly effective exercise strategy to keep you active and improve your quality of life, putting you in control of your physical health. Effective exercise can also help you to:
* Prevent Injury.
* Live longer.
* Live more healthily.
* Minimise pain.
* Be happier.

WHY EXERCISE?

Most people have a negative picture of exercise – picturing heavy exertion in a gym – and they often only link this with weight loss. However, numerous studies have shown that even minor effort, such as walking 30 minutes a day, can drastically reduce your risk to disease and premature death.

The statistics are overwhelming. Many of today's diseases are preventable – cancer, heart disease, diabetes, and osteoporosis just to name a few – and exercise is a key component of prevention. Similar studies have recorded there being just as much benefit for mindset.

Exercise stimulates the release of endorphins – our body's natural painkiller – and it is many times stronger than morphine. Endorphins also give a natural 'feel good' response. Regular exercise has been shown to reduce stress, anxiety, and depression. A huge fear amongst many is Alzheimer's or dementia in later life, and one study on over 65's recorded a 50% decrease in Alzheimer's amongst those who exercised regularly. Exercise has also been shown to improve memory and reduce dementia.

Lastly, exercise will help reduce weight. This in itself has huge beneficial implications to physical health and mindset.

RESOURCES

My clinic now has specialist software that enables us to directly email exercise programs to you after your treatment. Through a partnership with Physio Tec, we are able to offer you the ability to review your exercise program in detail as many times as you like from the comfort of your own home. The Physio Tec software enables a physiotherapist to select specific exercises from an extensive library and prescribe them to the patient.

MEDICATION FOR PAIN RELIEF

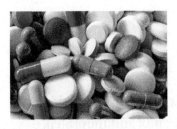

Various medications

With some conditions it is often not possible to effectively treat them with medication. Whilst my clinic provides this information for general purposes, it is always important to consult with the prescribing doctor before taking any medication. When prescribing medication, there are often a number of routes that it is possible to take.

ANALGESICS

More commonly known as 'painkillers', this group of medication works by interrupting the pain signals in the nervous system, which has the effect of blocking the pain and therefore reducing its effects. Some of the most common analgesics used include:

- Paracetamol.
- Co-Codamol.
- Tramadol.
- Dihydrocodeine.
- Morphine.

Whilst morphine is occasionally prescribed for extreme cases, Paracetamol at full strength is often sufficient for most problems. Some antidepressants – such as Amitriptyline, which can sometimes be used at low doses – have been found to help relieve certain types of pain. For example, taken at night, Amitriptyline is used to treat chronic (persistent) pain.

Specific nerve pain symptoms are sometimes treated with Pregabalin.

NON-STEROIDAL ANTI-INFLAMMATORIES

This group of medication works to reduce pain by reducing the inflammation that is causing it. Often, the pain is caused by the inflammation process itself. Some example of anti-inflammatories are:

- Ibuprofen.
- Diclofenac.
- Naproxen.

Anti-inflammatories are often highly effective when used in combination with analgesics, such as a combination of Paracetamol and Ibuprofen.

MUSCLE RELAXANTS

Some muscle relaxants – such as Diazepam – can be used to help relax muscles which are in spasm. In more severe cases, muscle relaxants such as Botulinum Toxin (Botox) can be injected directly into the muscle to release the spasm.

INTRAMUSCULAR STIMULATION

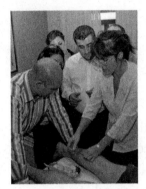

Nicky Snazell IMS

Many people suffer from chronic pain and are unable to find an effective long-term treatment to relieve it. Intramuscular stimulation provides an alternative, effective treatment for the relief of chronic pain. It has been proven to effectively:

- Make chronic pain history.
- Help you play sport at your best.
- Help you stop taking drugs.
- Prevent surgery.

The fact is that many of these problems can be symptoms – with the cause being in the spine – the trouble being that you can go on treating symptoms forever and still be in pain or restricted in movement.

Think of your car: if your headlight bulb keeps blowing because of a faulty wire in the fuse box, then you need to fix the fuse box, not keep replacing the headlight bulb.

The way that human anatomy is formed in the womb means that the limbs can be considered an extension of the spine. So, specific parts of the body are controlled by specific nerves, their roots emerging at the spine. Just as in the car analogy, you could have pain in your foot because of a nerve problem in your back, or an elbow problem because of a nerve problem in the neck.

Many spinal problems can be linked to muscular problems and the facts are that neither MRI nor X-ray can see such problems. IMS will find and treat muscular-related nerve (neuropathic) problems, and is used as part of a wider treatment by a physiotherapist. For neuropathic problems, IMS is unsurpassed.

WHAT IS GUNN IMS?

Professor Chan Gunn

Many people who suffer from chronic pain become frustrated and depressed when their doctor cannot help. Some try medications and physical therapies – such as massage, physiotherapy, manipulations, and even surgery – and do not find lasting relief.

Chronic pain is a form of pain that lasts for a prolonged period. This timescale can range from several weeks to many years, and the pain worsens over time. Chronic pain can significantly affect quality of life, and can lead to many secondary conditions, including depression. This cycle can be difficult to break out of.

Nicky Snazell

Have you suffered months, or even years, of pain and have you tried everything, but nothing seems to help? Are you on a cocktail of drugs to control your pain, are concerned about the possible side effects of the drugs, and do not want to be on the drugs forever? Have you suffered years of pain but nobody seems to know what it is?

If this is you, then it could be that you have a neuropathic problem, which conventional scans such as X-ray and MRI simply cannot see. This is where Gunn IMS excels, as it is unsurpassed in diagnosing and then treating such problems. That's why so many people come to this clinic from all over the UK, from Europe, the Middle and Far East, and the Caribbean. Gunn IMS succeeds where other treatments fail, and is used as part of a wider physiotherapy treatment.

GUNN IMS FOR SPORTS INJURIES

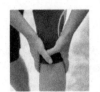

Sports injury

Complex sports injuries are often not resolved by conventional physiotherapy techniques. In part this is because many sports injuries have a neuropathic origin. Gunn IMS works by treating the root cause of the problem.

Athletes have been shown to recover far more quickly from their injuries when Gunn IMS has been used in their treatment, and some national teams and Olympic squads require IMS practitioners to be part of their core therapy team.

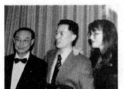

Pictured here in Vancouver, with Prof Gunn and Prof Aung, Nicky as an 'Honorary Fellow' speaking about pain advances and IMS in the UK.

IMS Pain Article: NICKY SNAZELL AUTHOR listed in 'Neurological', originally published in issue 111 - May 2005.

"Which Animal Are We Chasing?

Would you like to learn about an effective drug and surgery free treatment for pain relief? If the answer is a sceptical 'yes', then please read on.

This article will hopefully whet your appetite and get you to embark on a journey of discovery into the jungle of human pain. In this jungle, met-aphorically speaking, there are many different animals. Pain can disguise itself in many forms. The secret of killing pain is in knowing which animal you are dealing with before choosing your weapon.

My background is in human and animal physiology, physiotherapy, and musculoskeletal Acupuncture. I have collected rows of certificates in my search, and until I studied Intramuscular Stimulation (IMS), none of them allowed me to catch this elusive animal that I now come to realise is 'neuropathic pain'.

There are, broadly speaking, three types of animals in the jungle, but we are concerned here with only one. The animals we are not concerned with are:

1. Those described as pain due to acute injury or inflammation.
2. Those related to psychogenic disorders, including severe depression.

We are going to take a closer look at the more puzzling third group, exhibited by conditions such as tennis elbow, back pain, repetitive strain, frozen shoulder, whiplash, and fibromyalgia. These are all the result of the same type of pathology called neuropathy. You cannot kill this pain by cutting it out with surgery and it cannot be hidden by drugs. The only way to deal with this animal is by desensitising it by relieving the irritation at its source. Invariably this is at the nerve root.

Significantly, every one of us will see this animal at some time in our lives. But the camouflage is so effective it takes a special kind of hunter to find its cause. Professor Gunn, a world guru and Clinical Professor in pain relief, spent years mapping out muscle activity using EMG (Electromyography). He related this to physical signs, muscle shortening being the most important to the understanding of this third type of painful condition.

In 1996, Prof Gunn founded iSTOP (Institute for The Study and Treatment of Pain) in Vancouver, Canada, to promote IMS across the world and ensure its development. After many exciting trips to this clinic, and then to the rapidly evolving centre of excellence in Seoul, South Korea, my ability to hunt and kill this elusive animal improved immeasurably.

NEUROPATHIC PAIN

The treatment of chronic pain has always been a bone of contention, and I do not wish to debate as to which aspect is truly a new invention and which aspect is thousands of years old. My concern is to convey the truly amazing results that I have both witnessed and achieved through IMS, the latter being a fusion of oriental acupuncture with western concepts of neurophysiology.

Prof Gunn theorises that many patients with chronic pain have tender shortened muscles, because of neuropathy of the segmental nerves that supply them. His theory embraces the sound physiological principles of super sensitivity by Cannon and Rosenblueth. Their research explained the problems of super sensitivity when nerves themselves were sick, and this can be likened to a house alarm whose sensing system is too sensitive and hence normally innocent activities cause the alarm to go off – in the same way that a supersensitive nerve reacts abnormally to innocuous signals.

Aging, accidents, and poor posture all injure the nerves. Normal electrical signals are interrupted and the muscles become over-reactive to very small traces of a chemical called acetylcholine. Prof Gunn states, "It's like driving a car with the brakes on." Tight muscles lead to neuropathy in which poor blood circulation will make the area feel cold. This neuropathy also changes the skin surface, appearing pitted with reduced hair growth in the affected dermatome. Joint range is often restricted.

The disaster continues. Shortened muscles pull on tendons, creating conditions like Achilles tendonitis or Golfer's elbow. They compress spinal discs and hence the nerves, leading to sciatica and facet joint osteoarthritis. It accelerates the osteoarthritic changes in major joints. Lengthy problems can lead to permanent scarring, and this is why it is imperative that both GPs and physiotherapists recognise this type of animal and intervene early.

IMS TREATMENT

The programme of treatment can include gentle acupuncture, laser, and stretching prior to IMS. IMS is a dry needling technique using needles varying between 0.25 and 0.35mm gauge. The technique is most effective when the needle is placed within a plunger, a device that both enables extremely accurate control of the needle and significantly increases the amount of needling attainable within any amount of time. Ultimately the plunger, a device developed by Prof Gunn, allows the needle to be used as a micro surgical tool, preventing the need for surgery. Having equipped yourself with this formidable weapon, you can hunt down this neuropathic problem and kill the pain.

The insertion of the needle into the shortened muscle causes an instantaneous shock to that muscle, measurable with EMG, facilitating release. Locally it causes bleeding, attracting blood clotting platelets and growth factors to promote healing.

The implication of the muscle release is that it restores transmission along dormant nerve pathways, ultimately curing the condition. This can be seen objectively with changes to neuropathic signs and subjectively with the absence of pain.

ASSESSMENT OF NEUROPATHIC SIGNS

Evidence needs to be found, not only with questioning, but most importantly by carrying out many physical tests, to hunt out which animal we are dealing with and where is it hiding. This must include questions relating to internal organs, as well as musculoskeletal issues. The presence of neuropathic pain has to be confirmed before moving on to IMS treatment. Visible signs of a dysfunctional nerve and its corresponding spinal levels can be pieced together like a jigsaw puzzle. The visible neuropathic signs can be grouped into sensory, motor, autonomic, and trophic.

Sensory changes:
- Muscle tenderness.

- Exaggerated sensitivity.
- Numbness.

Motor changes:
- Shortened muscles and restricted joints.
- Thickened palpable muscle bands.

Autonomic features:
- Coldness.
- Excessive perspiration.
- Goosebumps.
- Excessive fluid in the subcutaneous tissue called trophoedema (skin rolling and matchstick tests).

Trophic Changes:
- Localised hair loss.
- Brittle nails.
- Abnormal skin, i.e. psoriasis.

Some of these signs might at first appear insignificant, but I cannot emphasise enough the benefits of learning to understand easily recognisable signs, which clearly indicate a problem and its location. To help illustrate, here are two case studies.

CASE STUDY 1 – DRUGS ELIMINATION

This patient worked in a physically demanding job when his 'back went'. He staggered into the clinic like a drunk, as a result of being prescribed a huge cocktail of pain killers from his GP, who could offer no help other than 'take drugs and wait for the pain to go away'. His speech was incoherent and the pain was so severe that assessment had to rely on neuropathic signs.

On flexing the patient forward and palpating the spinous processes, the tip of L4 (Lumbar 4) was thickened and prominent, indicating a problem in the disc below. This assessment was further supported by a damp strip at L4 and orange peel effect, indicating trophoedema. Sliding my hand down the legs, the L4 dermatome was cold on both legs and there was visible hair loss.

I found thickened superficial shortened muscles between L4 and L5. On deep needling with the plunger, both multifidus and rotators were gripping the left L4/5 disc and left sciatic nerve with a vengeance. He returned three days later and declared he was 50% better and had already cut back on the drugs, to the extent that he was coherent. Following the second session he said he felt 100% better and had stopped taking all the drugs. On the third visit he was doing well, although some calf pain had reappeared. The needle still grabbed at L4/5 indicating that the problem had not been fully resolved. One week later he still had an ache in his calf, although not bad enough to need even mild painkillers. Another week on and he was pain free with no needle grab. He was discharged after five treatments.

CASE STUDY 2 – SURGERY AVOIDANCE

This lady was referred to the clinic by an insurance company who indicated that she needed immediate help prior to a knee operation. She had severe pain in the knee and was unable to walk. All the tests for the knee ligaments and menisci were negative. The knee appeared normal but the erector spinae muscles in her back were in spasm. On palpation there was a thickened nodule on the right of L3, which related to the pain in the knee area. My hand skidded on damp skin at L3, which also exhibited the orange peel effect. The dermatome L3 over the lower aspect of her thigh had hair loss and was cold.

I commenced treatment by desensitising the area with laser and Acupuncture, covering the area between L2 and L5. Two days later the patient still struggled to walk. I laid her on her side, used laser as preparation and then needled once, with the help of the plunger, at L4 level, releasing tight muscle fibres. She yelped and said, "that's my knee pain". Four days later the pain had centralised to her buttock, which was an excellent improvement, and with further IMS I released the remaining tight multifidus fibres. A review eight days later showed full pain free movement and she was discharged with no further problems and no need for a knee operation.

FREQUENTLY ASKED QUESTIONS

What conditions respond well to IMS?

Sciatica responds brilliantly. In days we have got people back to work and sports. With the pressure taken off sensitive structures within the spine – such as nerve roots, prolapsed discs, and facet joints – they all have the best possible chance to heal without surgical involvement. It is then important to restore the stability with exercise.

In the cervical area, carpal tunnel nerve entrapment can be relieved by this method if treated early enough. RSI (Repetitive Strain Injury) can be helped greatly with IMS and changes to the workstation.

For the sports-oriented, chronic muscle shortening in the forearm causes conditions such as tennis and Golfer's elbow. These can be cured by needling the lower cervical and specific arm muscles.

Frozen shoulder, for those of us in our 40s, can be extremely debilitating. Current treatment options are long-term physical therapy and corticosteroid injections, with pain usually not resolved for up to 18 months. IMS can resolve this in many cases in days or weeks by needling the cervical and rotator cuff muscles.

Hamstring injuries are a major problem within football. IMS has demonstrably resolved these problems with lumbar needling and is now being used within the premier league.

Achilles tendonitis can cause major layoffs for runners. With IMS treatment, gentle training can continue and the problem can be resolved within days.

The knee is always vulnerable to overexertion and twisting. Sports injuries to the knee can respond quickly and chronic anterior knee pain can be a thing of the past. Numerous Olympic athletes are now being treated with IMS.

Is IMS the same as Acupuncture?

Acupuncture is an amazing ancient philosophy, its diagnosis and practice being based on oriental medicine originating many thousands of years ago. IMS is based on western medical knowledge and is aimed at treating neuro-pathic pain. IMS can only be administered by chartered physiotherapists or MDs who have a background in Acupuncture and who have been trained by an authorised IMS instructor.

I hate needles. Will it hurt?

When the muscle is normal, you should not feel anything at all, other than possibly a mild prick as the needle enters the skin. The needle is much thinner than the hollow needles used for injections or taking blood. However, if the muscle is supersensitive and in spasm, there is a very short but unpleasant cramping pain. This is due to the needle being grabbed by the muscle.

Why don't I feel the same unpleasant sensations with Acupuncture?

Acupuncture does not seek out the centre of muscles in spasm that elicits the grab at the heart of the super sensitivity. Acupuncture is based on inserting needles according to meridian points that form a map based on traditional Chinese medicine. This can often help a lot, especially if the problem is not severe. With mild cases, up to 70% of the problem can be treated with Acupuncture and laser alone. If the problem is neuropathic, traditional Acupuncture will not cure it.

What is the Plunger?

The Plunger developed by Prof Gunn turns dry needling into microsurgery. It transforms the use of the needle into a precision instrument, enabling many tiny incisions and literally cutting away the problem with a 0.25mm cutting edge.

Why does IMS feel more comfortable after using a laser?

The benefit of the laser is that it has an analgesic effect on the area and starts the healing process before the needle is inserted.

I am pain free, do I need to keep coming?

Once treated there is no need for top-ups.

I have severe osteoarthritis with bone erosion. Can IMS help?

IMS cannot change structural defects.

Could early IMS treatment have helped to arrest osteoarthritis development?

Yes. Unwell nerves equals shortened muscles, equals tight tendons, equals accelerated bone erosion.

How many treatments do I need and how often?

The number of treatments depends on many factors: age, stress, nutrition, general health, the severity and duration of the condition, and the degree of fibrosis. Furthermore, any previous surgery complicates the picture.

Typically my clinic aims to see an improvement within two treatments, or we would question why. Normally, five to six treatments will resolve it, though complex cases require more. The frequency of treatment depends on the individual's ability to heal. Treatments can be as often as weekly or as infrequent as monthly. IMS cures cumulatively, rather than offering temporary help, therefore leaving longer gaps between treatments is not an issue.

Can IMS cure me?

IMS is unequalled in the treatment of pain of a neuropathic origin. However, it is just one tool in the box to be used in combination with the many other tools available to fight pain.

How do I find IMS practitioners who are correctly trained?

The best source is the iSTOP website, www.istop.org. It lists all approved IMS practitioners and their level. At the moment IMS is still in the pioneering phase and there are not many practitioners available.

It is best to ask questions as to the amount of training any practitioner has had and if they have passed the exams. They should have also attended several days of internships with a recognised IMS instructor, which is imperative to assess practical skills in the use of a plunger.

SUMMARY

I have been fortunate enough to be taught how to identify the signs associated with neuropathy. The results that I have achieved by correct diagnosis and the use of IMS have been amazing. Surgery and drugs are not the answer with neuropathic pain.

Read the signs, identify the animal, and use the Gunn."

REFERENCES

1. Gunn CC. *The Gunn Approach to the Treatment of Chronic Pain*. Churchill Livingstone. ISBN 0-443-05422-3.
2. Gunn CC. *Pain, Acupuncture and IMS*. ISTOP. January 2004.
3. Cannon WB and Rosenblueth A. *The Super sensitivity of Denervated Structures. Macmillan*. 1949.

MASSAGE FOR INJURIES

Massage in this country tends to be thought of as a luxury indulgence, whereas in many countries it is perceived as a fundamental part of treatment, and may even be the prescribed first line of treatment. The difference perhaps lies in the more common UK leaning towards gentle massage, which has little, if any, therapeutic benefit.

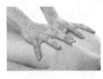

Back massage

SPORTS MASSAGE

Sports massage is applied with more pressure, and to be effective, the masseur must have a good understanding of anatomy. Massage is widely used with athletes and in the treatment of sports injuries. It is an essential part of sports rehab, assisting the speed of recovery.

If you have a sports injury – or an injury from an accident or just from normal daily living – a sports massage can help. Your normal pliable body tissue may have been replaced by scar tissue, which can bind other tissues together, causing loss of pliability and strength. Adhesions can occur in joints and ultimately become part of joint tissue. In such cases, ongoing stress or overuse will more likely cause you repeated injury.

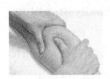

CALF MASSAGE

Sports massage can help you by breaking down scar tissue and helping its re-absorption, encouraging normal tissue to be laid down.

Deep tissue massage – which is more common in the east – is based on understanding the links in the body, as developed by Brandon Raynor, so that the cause of the pain can be treated rather than where it hurts. For some, there may be deep-seated causes, which will need excavation. This in turn may lead to emotional release.

AROMATHERAPY

This is a very relaxing, soft, gentle treatment. Aromatherapy uses plant materials and aromatic plant oils – including essential oils, and other aroma compounds – for the purpose of altering one's mood or physical well-being. It can be offered as a complementary therapy.

MINDSET THERAPY

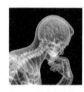 *Mindset*

- Healthy body.
- More happiness.
- Deeper meaning of life.

At my clinics, we encourage you to take control of your destiny in a more fulfilling and positive way, and this mindset change starts by developing a healthy body.

The mind has a powerful control of how we feel, both mentally and physically. Our behaviour is a result of our history of emotional experiences, which formed our learnt belief system. Provoking memories can yield to an instant response to past emotions, causing either pleasurable feelings, or irrational behaviour and physical pain.

It is no surprise, then, that a physical pain linked to a painful emotional experience can go on for years. In some cases treatment of the physical manifestation brings on a huge emotional response, with deeply buried memories flooding to the forefront.

Only by dealing with these past memories can a person move on and let go of their physical pain.

NLP

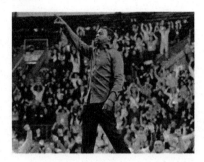

The Sports Sandwich, Stafford FM, Nicky talking about the mind.

Neuro-linguistic programming (NLP) is an approach to communication, personal development, and psychotherapy created by Richard Bandler and John Grinder in the United States in the 1970s. I thoroughly enjoyed a two-week course with Richard Bandler, and it did wonders for any nerves I feel before public speaking. We spent a lot of time in trance where learning is accelerated.

NLP's creators cleverly work on the connection between the neurological processes (*neuro-*), language (*linguistic*), and behavioural patterns learned through experience (*programming*). Changing these connections can enable you to lessen your fear and achieve your specific goals in life.

ORTHOPAEDIC SURGEON CONSULTATION

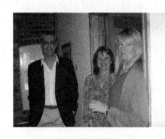

Vinod Kathuria
• Rapid access means you don't have to wait months.
• Highly skilled diagnosis gives peace of mind.
• Decision on need for surgery clarifies your plans.
• Diagnostic testing prescription.
• Qualified reading of scans within 48 hours of having scan.
• Rapid access to MRI within 48 hours of consultation.

Orthopaedic Surgeons use surgical and non-surgical means to diagnose and treat musculoskeletal trauma, sports injuries, arthritis, wear and tear, infections, and tumours. They can authorise MRI, ultrasound, X-ray, and bloods, then can interpret the results to fine-tune the diagnosis.

PHYSIOTHERAPISTS

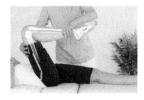

Physiotherapy

- Re-ignite your motivation for life.
- Feel more attractive and confident.
- Move towards a pain free life.
- Give yourself a slimmer, more flexible and active body.
- Recover more quickly and more fully following surgery.

WHAT IS PHYSIOTHERAPY? A BRIEF HISTORY

Physiotherapy's origins date back to 1813 in Sweden, when massage manipulation and exercise were used to treat gymnasts. As a profession, however, physiotherapy wasn't founded until 1894, by four nurses through the Society of Trained Masseuses. By 1900 it was recognised as a professional organisation and later, in 1920, it was awarded a royal charter, forming the Chartered Society of Massage and Medical Gymnastics. By 1944 the society became the Chartered Society of Physiotherapy (CSP).

"Physiotherapy is a science-based healthcare profession concerned with human function, movement and maximizing potential," (CSP). As a professional body it is regulated by the Chartered Society of Physiotherapy, and the Health and Carers' Profession Council (HCPC).

As each case is unique, a physiotherapist clinical diagnosis is based upon an assessment of previous medical history, work, and lifestyle, and it also takes into account psychological, cultural, and social factors. Physiotherapy training is comprehensive and physiotherapists' skills are endorsed by

GPs. This means you can trust that you will receive a skilled and informed diagnosis of your problem.

HOW DOES PHYSIOTHERAPY TREAT MY CONDITION?

At my clinic, we focus on a holistic approach, providing information on healthy lifestyle, weight targets, and diet and nutrition.

We have very senior, experienced Grade 7 neuromusculoskeletal physiotherapists with a keen interest in sports injuries, and our ultimate goal is to establish your maximum functional independence. Our physiotherapists develop a personalised program to move you towards optimum musculoskeletal health. To achieve this, we combine our diagnostic listening skills with hands on treatment, supported by our broad range of technology. Physiotherapists prescribe and monitor a lifestyle and exercise program with realistic and attainable goals.

RICE THERAPY

This is now more often called MICE movement, and we offer advice on this home treatment.

RICE is an acronym for **R**est, **I**ce, **C**ompression, and **E**levation, and is an important first aid treatment for immediate post-injury use, to help reduce swelling and pain and prevent further complications. Soft tissue injuries to muscles, tendons, and ligaments often occur in sports, and can also occur in normal daily life from a trip or fall. In many cases the injured area will swell and bruise from internal bleeding and become tender. Early first aid treatment with RICE can reduce the swelling and make the injury heal faster.

Although not part of the official RICE acronym, it is important to protect the injured area as quickly as possible from further injury, by using:

Rest: Stop all aggravating activity and make sure the injury is not weight bearing.

Ice: Apply ice (a frozen pack of peas works well) to the area for 15 to 20 minutes, but always with a towel or similar between the skin and ice, to prevent frostbite – never leave on for more than 20 minutes to avoid frostbite. Also, allow sufficient time between applications for the skin to warm up, typically 45 to 60 minutes. Ice is used to lower the blood supply to the injury and thus restrict swelling. It also helps reduce the pain level.

Compression: This aids the ice in reducing the swelling and can also help with pain relief. Compression can be achieved with a simple bandage wrap, or an elasticated wrap. It is important not to wrap too tightly, however, as this can promote swelling and pain. If this occurs, just reapply the wrap a little looser.

Elevation: Try to elevate the injured area above heart level to help reduce swelling.

SPORTS INJURY REHABILITATION

Recent research has shown that around 30% (that's a staggering 22 million people) of the population of the UK suffer a sporting injury every year. So, the chances are high that most sports people will suffer multiple injuries over their sporting careers. On average, a person participating in sport will:
- Pick up 1-2 injuries per year.
- Take up to 5 days off work every year.

Even worse, of all the people injured, 25% will not be able to carry on playing sport as a direct result of the sporting injury.

If you love your sport, want to keep playing, and can't afford the risk of time off work, then you need to be proactive and make sure you know how to be as well prepared as you can be. You should also know where to get the best treatment, so that if you are injured, you can get yourself back to full fitness as quickly as possible.

Chartered physiotherapists will make an enjoyable exercise programme for self-analysis. This will enable you to recover from an operation, return to sport, or simply improve everyday life.

Benefits of one of our rehab programmes include:
- Resolution of neck or back pain.
- Reduction in joint pain.
- Greater strength and tone.
- Less stress and fewer headaches.
- Improved looking, firmer, more supple body.
- Better posture and gait.
- Increased bone density.
- A return to sport with fewer injuries.
- Improved circulation and immune system.

Your road to recovery following an injury will be a lot more effective and enjoyable when guided by specialists.

ENERGY MEDICINE

REIKI

June, my beloved Reiki Master, who passed over last March.

Reiki was developed in 1922 by a Japanese Buddhist called Mikao Usui. Universal energy or Chi is said to be channelled through the hands of the healer to the patient. The name means 'mysterious atmosphere' or 'miraculous sign', and was first recorded in AD 1001.

MAGNETIC RESONANCE TREATMENT

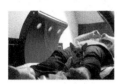 All of our information regarding Magnetic Resonance Treatment and MBST has now been transferred to our specialist website, which also provides details of our specialist magnetic resonance treatment centre, if you'd like to find out more about this: WWW.MRTCENTRE.CO.UK

WHAT IS MRT (MBST)?

Magnetic Resonance Treatment (MRT) is provided on MBST technology made by MedTec in Germany. In that respect, MRT and MBST are equivalent in terms of meaning.

MRT is a cellular regeneration treatment for osteoarthritis, osteoporosis, bone fractures, spinal discs, and sports injuries to ligaments and tendons. Traditional treatment is either a cocktail of drugs or surgery, but now we can offer you a third and more attractive option.

- Increase your physical activities capability.
- Improve your joint flexibility.
- Enhance your sleep quality.
- Reduce your reliance on drugs.
- Delay or eliminate your need for surgery.
- Minimise your risk of bone fracture.
- Significantly speed bone fracture healing.
- Increase rate of recovery from sports injuries to tendons and ligaments.

Osteoarthritis is mainly caused by a loss of cartilage, leading to painful bone-on-bone contact. MRT can stimulate the growth of new cartilage. So, for example, for those suffering knee arthritis, a treatment would be given to target the cartilage in the knee. This stimulates the thickening of the cartilage and typically, a reduction in pain would be felt within days. Cell regeneration starts with treatment, but then continues afterwards, with further improvements felt for up to six months after treatment. The latest research from Germany indicates that patients feel significant benefits more than four years later.

Most joints in the body can be treated, including:
- Shoulder, elbow, wrist, and hand.
- Hip, knee, ankle, and foot.
- Spinal facet joints.

Spinal discs, particularly in the lumbar region, are prone to damage from normal daily activities and can become frayed, weakened, or torn. MRT can help treat these conditions by stimulating spinal disc regeneration.

Osteoporosis is a silent disease that many people suffer from with no awareness until the bones start breaking or crumbling. The pain associated with this condition can be severe and can effectively destroy any quality of life. One in three women and one in twelve men over 50 suffer from osteoporosis.

MRT can be used to stimulate the growth of new bone, causing the bones to regenerate and become both thicker and stronger. In the same way, bone fractures can be stimulated to heal more quickly.

Soft tissue injuries to ligaments and tendons – typical in sports injuries – can linger longer than bone fractures. MRT can be used to speed the recovery of damaged tissue.

PREVENTATIVE TREATMENT

The careers of professional sports athletes are reliant on joint quality. In football, for example, wear and tear on knee joints alone has led to significant injury time and has cut many careers short; many retired football players end up needing new knees. MRT offers a risk free, painless option to preventatively treat such conditions, potentially extending careers and avoiding the need for later surgery.

MRT was developed directly from Magnetic Resonance Imaging (MRI) by German scientists in the 1990s. MRI was the state of the art diagnostic image producing procedure, which used very expensive, highly complex technology to produce clear internal body scans. Prompted by the fact that some patients claimed a therapeutic benefit from the MRI scan, it was clear that a new state-of-the-art therapeutic treatment was feasible.

The key to MRT success was in the understanding of the therapeutic mechanism of MRI, and enhancing this in a cost effective solution. MRT uses a complex triple independent energy field to deliver energy to the targeted human tissue, whether it is bone or cartilage.

In simple terms, MRT is able to target specific body tissue and saturate that tissue with energy, stimulating cell growth. In practical terms, this means we can heal bone and soft tissue injuries considerably quicker.

FOR THOSE WHO WANT A MORE SCIENTIFIC UNDERSTANDING

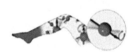 Hydrogen nuclei behave like small magnets, which spin around their own polar axes. The positions of these spin axes in space are usually random, so that molecules containing hydrogen do not exhibit external magnetic characteristics.

However, when such molecules – for example, cartilage tissue in the human body – are subjected to a nearly homogenous static magnetic field, the spin axes of the hydrogen nuclei (protons) align parallel to the magnetic field and precess at a frequency (known as the Larmor frequency), which depends on the strength of the external magnetic field.

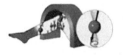 If the hydrogen atom is subjected to an electromagnetic field that oscillates at the Larmor frequency, the field can transfer energy to the proton by inverting its spin direction. When the field is turned off, the proton spin decays back to its original direction and gives off the acquired energy to the surrounding tissue, resulting in the following recurrent action: the electromagnetic energy of the therapeutic appliance raises the energy of the hydrogen protons. These pass energy on to their environment as the energy falls back to the initial (ground state) value.

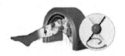 In this way, information for renewed synthetic activity can be transferred from the MBST appliance to the cartilage tissue. It is the resonance between the proton spin precession frequency and the electromagnetic field frequency in the MBST device that allows the highest possible quantity of therapeutic energy to be transferred accurately into human tissue.

MBST technology – which provides MRT – was developed in the 1990s in Germany and has had substantial interest and use, initially in Germany and Austria, and more latterly around the world. This has stimulated a lot of academic interest and various studies have been completed on the subject. Perhaps of most significance is the 10 year study of over 4,500 patients, published in early 2013, as this gives the most comprehensive real world data on the efficacy of MBST.

WHAT IS MRT?

MRT uses the same magnetic resonance technology principles as MRI, but uses it for therapy instead of imaging.

WHAT HAPPENS IN TREATMENT?

MRT works by applying a stimulating and regenerative magnetic field directly to the affected area.

IS MRT THE SAME AS MAGNETIC FIELD THERAPY?

No. MRT differs fundamentally from magnetic field therapy due to its unique use of magnetic resonance technology.

IS MRT EFFECTIVE?

Its effectiveness in stimulating cells to regenerate has been proven in a number of scientific studies and by more than 180,000 successfully treated patients.

HOW CAN YOU BE CONFIDENT IN MRT?

MRT is currently used in over 290 centres around the world. In Germany and Austria alone – countries with very high medical standards – there are over 150 orthopaedic consultants trusting and using MRT.

WHY HASN'T MY GP HEARD OF MRT?

MRT is still fairly new to the UK, with only four sites offering this technology. To be fair to your GP, there is little chance they would have any knowledge of something so new to the UK. However, the fact that over 150 orthopaedic consultants trust in this technology in countries with very high medical standards should give you confidence. We will happily send your GP an information pack if requested.

HOW LONG DOES MRT TAKE?

MRT requires seven hours for osteoarthritis (nine for osteoporosis) in one-hour sessions each day, except weekends. Patients who travel, or who would prefer treatment completed in five days, can have two treatments per day, provided there are eight hours or more between the sessions.

HOW LONG IS MRT EFFECTIVE FOR?

Controlled clinical studies have found MRT to be effective over 12 months, though latest research indicates significant benefits with some patients for more than four years. An annual top up of three sessions is recommended to maintain the benefits. For those who would prefer to wait until symptoms return, a full seven-hour treatment would be required.

WHAT DOES IT MEAN FOR YOU?

You will be receiving treatment specifically designed for the joints and tissues causing you pain. The treatment device is programmed specifically for you using controlled software, targeting the underlying cause of pain.

WILL MRT BE EFFECTIVE FOR YOU?

Most probably. MRT's success rate is around 80% for reducing pain, improving function, and increasing cartilage thickness. MRT nearly always works, alleviates pain, improves mobility, and makes a significant improvement to quality of life.

DOES MRT HURT?

No. MRT is not painful, and in some cases there is a pleasant feeling of warmth in the joint treated. In rare cases, pain may briefly increase before rapidly declining. However, this is a sure sign that the treatment is working for you.

ARE THERE ANY SIDE EFFECTS?

No. MRT has never produced any side effects in over 180,000 treatments or any clinical trials.

WHAT ARE THE CONTRAINDICATIONS FOR MBST?

All types of electrical implants located in the area to be treated. Pregnancy, bacterial inflammations within the area to be treated, tumours, leukaemia, or HIV. Patients who have had cancer must have been clear for a minimum of five years.

CAN MRT BE USED WITH METAL IMPLANTS?

Yes. Metal implants are of no concern at all. This is because the energy pulses used in MRT are tiny, i.e. only 1/30,000 of those used in MRI.

WHAT DO YOU NEED TO DO?

Make sure you drink at least 1.5 to 2 litres of water a day, starting at least one week before and during treatment. Avoid excessive exercise. Eat healthily, ensuring good nutrition.

HOW DO YOU BOOK MRT?

You cannot self-refer for MRT. It is most important to be first assessed by a qualified physiotherapist to determine your condition and make sure MRT is right for you. The physiotherapist will evaluate your condition, your physical and mental health, lifestyle, fitness, and diet. The features and benefits of MRT will be reviewed and your questions answered.

WHAT HAPPENS DURING MRT?

MRT treatment will require you to lie on the bed for one hour for each session. We can prop you up a bit, but not into a sitting position. You will be assisted getting on and off the bed, but otherwise left alone throughout the treatment. Some patients like to book additional sessions with their therapist for associated treatment and to answer further questions.

You can read, listen to music, just relax, or sleep. You can move during the treatment, provided you keep the joint being treated within the coil, and should you need assistance during the treatment, there is an intercom directly to reception. Please be aware that your therapist may be treating other patients during your treatment and may not be available to answer your questions.

WHAT HAPPENS AFTER TREATMENT?

MRT stimulates the growth of the targeted tissues, and for most patients there will be a noticeable difference at the end of the treatment. The stimulation process continues after treatment, with further improvements being noticeable after two months. Growth stimulation continues, but at a reducing rate up to six months after treatment.

IS THERE POST-TREATMENT FOLLOW UP?

Yes. You will be called to see how you are progressing in the first three months after treatment.

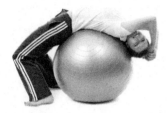

ESSENTIAL LUMBAR STABILITY DRILL AND CORE EXERCISES

These show you how to isolate and engage the deep stabilising muscles of the pelvis and spine, the transversus abdominis, the pelvic floor, and the multifidus muscles. To get the best stability, either brace your core, dig your fingers into your ribs and push the muscles of your trunk up against them, or contract the pelvic floor at the same time as pulling the tummy button in to the spine (called hollowing) in order to engage the transversus abdominis. It is important to practice spinal stability drills if engaging in Pilates or Yoga classes.

Please see chapter six in this book for yoga and McGill exercises, and also my first book, *The 4 Keys To Health*.

Glossary

"I grow old ... I grow old ...
I shall wear the bottoms of my trousers rolled."

–T.S. Eliot

Some of the following information has been gathered from various places on the internet, from sites such as Wikipedia.

ACUPUNCTURE: A key part of Chinese Medicine that treats using needles and herbs. It involves inserting thin needles into Acupuncture points and it now has a big part to play in western physical therapy.

ALCOHOLISM: A broad term for addictive drinking that is over the safe limits and can result in social, personality, and health issues.

ALLODYNIA: I used this term when discussing IMS dry needling. It refers to central pain amplification of innocuous stimuli. Just massaging or the touching of clothes on the skin can elicit pain.

ALZHEIMER'S: A chronic neurodegenerative disease, a deterioration in cognition, memory, and general thinking. It accounts for 70% of dementia cases.

AORTIC VALVE: This sits between the left ventricle and the aorta heart chambers. The other semilunar valve is the pulmonary valve. The other two valves are the mitral and tricuspid.

ATRIA: One of two blood collection chambers in the heart, the plural being atrium.

ATRIOVENTRICULAR NODE: This is part of the heart's electrical conduction system. It electrically connects atrial and ventricular chambers.

ARTERIOLE: A small, thin blood vessel in the microcirculation going from the arteries to the capillaries.

ARTHRITIS: A joint disorder involving inflammation and pain. There are many different types.

ATP [Adenosine Triphosphate]: A coenzyme used as an energy carrier in the cells.

AUTONOMIC NERVOUS SYSTEM (ANS): A division of the peripheral nervous system that affects the internal organs unconsciously in order to control sex drives, digestion, heart rate, eye dilation, and urination. It is also known for its key role in fight or flight.

CENTRAL NERVOUS SYSTEM (CNS): The part of the nervous system that is the brain and the spinal cord. It integrates information it receives and then centrally coordinates and influences the outcome of everything.

CANCER: An abnormal cell growth that can invade or spread to other parts of the body. Not all tumors are cancerous; benign tumors do not spread to other parts of the body.

CERVICAL GANGLIONS, INFERIOR AND SUPERIOR: Nerves of the cervical/neck and part of the sympathetic nervous system. Nerves from the thoracic spinal cord enter into the cervical ganglions and synapse (join) with its postganglionic fibers. The cervical ganglion has three paravertebral (spinal) ganglia:
- Superior cervical ganglion – adjacent to Cervical 2 & Cervical 3, targets the heart, head, and neck via the carotid arteries.
- Middle cervical ganglion – adjacent to Cervical 6, looks to the heart and neck.
- Inferior cervical ganglion (fused with the stellate ganglion) – adjacent to Cervical 7 at the base of neck, and transmits to the heart, lower neck, arm, and posterior cranial arteries.

Nerves emerging from cervical sympathetic ganglia contribute to the cardiac plexus, among other things.

CELIAC PLEXUS AND GANGLION: The celiac/coeliac/solar plexus is a complex network of nerves (a nerve plexus) located in the abdomen. It is behind the stomach and in front of the diaphragm, on the level of the first lumbar vertebra.

CHIROPRACTOR: Specialising in the diagnosis, treatment, and prevention of disorders of the neuromusculoskeletal system, and the effects of these disorders on general health. They predominately manipulate the spine in order to improve general health as well as reducing spinal subluxations.

CHROMOSOME: This contains most of the DNA of a living organism – the hard drive. It is a structure wrapped around protein complexes called nucleosomes, which consist of histones. The DNA in chromosomes is also associated with the transcription (copying) of genetic sequences factors. During most of the duration of the cell cycle, a chromosome consists of one long double-stranded DNA molecule. The chromosome gets replicated, like a photocopy resulting in an 'X'-shaped structure called a metaphase chromosome. Both the original and the newly copied DNA are now called chromatids. The two 'sister' chromatids join together at a protein junction called a centromere. During a sequence of mitosis known as metaphase, they are attached to the mitotic spindle and prepare to divide.

CROHNS DISEASE: A type of inflammatory bowel disease (IBD) that may affect any part of the gastrointestinal tract from mouth to bottom.

CYTOPLASM: This comprises of cytosol (the gel-like substance within the cell membrane) and the organelles – the cell's sub-structures.

DERMATOME: An area of skin that is supplied by a single pair of dorsal spinal nerve roots.

DIABETES: A metabolic disease in which there are high blood sugar levels over a prolonged period of time.

DISC: Each intervertebral disc forms a fibrocartilaginous joint to allow movement, and ligaments hold the spine together. Their role as shock absorbers in the spine is crucial.

DISC HERNIATION: Another name for this is a 'slipped disc' and it happens when the outer fibrous ring of the disc allows the soft central bit to bulge out of the fibrous rings. The annulus fibrosus gets more fragile with impacts and age, and the tears are nearly always posterolateral (back and to the side). The tear can result in a leak of chemicals that cause pain, and also the disc tear can cause nerve root compression.

DISC PROTUBERANCE: When the outermost fibers are intact and the central bit does not escape but the disc bulges under pressure. This is less serious than a herniation.

DEOXYRIBONUCLEIC ACID (DNA): Nucleic acid carrying our genetic blueprint for function and reproduction. The two DNA strands are made of nucleotides – cytosine, guanine, adenine, or thymine – as well as a sugar, deoxyribose, and a phosphate group. They pair up, A with T and C with G.

ECHOCARDIOGRAM: Often referred to as a 'cardio echo', this is a sonogram of the heart.

ENDOPLASMIC RETICULUM (ER): This is a type of organelle in cells that forms an interconnected network of membrane-enclosed tube-like structures, continuous with the outer nuclear membrane, rough and smooth. The outer face of the rough endoplasmic reticulum is studded with ribosomes that are the sites of protein synthesis.

SMOOTH ENDOPLASMIC RETICULUM: This lacks ribosomes and functions in lipid metabolism, as well as the production of steroid hormones and detoxification.

ENERGY MEDICINE: Also 'spiritual healing', these are branches of alternative medicine. The healers can channel healing energy into a patient, and there are several methods: hands-on, hands-off, and distant, where the patient and healer are in different locations.

GENES: This is a region of DNA that encodes a functional RNA or protein, and is the unit of heredity. The transmission of genes to an organism's offspring is the basis of the inheritance.

GLUTEUS MUSCLES: These are a group of three muscles which make up the buttocks: the gluteus maximus, gluteus medius, and gluteus minimus. The three muscles originate from the ilium (pelvic bone) and sacrum (pelvic central posterior triangular bone) and insert on the femur. The functions of the muscles include extension, abduction (outward movement of hip), external rotation, and internal rotation of the hip joint.

GUNN IMS: A dry needling technique taught by Professor Gunn after a qualification in understanding and treating neuropathic pain.

EXTENSOR DIGITORUM BREVIS AND LONGUS (EDB): A muscle on the upper surface of the foot that helps extend digits 2 through 4.

FACET JOINTS (or Z joints, zygapophyseal, or apophyseal): These are a set of synovial plane joints between the articular processes of two adjacent vertebrae. There are two facet joints in each spinal motion segment and each facet joint is innervated by the recurrent meningeal nerves.

FASCIA: A sheet of connective tissue – collagen – under the skin that attaches, encloses, and separates muscles and other internal organs.

HISTAMINE: A nitrogenous compound involved in immune responses and physiological control in the gut, it also acts as a neurotransmitter.

HORMONE: A signalling juice produced by glands, and carried by the circulatory system to target distant organs in order to regulate physiology.

HYPERALGESIA: A temporary increased sensitivity to pain, which may be caused by damage to nociceptors or peripheral nerves.

INFLAMMATION: A biological response of body tissues to harmful stimuli – such as pathogens, damaged cells, or irritants – this is a protective response involving immune cells, blood vessels, and specific juices. Inflammation clears out dead cells damaged from the trauma, ready to initiate tissue repair.

INFERIOR MESENTERIC GANGLION: Located near to where the inferior mesenteric artery branches off from the abdominal aorta.

IRRITABLE BOWEL SYNDROME: Abdominal pain and changes in the pattern of bowel movements, these symptoms occur over a long time, often years.

KYPHOSIS: Convex (bent over) curvature of the spine as it occurs in the thoracic and sacral regions.

LEVATOR SCAPULA: A muscle situated at the back and side of the neck, its main function is to lift the scapula.

LORDOSIS: This refers to the normal healthy inward curvature of the lumbar and cervical regions of the spine. Excessive curvature of the lower back is known as lumbar hyper lordosis, commonly called sway back.

MAGNETIC RESONANCE TREATMENT: This is based on the physical principle of magnetic resonance imaging, and it aims to activate repair and regeneration processes in specific cells and tissues such as bone and cartilage.

MAST CELL: A type of white blood cell. It is a type of granulocyte that is a part of the neuroimmune system and contains many granules rich in histamine and heparin. As well as their role in allergic reactions, mast cells play an important protective role in wound healing, defense against pathogens, and blood–brain barrier function.

MERIDIANS: These are channels of life-energy known as 'Qi'.

MECHANICAL BACK/NECK PAIN: This is classified by the underlying cause of pain as either mechanical, non-mechanical, or referred pain. The symptoms of mechanical low back pain usually improve within a few weeks. It refers to the pain being to do with the structures of the spine, not involving nerve root compression or any more serious/sinister cause.

MITOCHONDRIA: These organelles (structures inside the cell) are described as 'the powerhouse of the cell' because they generate most of the cell's chemical energy called adenosine triphosphate (ATP). Other roles include: signalling, cellular differentiation (cells changing to different cells), and cell death for cancerous and old cells, as well as controlling cell division and cell growth.

MOTOR NEURONE DISEASE: This can refer to any of five neurological disorders that selectively affect the motor neurons (brain to muscle/gland), the cells that control voluntary (conscious) muscles. There are five conditions, all neurodegenerative in nature and that all cause muscle wasting, increasing disability, and eventually, death. The names of the five conditions are: amyotrophic lateral sclerosis (Lou Gehrig's Disease), primary lateral sclerosis, progressive muscular atrophy, progressive bulbar palsy, and pseudobulbar palsy.

MRI (magnetic resonance imaging): A medical non-invasive imaging technique used in radiology to image the anatomy in order to look for damage and disease. MRI scanners use strong magnetic fields, radio waves, and field gradients to form images of the body.

MUSCLE: This contains protein filaments of actin and myosin that slide past one another in healthy muscle, producing a contraction that changes both the length and the shape of the cell. Muscle contractures are fixed and sore and are targeted by dry needling. The muscle's role is to produce force and movement, and they are primarily responsible for maintaining and changing posture, running, walking, writing, and eating, as well as the contraction of the heart and the movement of food through the digestive system.

MUSCULOSKELETAL: Involving both muscles and bones, hence the musculoskeletal system.

NERVE: This is an enclosed, cable-like bundle of axons (nerve fibers, the long thin projections of neurons/nerve cells) in the peripheral nervous system. A nerve provides a roadway for electrochemical nerve impulses/messages that are transmitted along each of the axons/nerve fibers to the peripheral organs.

NEUROPATHIC: This is damage to or a disease affecting nerves, which may impair sensation, movement, and gland or organ function. It may lead to unpleasant pain. Learning to read the physical signs of its presence can lead to treatment.

NEUROENDOCRINE: Cells receive messages from neurotransmitters released by nerve cells or neurosecretory cells, and in return, they release message molecules (hormones) to the blood. In this way they bring about a conversation or integration between the nervous system and the endocrine (hormones) system, through a process known as neuroendocrine integration.

NEURITIS: This is a general term for the inflammation of a nerve in part of or all of the peripheral nervous system. Physical signs depend on the severity and the nerves involved, but they may include pain, paresthesia (pins-and-needles), paresis (weakness), hypo aesthesia (numbness), anaesthesia (no feeling), paralysis (no movement), muscle wasting, and reflex (automatic response to stimuli) being absent on testing.

NOCICEPTOR: This is a sensory neuron (nerve cell) that responds to touch/pressure on the body in response to potentially damaging stimuli by sending signals to the spinal cord and brain. A kick or slap fires off these receptors/nerve endings, and this process, called nociception, causes the perception of pain in the brain.

NUCLEUS: This is a membrane-enclosed organelle (inside the cell). Human cells have a single nucleus, but a few cell types have no nuclei, and others many. It houses the 'blueprint', or the map of life – the genetic material in the form of DNA. Proteins called histones make up the chromosomes, and these paired snake-like structures carry the genome – which is the encoded genetic material – while the nucleus provides a safe house for these precious jewels. The cell membrane allows material into the cellular cytoplasm that could affect the gene expression of these guys. Therefore, there is a nuclear envelope, a double membrane that encloses the nucleus and isolates its contents from the cellular cytoplasm, and the nucleoskeleton (cell structure).

ORTHOPAEDIC: This word derives from 'ortho', which is the Greek for 'straight', and 'pais' for 'child'. Years ago, orthopaedists used braces to make a child 'straight', and bone setters worked on joints. Today, orthopaedic medicine means the treatment of musculoskeletal trauma, spinal discs, the wear and tear of the spine, osteoarthritic joints, sports injuries, and bone or muscle tumors. Treatments are carried out by orthopaedic surgeons and chartered physiotherapists.

OSTEOARTHRITIS: This is a wear and tear problem, a joint disease, also called 'osteoarthrosis'. Aging and use wears down the cartilage and underlying bone, leading to stiffness and then pain in the joints. This is initially due to overexertion, then being at rest at night.

OSTEOPAENIA: A condition in which bone mineral density is lower than normal, a precursor to osteoporosis (brittle bones). However, not everyone with osteopaenia will develop osteoporosis, and physiotherapy will help prevent the next stage. Osteopaenia is defined as having a bone mineral density T-score between -1.0 and -2.5.

OSTEOPOROSIS: A disease where bone weakness increases the risk of a broken bone, it is more common in post-menopausal women. Bones may weaken to such a degree that a break may occur with minor stress, a mild fall, or just a sneeze. The bones become painful and tender to the touch, made worse by microfractures and full blown fractures. Diet, supplementation, and weight bearing exercise helps.

OSTEOPATHY: A type of treatment that involves hands-on soft tissue massage and manipulation for musculoskeletal problems.

PELVIC PLEXUS/INFERIOR HYPOGASTRIC PLEXUS: A plexus of nerves that supplies the organs of the pelvic cavity. It is a paired structure on the side of the rectum in the male, and at the sides of the rectum and vagina in the female.

PERIPHERAL NERVOUS SYSTEM (PNS): This is outside of the brain and spine, and communicates with the central nervous system back and forth to the extremities.

PEPTIDES: These are short chains of amino acid monomers linked by peptide bonds.

PIEZOELECTRIC: A static electric charge that accumulates in certain materials like a crystal: bone, DNA, and proteins. It is electricity from pressure.

PILOMOTOR: Goosebumps are the bumps that appear (unconsciously/involuntarily) on a person's skin at the base of their body hairs when a person is cold or experiences strong emotions such as excitement, fear, euphoria, or sexual arousal. It is also present in a dermatome affected by a neuropathic nerve.

PHYSIOTHERAPY: A physical medicine and rehabilitation specialty that diagnoses and treats physical disability, pain, sports injuries, neurological conditions (like strokes), and respiratory illness. This career is all about promoting preventative health and physical activities such as mobility, function, and quality of life, through examination, diagnosis, prognosis (outcome), and physical intervention, using specific medical technology,hands-on treatment, and exercise and lifestyle prescription.

PLANTAR FASCITIS: Sole pain, especially under the heel, the pain being most severe with the first steps of the day or following a period of rest.

PIRIFORMIS: a muscle in the gluteal region (bottom), it is one of six muscles that turns the hip out and can cause sciatica.

POSTURE: Correct body alignment with a neutral spine.

POSTURAL DYSFUNCTION: biomechanical malalignment.

PROSTRATE: An exocrine gland of the male reproductive system

RADICULOPATHY: Nerve root entrapment at the spinal cord, which, according to the level, can cause pain and weakness down a limb, be it the arm or the leg.

REIKI: A form of alternative medicine developed in 1922 In Japan, by Japanese Buddhist Mikao Usui. Reiki has been taught in different ways across varying cultural traditions, and it uses hands-on-healing. Through the use of this technique, practitioners believe that they are transferring 'universal energy' through the palms of the practitioner, which they believe encourages healing.

RHEUMATOID ARTHRITIS (RA): A long-lasting autoimmune disorder (where the body attacks itself) that most significantly affects joints – you get swollen, stiff, and painful joints, and pain and stiffness often worsen after rest. Most commonly, it firstly affects the wrist and hands, with typically the same joints being involved on both sides of the body. The back can also ache without being diagnosed as RA, and the disease may affect other parts of the body too. This may result in low red blood cells, and inflammation around the lungs and heart. Fever and low energy also comes with flare ups. Rheumatologists run repeated specific tests in order to diagnose.

RIBOSOME: This serves as the site of biological protein synthesis (translation) inside cells. Ribosomes link amino acids (the building blocks of proteins) together in the order specified by messenger RNA (mRNA) molecules. Ribosomes consist of a reader of the RNA, and a joiner together of amino acids in order to form a polypeptide chain.

RIBONUCLEIC ACID (RNA): This is involved in coding, decoding, regulation, and the expression of genes, which is essential for all known forms of life. Like DNA, RNA is assembled as a chain of nucleotides, but unlike DNA, it is a single-strand folded onto itself, rather than a paired double-strand. Messenger RNA (mRNA) convey genetic information (using the letters G, U, A, and C to denote the bases guanine, uracil, adenine, and cytosine) that directs synthesis of specific proteins.

SCIATICA: Also known as lumbar radiculopathy, this is when pain is felt going down the back, outside, or front of the leg. Typically, symptoms are only on one side of the body, but occasionally on both sides. Lower back pain is sometimes present, and a weakness, numbness, or tingling may occur in parts of the leg and foot.

SCHEUERMANN'S DISEASE: A disorder of a child's spine where the vertebral endplates and discs are believed to have an autoimmune problem, causing damage. This results in an idiopathic juvenile kyphosis of the spine (a hunchback shape, and this uneven growth results in the signature 'wedging' shape of the vertebrae, causing this posture.

SHIATSU: A physical therapy that supports and strengthens the body's natural ability to heal and balance itself. It works on the whole person; the physical, psychological, emotional, and spiritual aspects of being. Shiatsu originated in Japan from traditional Chinese medicine, with influences from more recent western therapies. It means 'finger pressure' in Japanese. As well as fingers, hands and elbows give comfortable pressure, and manipulative techniques adjust the body's physical structure and balance its energy flow. It is a deeply relaxing experience, and regular treatments can alleviate stress and illness and maintain health and well-being.

SENSORY NEURONS: Nerve cells that transmit sensory info like sound or touch.

SPONDYLOSIS DEFORMANS: A disease of the spine. Some think it is osteoarthritis of the spine but since spondylosis deformans does not involve active arthritis in joints, it is a degenerative disease of the discs of the spine that in turn causes wear on the bones. It comes from the annulus fibrosus of the disc bulging against connective tissue and causing traction on the bony attachment of the vertebrae causing osteophyte (bony spurs) on the front and side of the vertebral body. The traction causes osteophytes to rise several millimetres from the end-plates that may bridge the disc spaces, then at times, may cause nerve problems.

SPONDYLOLISTHESIS: The forward displacement of a vertebra, most often the fifth lumbar vertebra, and often after a fracture. Backward displacement is referred to as a retrolisthesis, a posterior displacement of one vertebral body with respect to the adjacent vertebrae to a degree less than a luxation (dislocation).

STEM CELL: Undifferentiated (undecided on what they will be) biological cells that can differentiate into specialised cells and can divide (through mitosis) to produce more stem cells. There are two broad types of stem cells: embryonic stem cells, which are isolated from the inner cell mass of blastocysts, and adult stem cells, which are found in various tissues.

STROKE/CEREBROVASCULAR ACCIDENT (CVA): When poor blood flow to the brain results in cell death. There are two main types of stroke: ischaemic, due to a lack of blood flow because of a clot, and a bleed. They both result in part of the brain not functioning properly.

SUBLUXATION: This may have different meanings, depending on the medical specialty involved, but it basically implies the presence of a partial dislocation of a joint. The World Health Organization (WHO) defines both the medical subluxation and the chiropractic subluxation, contrasting the two and stating in a footnote that a medical subluxation "is a significant structural displacement, and therefore visible on static imaging studies. In chiropractic, vertebral subluxation is a set of signs and symptoms of the spinal column." Those chiropractors who assert this concept also add a visceral component to the definition; chiropractors maintain that a vertebral subluxation complex is a dysfunctional biomechanical spinal segment which is fixated.

SUDOMOTOR: The cholinergic innervation of the sympathetic nervous system prominent in sweat glands, which causes perspiration to occur via activation of muscarinic acetylcholine receptors.

TRAPEZIUS: One of two large superficial muscles that extend from the occipital bone (skull) to the lower thoracic vertebrae and to the shoulder blade. Its functions are to move the scapulae and support the arm, and it is usually tense, both emotionally and physically.

TENDINITIS: The inflammation of a tendon.

TENOSYNOVITIS: The inflammation of the fluid-filled synovium that surrounds a tendon. Symptoms include pain, swelling, and difficulty moving the joint.

TROPHEDEMA: A pitting appearance in skin above the neuropathic nerve.

VACUOLE: A membrane-bound organelle.

VESICLE: A small fluid-filled structure within a cell, enclosed by a lipid bilayer. Vesicles form during secretion (exocytosis), uptake of garbage (phagocytosis and endocytosis), and the transport of materials within the cytoplasm.

VASOMOTOR: This refers to actions upon a blood vessel that alter its diameter. More specifically, it can refer to vasodilator action and vasoconstrictor action.

VASOCONSTRICTION: The narrowing of the blood vessels resulting from the contraction of the muscular wall of the vessels. The process is the opposite of the widening (dilating) of the blood vessels. On a larger level, vasoconstriction and dilation is one mechanism by which the body regulates and maintains arterial pressure.

VENTRICLE: The pumping chambers of the heart.

X-RAY: Composed of radiation, this is a form of electromagnetic radiation. Most X-rays have a wavelength ranging from 0.01 to 10 nanometers.

Bibliography

"Spring passes and one remembers one's innocence.
Summer passes and one remembers one's exuberance.
Autumn passes and one remembers one's reverence.
Winter passes and one remembers one's perseverance."

– *Yoko Ono*

CHAPTER ONE

Barnes, John F. *Healing Ancient Wounds: The Renegade's Wisdom*. Malvern, Pennsylvania, RSI T/A MFR Treatment Centers and Seminars, 2000.

Barnes, John F. *Myofascial Release: The Search For Excellence*. Malvern, Pennsylvania, RSI T/A MFR Treatment Centers and Seminars, 1990.

Bernhard, H.R et al., 2008. 'A randomised controlled trial of spinal manipulative therapy in acute low back pain'. *Annals of the Rheumatic Diseases*, 68: 1420-1427.

Bogduk, N. *Clinical Anatomy of the Lumbar Spine and Sacrum, 3rd Ed*. Churchill Livingstone, 1997.

Broadhurst, N.A & Bond, M.J, 1998. 'Pain provocation tests for the assessment of sacroiliac joint dysfunction'. *Journal of Spinal Disorders*, 1998, 11(4):341-5.

Cao, T et al., 2015. 'Duration and Magnitude of Myofascial Release in 3Dimensional Bioengineered Tendons: Effects on Wound Healing'. *American Osteopathic Association*, 115(2): 72-82.

Carvalhais, V et al., 2013. 'Myofascial force transmission between the latissimus dorsi and gluteus maximus muscles: An in vivo experiment'. *Journal of Biomechanics*, 46: 1003–1007.

Chaitow, L. *Modern Neuromuscular Techniques*. Churchill Livingstone, 2011.

Cochrane, C.G, 1987. 'Joint Mobilisation Principles: Considerations for Use in the Child with Central Nervous System Dysfunction'. *Physical Therapy*, 1105-1109.

Colquhoun, D, 2008. 'Doctor Who? Inappropriate use of titles by some alternative 'medicine' practitioners'. *The New Zealand Medical Journal*, 121 (1278): 6-10.

Cyriax, J.H. *Cyriax's Illustrated Manual of Orthopaedic Medicine*. Butterworth & Heinemann, 1993.

Di Fabio, R.P, 1999. 'Manipulation of the Cervical Spine: Risks and Benefits'. *Physical Therapy*, 79(1): 50-65.

Egan, D, Cole, J, and Twomey, L, 1996. 'The standing forward flexion test: an inaccurate determinant of sacroiliac joint dysfunction'. *Physiotherapy*, 82(4): 236-242.

Ernst, E, 2007. 'Adverse effects of spinal manipulation: a systematic review'. *Journal of the Royal Society of Medicine*, 100 (7): 330-8.

Ferguson, F, Holdsworth, L and Rafferty, D, 2010. 'Low back pain and physiotherapy use of red flags: the evidence from Scotland'. *Physiotherapy*, 96, 4; 282-288.

Fields, H.L and Basbaum, A.I, 1999. 'Central Nervous System Mechanisms of Pain Modulation'. *Textbook of Pain*, 309-330.

Freburger, J.K and Riddle, D.L, 1999. 'Measurement of sacroiliac dysfunction: a multicenter intertester reliability study'. *Physical Therapy*, 79(12): 1134-41.

Frese, E.M, Richter, R.R and Burlis, T.V, 2002. 'Self-reported measurement of heart rate and blood pressure in patients by physical therapy clinical instructors'. *Physical Therapy*, 82(12): 1191-1200.

Fryer, G, 2000. 'Muscle Energy Concepts - A Need for Change'. *Journal of Osteopathic Medicine*, 3 (2). pp. 54-59.

Fryer, G and Fossum, C, 2009. 'Therapeutic Mechanisms Underlying Muscle Energy Approaches'. *Physical Therapy for tension type and cervicogenic headache*. Jones & Bartlett, Boston.

Goldberger, L and Breznitz, S. *Handbook of Stress*. MacMillan, 1982.

Greene, K, 2015. 'An Overview of the 13th International MDT Conference: Supporting Clinical Observations'. *The McKenzie Institute® International*, Vol. 4, No. 3.

Grod, J.P, Sikorski, D and Keating, J.C, 2001. 'Unsubstantiated claims in patient brochures from the largest state, provincial, and national chiropractic associations and research agencies'. *Journal of Manipulative and Physiological Therapeutics*, 24 (8): 514–9.

Gunther Brown, Candy, 2014. 'Chiropractic: Is It Nature, Medicine or Religion?' *The Huffington Post*, July 7.

Harrison, D.E, Harrison, D.D and Troyanovich, S.J, 1997. 'The Sacroiliac Joint: a Review of Anatomy and Biomechanics with Clinical Implications'. *Journal of Manipulative and Physiological Therapeutics*, 20(9): 607-617.

Hengeveld, E. and Banks, K. *Maitland's Peripheral Manipulation*. Elsevier: London, 2005.

Hicks, M et al., 2012. 'Mechanical strain applied to human fibroblasts differentially regulates skeletal myoblast differentiation'. *Journal of Applied Physiology*, 113(3): 465-472.

International Maitland Teachers Association. 'A tribute to the life and work of G.D. Maitland, 1924-2010'. *Manual Therapy*, 2010.

Jacob, H.A.C and Kissling, R.O, 1995. 'The mobility of the sacroiliac joints in healthy volunteers between 20 and 50 years of age'. *Clinical Biomechanics*, 10: 352-361.

Jaroff, Leon, 2002. 'Back Off, Chiropractors!' *Time*, 7 June.

Jarvis, W.T, 1992. 'Quackery: a national scandal'. *Clinical Chemistry*, 38 (8B Pt 2): 1574-86.

Jenkins, G, Kemnitz, C, and Tortora, G. *Anatomy and Physiology: From Science to Life*. John Wiley & Sons, Inc, 2007.

The John F. Barnes Myofascial Release Approach MASSAGE Magazine, June 2007.

Kaptchuck, T.J and Eisenberg, D.M, 1998. Chiropractic: orgins, controversies, and contributions'. *Archives of Internal Medicine*, 158 (20): 2215-24.

Keating, Jr., Joseph, 2015. 'D.D. Palmer's Lifeline'. *The Chiropractic Resource Organization*, Feb 22.

Keating, Jr., Joseph C, 1991. 'Quackering in Chiropractic'. *Dynamic Chiropractic*, vol 09, issue 4.

Kessler R and Hertling, D. *Management of Common Musculoskeletal Disorders: Physical Therapy, Principles and Methods*. Lippincott Williams and Wilkins, 1983.

Kimbrough, M.L, 1998. 'Jailed chiropractors: those who blazed the trail'. *Chiropratic History*, 18 (1): 79 – 100.

Langevin, H et al., 2005. 'Dynamic fibroblast cytoskeletal response to subcutaneous tissue stretch ex vivo and in vivo'. *American Journal of Physiology*, 288: C747–C756.

Lederman, E. *The Science and Practice of Manual Therapy*. Elsevier: London, 2005.

Levangie, P.K, 1999. 'Four clinical tests of sacroiliac joint dysfunction: the association of test results with innominate torsion among patients with and without low back pain'. *Physical Therapy*, 79(11): 1043-1057.

Levangie, P.K, 1999. 'The association between static pelvic asymmetry and low back pain'. *Spine*, 24(12): 1234-42.

Levangie, P and Norkin, C. *Joint Structure and Function: a Comprehensive Analysis*. F.A. Davis Company, 2001.

Lynch, G, McGaugh, J, and Weinberger, N. *Neurobiology of Learning and Memory*. Guilford Press, 1984.

Maigne, J.Y, Aivaliklis, A and Pfefer, F, 1996. 'Results of sacroiliac joint double block and value of sacroiliac pain provocation tests in 54 patients with low back pain'. *Spine*, 21(16): 1889-92.

Manipulation Association of Chartered Physiotherapists. 'Tribute to Geoffrey Maitland (1924-2010)'. *Manual Therapy*, 2010.

Martini, F.H, and Nath, J.L. *Fundamentals of Anatomy and Physiology*. Pearson, 2009.

McConnell, C. *Osteopathic Institute of Applied Technique Yearbook*. London, 1962.

Melzack, R and Wall, P.D, 1965. 'Pain Mechanisms: A New Theory'. *Science: New Series 150*, 971-979.

Mitchell, F.L, Moran, P.S and Pruzzo, N.A. *An Evaluation and Treatment Manual of Osteopathic Muscle Energy Procedures*. Institute for Continuing Education in Osteopathic Principles, Missouri, 1979.

Murphy, D.R, Schneider, M.J, Seaman, D.R, Perle, S.M and Nelson, C.F, 2008. 'How can chiropractic become a respected mainstream profession? The example of podiatry'. *Chiropractic & Osteopathy*, 16:10.

Nelso, C.F, Lawrence, D.J, Triano, J.J, Bronfort, G, Perle, S.M, Metz, R.D, Hegetschweiler, K and Labrot, T, 2005. 'Chiropractic as spine care: a model for the profession'. *Chiropractic & Osteopathy*, 13: 9.

Norkin, C.C and Levangie, P.K. *Joint Structure and Function: a Comprehensive Analysis*. F.A. Davis Company, 1992.

O'Haire, C, and Gibbons, P, 2000. 'Inter-examiner and intra-examiner agreement for assessing sacroiliac anatomy using palpation and observation: pilot study'. *Manual Therapy*, 5(1): 13-20.

Ombregt, L. *A System of Orthopaedic Medicine*. WB Saunders Company Ltd., 1995.

Palmer, Daniel, 1911. 'D.D. Palmer's Religion of Chiropractic'. *The Chiropractic Resource Organization*, Feb 22.

Parmar, S et al., 2011. 'Effect of isolytic contraction and passive manual stretching on pain and knee range of motion after hip surgery'. *Hong Kong Physiotherapy Journal*, 29: 25-30.

Pavan, P.G et al., 2014. 'Painful connections: densification versus fibrosis of fascia'. *Current Pain Headache Reports*, 18(8): 441.

Rossi, E.L, 1987. 'From mind to molecule: a state-dependent memory, learning, and
behaviour theory of mind-body healing'. *Advances*, 4(2): 46-60.

Selye, H. *The stress of Life*. McGraw-Hill, 1976.

Sibby, George Mathew, Narasimman, Kavitha Vishal, 2009. 'Effectiveness of integrated neuromuscular inhibitory technique and LASER with stretching in the treatment of upper trapezius trigger points. *Journal of Exercise Science and Physiotherapy*, volume 5, issue 2.

Singh, S and Ernst, E, 2008. 'The truth about chiropractic therapy'. *Trick or Treatment: The Undeniable Facts About Alternative Medicine*. W.W. Norton, 145-90.

Slipman, C.W, Sterenfeld, E.B, Chou, L.H, Herzog, R and Vresiliovic, E, 1998. 'The predictive value of provocation sacroiliac joint stress maneuvers in the diagnosis of sacroiliac joint syndrome'. *Archives of Physical Medicine and Rehabilitation*, 79: 288-292.

Smith-Cunnien, Susan L. *A Profession of One's Own: Organized Medicine's Opposition to Chiropractic*. University Press of America, 1997.

Spoonemore, S. *Cervical Manipulation Risk vs Reward*, 2015 (Video).

Stamford, J, 1995. 'Descending Control of Pain'. *British Journal of Anaesthesia*, 75: 217-227.

Standley, P and Meltzer, K, 2008. 'Effects of Repetitive Motion Strain (RMS) & Counter-Strain (CS), on fibroblast morphology and actin stress fiber architecture'. *Journal of Bodywork and Movement Therapies*, 12(3): 201-203.

Stecco, A et al., 2013. 'The anatomical and functional relation between gluteus maximus and fascia lata'. *Journal of Bodywork and Movement Therapies*, 17(4): 512-517.

The Stroke Association. 'Millions at risk from 'silent killer''. (Online) available from: www.stroke.org.uk/media_centre/press_releases/millions_at_risk.html. 2011.

Squire, S. and Butters, N. *Neuropsychology of Memory*. Guilford Press, 1984.

Toussaint, R, Gawlik, C.S, Rehder, U, and Ruther, W, 1999. 'Sacroiliac dysfunction in construction workers'. *Journal of Manipulative and Physiological Therapeutics,* 22(3): 134-8.

Tullberg, T, Blomberg, S, Branth, B, and Johnsson R, 1998. 'Manipulation does not alter the position of the sacroiliac joint'. *Spine,* 23(10): 1124-8.

Vincent-Smith, B and Gibbons, P, 1999. 'Inter-examiner and intra-examiner reliability of the standing flexion test'. *Manual Therapy,* 4(2): 87-93.

Weppler, C.H and Magnusson, S.P, 2010. 'Increasing Muscle Extensibility: A Matter of Increasing Length or Modifying Sensation?' *Physical Therapy,* 90:438-449.

WHO guidelines on basic training and safety in chiropractic, 2005.

CHAPTER TWO

Baer, Hans. *Toward an Integrative Medicine: Merging Alternative Therapies with Biomedicine.* Rowman AltaMira, 2004.

Baggoley, C, 2015. 'Review of the Australian Government Rebate on Natural Therapies for Private Health Insurance'. *Australian Government – Department of Health.*

Berisio, R, Vitagliano, L, Mazzarella, L and Zagari, A, 2002. 'Crystal structure of the collagen triple helix model'. *Protein Science,* 11, 2, 262-270.

Beyerstein, Barry, 1995. 'Distinguishing Science from Pseudoscience'. *Victoria, BC: Center for Curriculum and Professional Development.*

Carew, J.S and Haung, P, 2002. 'Mitochondrial defects in cancer.' *Molecular Cancer,* 1. 9.

Cassar, Mario-Paul. *Handbook of Clinical Massage: A Complete Guide for Students and Practitioners*. Churchill Livingston, 2004.

Cohen, S and Popp, F.A, 2003. 'Biophoton emission of the human body'. *Indian Journal of Experimental Biology*, 41, 440-445.

Considine, Austin, 2010. 'Rolfing, excruciatingly helpful'. *New York Times*, 6 October.

Cordón, Luis. *Popular Psychology: An Encyclopedia*. Greenwood Press, 2005.

Daniels, Rick and Nicoll, Leslie, 2011. 'Ch. 14: Complementary and Alternative Therapies'. *Contemporary Medical-Surgical Nursing*, 1, 306.

Deutsch, Judith E. *Complementary Therapies for Physical Therapy: A Clinical Decision-Making Approach*. Saunders, 2008.

Dunster, Christine, 2012. 'Treatment of Anxiety and Stress with Biofeedback'. *Global Advances in Health and Medicine*, vol 1, no. 4, 76-83.

Feng, J.F, Liu, J and Zhang, X.Z, 2012. 'Guided migration of neural stem cells derived from human embryonic cells by an electric field'. *Stem Cells*, 30, 2,349-355.

Fernandez, J.R, Garcia-Aznar, J.M and Martinez, R, 2012. 'Piezoelectricity could predict sites of formation/resorption in bone remodelling'. Journal of Theoretical Biology, 292, 86-92.

Gavura, S, 2015. 'Australian review finds no benefit to 17 natural therapies'. *Science-based Medicine*, 19 November.

Ginsberg, Jay P, Berry, Melanie E and Powell, Donald A, 2010. 'Cardiac coherence and post traumatic stress disorder in combat veterans'. *Alternative Therapies*, vol 16, no. 4, 52-60.

Hartig, M, Joos, U and Wiesmann, H.P, 2000. 'Capacity coupled electric fields accelerate proliferation of osteoblast like primary cells and increase bone extracellular matrix formation in vitro'. *European Biophysics Journal*, 29, 7, 499-506.

Jones, Tracey A, 2004. 'Rolfing'. *Physical Medicine and Rehabilitation Clinics of North America*, 15 (4): 799-809.

Knaster, Mirka. *Discovering the Body's Wisdom: A Comprehensive Guide to More Than Fifty Mind-Body Practices*. Bantam, 1996.

Levine, Andrew. The *Bodywork and Massage Sourcebook*. Lowell House, 1998.

Lipton, Bruce, 1986. *Planetary Association for Clean Energy Newsletter*, 5; 4.

Lipton, Bruce. *The Biology of Belief*. Cygnus, 2005.

McCraty, R and Shaffer, F, 2015. 'Heart Rate Variability: New Perspectives on the Physiological Mechanisms, and Assessment of Self-Regulatory Capacity and Health Risk'. *Global Advances in Health and Medicine*.

Minary-Jolandan, M and Yu, M.F, 2009. 'Nanoscale characterization of isolated individual type 1 collagen fibrils; polarization and piezoelectricity'. *Nanotechnology*, 20, 8.

Myers, Thomas. *Anatomy Trains*. Elsevier, 2009.

Myers, Thomas. *Fascial Release for Structural Balance*. North Atlantic, 2010.

Myers, Thomas W, 2004. 'Structural integration – Developments in Ida Rolf's 'Recipe''. *Journal of Bodywork and Movement Therapies*, 8 (2): 131-42.

Perls, Frederick. *In and Out of the Garbage Pail*. Real People Press, 1969.

Rolf, Ida. *Rolfing: Reestablishing the Natural Alignment and Structural Integration of the Human Body for Vitality and Well-Being.* Healing Arts Press, 1989.

Salvo, Susan G. *Massage Therapy: Principles and Practice.* Elsevier Saunders, 2012.

Schultz, Richard Louis and Feitis, Rosemary. *The Endless Web: Fascial Anatomy and Physical Reality.* North Atlantic Books, 1996.

Shapiro, Rose. *Suckers: How Alternative Medicine Makes Fools of Us All.* Vintage Books, 2008.

Sherman, Karen J, Dixon, Marian W, Thompson, Diana, and Cherkin, Daniel C, 2006. 'Development of a taxonomy to describe massage treatments for musculoskeletal pain'. *BMC Complementary and Alternative Medicine*, 6: 24.

Stillerman, Elaine. *Modalities for Massage and Bodywork.* Mosby, 2009.

Stirling, Isabel. *Zen Pioneer: The Life & Works of Ruth Fuller Sasaki.* Shoemaker & Hoard, 2006.

Takeda, M, Kobayahi, M, Takayama, M and Suzuki, S et al., 2004. 'Biophoton detection as a novel technique for cancer imaging.' *Cancer Science*, 95, 8, 656-661.

Thomas, Claire. *Bodywork: What Type of Massage To Get and How to Make the Most of It.* William Morrow and Company, 1995.

Tomaselli, V.P and Shamos, M.H, 1974. 'Electrical properties of hydrated collagen.' *Biopolymers*, 13, 12, 2423-2434.

Velugotla, Srinivas et al., 2012. 'Dielectrophoresis based discrimination of human embryonic In stem cells from differentiating derivatives'. *Biomicrofluidics*, 6 (4).

Woody, Bedell and Kaskine-Bettag, Marietta, 2010. 'Coherence and health care cost – RCA actuarial study: a cost-effectiveness cohort study'. *Alternative Therapies*, vol 16, no. 4, 26-31.

CHAPTER THREE

Axelsson, J and Thesleff, S, 1959. 'A study of supersensitivity in denervated mammalian skeletal muscle'. *The Journal of Physiology*, 174: 178.

Bradley, W.G, 1974. 'Disorders of Peripheral Nerves'. *Oxford, Blackwell Scientific Publications*, 129-201, 253-267.

Brown, M.J, Martin, J.R, and Asbury, A.K, 1976. 'Painful diabetic neuropathy'. *Archives of Neurology*, 33: 164-171.

Cannon, W.B and Rosenblueth, A. *The Supersensitivity of Denervated Structures*. The Macmillan Company, 1949.

Chapman, L.F, Ramos, A.O, Goodell, H, and Wolff, H.G, 1961. 'Neurohumoral features of afferent fibers in man'. Archives of Neurology, 4: 617-650.

Coers, C, 1953. 'Note sur une technique de prelevement des biopsies neuro-musculaires'. *Acta Neurol Phychiatr Belg*, 53: 750-765.

Coers, C, and Woolf, A.L, 1959. 'The technique of muscle biopsy. Chap 1. The Innervation of Muscle'. *Oxford, Blackwell Scientific Publications*, 1-41.

Cross, John. *Healing With the Chakra Energy System*. North Atlantic Books, 2006.

Denny-Brown, D, and Brenner, C, 1944. 'Paralysis of nerve induced by direct pressure and by tourniquet'. Archives of Neurology & Psychiatry, 51: 1-26.

Doupe, J, Cullen, C.H, and Chance, G.Q, 1944. 'Post-traumatic pain and causalgic syndrome'. *Journal of Neurology, Neurosurgery & Psychiatry*, 7: 33-48.

Dyck, P.J, Lambert, E.H, and O'Brien, P.C, 1976. 'Pain in peripheral neuropathy related to rate and kind of nerve fibre degeneration'. *Neurology*, 26: 466-477.

Fambrough, D.M, Hartzell, H.C, Powell, J.A, Rash, J.E and Joseph, N, 1974. *On differentiation and organization of the surface membrane of a post-synaptic cell-the skeletal muscle fibre. Synaptic Transmission and Neuronal Interaction*. Raven Press, 1974.

Fields, H.L. *Pain*. McGraw-Hill, 1987.

Gunn, Chan, 2000. 'Neuropathic Myofascial Pain Syndromes'. *Bonica's Management of Pain*.

Gunn, Chan, 2005. 'Acute Respiratory Distress Syndrome Successfully Treated with Low Level Laser Therapy'. *Journal of Complementary and Integrative Medicine*, 41: 2.

Gunn, C.C and Milbrandt, W.E, 1977. "Bursitis' around the hip'. *American Journal of Acupuncture*, 5: 53-60.

Gunn, C.C and Milbrandt, W.E, 1980. 'Dry needling of muscle motor points for chronic low-back pain: A randomized clinical trial with long-term follow-up'. *Spine*.

Gunn, C.C, and Milbrandt, W.E, 1978. 'Early and subtle signs in 'low back sprain''. *Spine*, 3: 267-281.

Gunn, C.C and Milbrandt, W.E, 1978. 'Tennis elbow and the cervical spine'. Canadian Medical Associaton Journal, 114: 803-809.

Gunn, C.C and Milbrandt, W.E, 1976. 'Tenderness at motor points - a diagnostic and prognostic aid for low-back injury'. Journal of Bone & Joint Surgery, 58A: 815-825.

Gunn, C.C and Milbrandt, W.E, 1977. 'Tenderness at motor points - an aid in the diagnosis of pain in the shoulder referred from the cervical spine'. The Journal of the American Osteopathic Association, 77: 196/75-212/91.

Gunn, C.C and Milbrandt, W.E, 1977. 'Utilizing trigger points'. The Osteo-Physician, 29-52.

Guth, L, 1968. "Trophic' influences of nerve on muscle. Physiological Reviews, 48: 645-687.

Hughes, J, Smith, T.W and Kosterlitz, H.W et al., 1975. 'Identification of two related pentapeptides from the brain with potent opiate agonist activity'. Nature, 258: 577-579.

Hughes, J, Kosterlitz, H.W, and Smith, T.W, 1977. 'The distribution of methionine-enkephalin and leucine-enkephalin in the brain and peripheral tissues'. British Journal of Pharmacology, 61: 639-647.

Katz, B, and Miledi, R. 'The development of acetylcholine sensitivity in nerve-free segments of skeletal muscle'. Journal of Physiology, 170: 389-396.

Klein, L, Dawson, M.H and Heiple, K.G, 1977. 'Turnover of collagen in the adult rat after denervation'. The Journal of Bone & Joint Surgergy, 59A: 1065-1067.

Kraus, H, 1973. 'Triggerpoints'. New York State Journal of Medicine, 73: 1310-1314.

Livingston, W.H. *Pain Mechanism. Physiological Interpretation of Causalgia and Its Related States.* The Macmillan Company, 1943.

Lomo, T, 1976. 'The role of activity in the control of membrane and contractile properties of skeletal muscle. Chap 10. Motor Innervation of Muscle'. *Academic Press.*

Melzack, R and Wall, P.D, 1965. 'Pain mechanisms: A new theory'. *Science*, 150: 971-979.

Melzack, R, Stillwell, D.M and Fox, E.J, 1977. 'Trigger points and acupuncture points for pain-correlation and implications'. *Pain*, 3: 3-23.

Noordenbos, W. *Pain*. Elsevier, 1959.

Purves D, 1976. 'Long-term regulation in the vertebrate peripheral nervous system'. *Neurophysiology II*, vol 10, 125-177.

Rosenblueth, A and Luco, J.V, 1937. 'A study of denervated mammalian skeletal muscle'. *American Journal of Physiology*, 120: 781-797, 1937.

Seddon, H.J, 1943. 'Three types of nerve injury'. *Brain*, 66: 237-288.

Shepard, G.M, 1978. 'Microcircuits in the nervous system'. *Scientific American*, 238: 93-103.

Snazell, Nicky, 2005. 'The Pain Jungle – Assessment and Treatment with Gunn Intramuscular Stimulation (IMS). *Neurological*, issue 111, May.

Snyder, S.H, 1977. 'Opiate receptors in the brain'. *New England Journal of Medicine*, 296: 266-271.

Sternschein, M.J, Myers, S.J, Frewin, D.B and Downey, J.A, 1975. 'Causalgia'. *Archives of Physical Medicine and Rehabilitation*, 56: 58-63.

Sunderland, S. *Nerve and Nerve Injuries*. E&S Livingstone, 1968.

Tower, S.S, 1939. 'The reaction of muscle to denervation'. *Physiological Reviews*, 19: 1-48.

Travell, J and Rrinzler, S.H, 1952. 'The myofascia genesis of pain'. *Postgraduate Medicine Journal*, 11: 425-434.

Wall, P.D, 1978. 'The gate control theory of pain mechanisms-a re-examination and re-statement'. *Brain*, 101: 1-18.

Wall, P.D, Waxman, S and Basbaum, A.I, 1974. 'Ongoing activity in peripheral nerve injury discharge'. *Experimental Neurology*, 45: 576-589.

Walthard, K.M and Tchicaloff, M. *Motor Points. Chap 6. Electrodiagnosis and Electromyography*. Waverly Press, 1971.

Wilkinson, J. *Cervical Spondylosis-Its Early Diagnosis and Treatment*. WB Saunders Company, 1971, 1-8.

Willis, W.D and Grossman, R.G. *Medical Neurobiology*. CV Mosby Company, 1973, 1-4, 53, 71.

Wolfe, F, 1993. 'Why it is Important, if You Have Been Diagnosed with Fibromyalgia, to Seek Examination by a True Expert in Myofascial Pain'. *Fibromyalgia – What have we created?*

Zimmerman, M: *Neurophysiology of Nociception*. Raven Press, 1979, 79-221.

CHAPTER FOUR

Blanks, R.H, 2009. 'Editorial: Reorganizational Healing: A Health Change Model Whose Time Has Come'. *Journal of Alternative and Complimentary Medicine*, 15 (5): 461-64.

Cannon, W.B and Rosenblueth, A. *The Supersensitivity of Denervated Structures*. The Macmillan Company, 1949, 1-22, 185.

Chaitow, Leon. *Modernneuromuscular Techniques*. Churchill Livingstone Elsevier, 2011.

Crosby, J, 2010. 'Promoting Dos: Words and medium change, but message stays the same'. *DO Magazine*.

Epstein, D.M, Senzon, S.A and Lemberger, D, 2009. 'Reorganizational Healing: A Paradigm for the Advancement of Wellness, Behavior Change, Holistic Practice, and Healing'. *Journal of Alternative and Complimentary Medicine*, 15 (5): 461-64.

Gibbons, Peter and Tehan, Philip. *Manipulation of the Spine, Thorax and Pelvis*. Church Livingstone Elsevier, 2014.

Gunn, Chan. *The Gunn Approach Of Chronic Pain*. Elsevier Science Limited, 2003.

Jonckheere, E.A, 2009. 'Letter to the Editor: Network Spinal Analysis'. *Journal of Alternative and Complimentary Medicine*, 15 (5): 469-70.

'Osteopathic Manipulative Treatment'. *NYU Langone Medical Center*, 2012.

'Osteopathy – NHS Choices'. *NHS UK*, 2011.

Still, A.T. *Osteopathy Research and Practice*. Kirksville Journal Printing Company, 1910.

'Style Guide for Reporting on Osteopathic Medicine'. *American Osteopathic Association*, 2012.

Vleeming, A, Mooney, V, Dorman, T, Snijders, C and Stoeckert, R. *Movement, Stability and Low Back Pain: The Essential Role of the Pelvis*. Churchill Livingstone, 1999.

CHAPTER FIVE

Abate, M, Silbernagel, K.G, Siljeholm, C, Di Iorio, A, De Amicis, D, Salini, V, Werner, S and Paganelli, R, 2009. 'Pathogenesis of tendinopathies: inflammation or degeneration?'. *Arthritis Research & Therapy*, 11 (3): 235.

Amagase, H and Nance, D.M, 2008. 'A randomized, double-blind, placebo-controlled, clinical study of the general effects of a standardized Lycium barbarum (Goji) Juice, GoChi'. *Journal of Alternative and Complementary Medicine*, 14 (4): 403-12.

Aviram, M et al., 2004. 'Pomegranate juice consumption for 3 years by patients with carotid artery stenosis reduces common carotid intima-media thickness, blood pressure and LDL oxidation'. Clinical Nutrition, 23 (3): 423-33.

Bahadoran, Z et al., 1996. 'Broccoli sprouts powder could improve serum triglyceride and oxidized LDL/LDL-cholesterol ratio in type 2 diabetic patients: a randomized double-blind placebo-controlled clinical trial'. *Diabetes Research and Clinical Practice*, 96 (3): 348-54.

Bannuru, R.R, Flavin, N.E, Vaysbrot, E, Harvey, W and McAlindon, T, 2014. 'High-energy extracorporeal shock-wave therapy for treating chronic calcific tendinitis of the shoulder: a systematic review'. *Annals of Internal Medicine*, 160 (8): 542–9.

Bell, R, Boniello, M.R, Gendron, N.R, Flatow, E.L and Andarawis-Puri, N, 2015. 'Delayed exercise promotes remodeling in sub-rupture fatigue damaged tendons'. *Journal of Orthopaedic Research*, 33 (6): 919–25.

Bennett, William F, 2014. 'Arthroscopic Supraspinatus Repair'. *Bennett Orthopedics & Sports Medicine.*

Berrington de Gonzalez, A, Mahesh, M, Kim, K-P, Bhargavan, M, Lewis, R, and Mettler, F, et al., 2007. 'Projected Cancer Risks From Computed Tomographic Scans Performed in the United States in 2007'. *Archives of Internal Medicine*, 169(22): 2071-7.

Boehm, K, Borrelli, F, Ernst, E, Habacher, G, Hung, S.K, Milazzo, S and Horneber, M, 2009. 'Green tea (Camellia sinensis) for the prevention of cancer'. *Cochrane Gynaecological, Neuro-oncology and Orphan Cancer.*

Ben-Arye, E et al., 2004. 'Wheat grass juice in the treatment of active distal ulcerative colitis: a randomized double-blind placebo-controlled trial'. *Scandinavian Journal of Gastroenterology*, 41(7): 716-20.

Cassidy, A, Mukamal, K.J, Liu, L, Franz, M, Eliassen, A.H and Rimm, E.B, 2013. 'Heart health and blueberries'. *Circulation*, 127 (2): 188-96.

Chambler, A.F, Pitsillides, A.A and Emery, R.J, 2003. 'Acromial spur formation in patients with rotator cuff tears'. *Journal of Shoulder and Elbow Surgery*, 12: 314-21.

Chen, A.L, Rokito, A.S and Zuckerman, J.D, 2003. 'The role of the acromio-clavicular joint in impinement syndrome'. *Clinical Sports Medicine*, 22 (2): 343-57.

Chopra, Deepak. *Ageless Body, Timeless Mind.* Rider, 2008.

Christiansen, B et al., 2010. 'Ingestion of broccoli sprouts does not improve endothelial function in humans with hypertension.' *PLOS One*, 27; 5 [8].

Cools, A, Dewitte, V, Lanszweert, F, Notebaert, D and Roets, A et al., 2007. 'Rehabilitation of scapular muscle balance'. *The American Journal of Sports Medicine*, 35 (10), 1744.

Di Castelnuovo, A, Costanzo, S, Bagnardi, V, Donati, M.B, Iacoviello, L, and de Gaetano, G, 2006. 'Alcohol dosing and total mortality in men and women: an updated meta-analysis of 34 prospective studies'. *Archives of Internal Medicine*, 166: 2437-45.

Di Guiseppe, Daniela et al., 2002. 'Long-term intake of dietary long-chain n-3 polyunsaturated fatty acids and risk of rheumatoid arthritis: a prospective cohort study of women'. *Scandinavian Journal of Surgery*, 37(4): 444-9.

Doll, R, 2004. 'Mortality in relation to smoking: 50 years' observations on male British doctors'. *BMJ*, 328: 1519-0.

Duenwald-Kuehl, S, Lakes R and Vanderby, R, 2012. 'Strain-induced damage reduces echo intensity changes in tendon during loading'. *Journal of Biomechanics*, 45 (9): 1607–11.

Duenwald, S, Kobayashi, H, Frisch, K, Lakes, R and Vanderby, R, 2011. 'Ultrasound echo is related to stress and strain in tendon'. *Journal of Biomechanics*, 44 (3): 424–9.

Du Toit, C, Stieler, M, Saunders, R, Bisset, L and Vicenzino, 2008. 'Diagnostic accuracy of power Doppler ultrasound in patients with chronic tennis elbow'. *British Journal of Sports Medicine*, 42 (11): 572–576.

Ebenbicher, G.R, Erdogmus, C.B and Resch, K.L et al., 1999. 'Ultrasound therapy for calcific tendinitis of the shoulder'. *New England Journal of Medicine*, 340 (20): 1533–8.

Epstein, Atman. *The 12 Stages of Healing*. Amber-Allen, 1994.

Ergun, Sahin et al., 2011. 'Telomere dysfunction induces metabolic and mitochondrial compromise'. *Nature*, 470; 359-365.

Fongemie, A.E, Buss, D.D and Rolnick, S.J, 1998. 'Management of shoulder impingement syndrome and rotator cuff tears'. *American Family Physician*, 57 (4): 667–74, 680–2.

Freedland, S.J. et al., 2013. 'A double-blind, randomized, neoadjuvant study of the tissue effects of POMx pills in men with prostate cancer before radical prostatectomy'. Cancer Prevention Research, 6 (10): 1120-7.

Freedman, N.D, Park, Y, Abnet, C.C, Hollenbeck, A.R and Sinha, R, 2012. 'Association of coffee drinking with total and cause-specific mortality'. *New England Journal of Medicine*, 366: 1891-904.

Freer, Amelia. *Eat. Nourish. Glow*. Harper Collins, 2015.

Fu, S.C, Rolf, C, Cheuk, Y.C, Lui, P.P and Chan, K.M, 2010. 'Deciphering the pathogenesis of tendinopathy: a three-stages process'. *Sports Medicine, Arthroscopy, Rehabilitation, Therapy & Technology*, 2: 30.

Gazielly, D.F, Gleyze, P and Thomas, T. *The Cuff*. Elsevier, 2014.

Gonzalez, Santander R, Plasencia, Arriba M.A, Martinez, Cuadrado G, Gonzalez-Santander Martinez, M and Monteagudo de la Rosa, M, 1996. 'Effects of "in situ" vitamin E on fibroblast differentiation and on collagen fibril development in the regenerating tendon'. *The International Journal of Developmental Biology*.

Harley, C.B, Futcher, A.B and Greider, C. W, 1990. 'Telomeres shorten during aging of human fibroblasts'. *Nature*, 345; 458-460.

Hartley, L, Flowers, N, Holmes, J, Clarke, A, Stranges, S, Hooper, L and Rees, K, 2013. 'Green and black tea for the primary prevention of cardiovascular disease'. *Cochrane Heart group*.

Haybittle, J.L, 1998. 'The use of the Gompertz function to relate changes in life expectancy to the standardized mortality ratio'. *International Journal of Epidemiology*, 1; 27(5): 885–9.

Ho, J.O, Sawadkar, P and Mudera, V, 2014. 'A review on the use of cell therapy in the treatment of tendon disease and injuries'. *Journal of Tissue Engineering*, 5.

Holford, Patrick. *Arthritis*. Piatkus Books, 2009.

Hoon, M.W, Johnson, N.A, Chapman, P.G and Burke, L.M, 2013. 'The effect of nitrate supplementation on exercise performance in healthy individuals: a systematic review and meta-analysis'. *International Journal of Sport Nutrition and Exercise Metabolism*, 23 (5): 522-32.

Horner, J, Maratos-Flier, E, and Depinho R, et al., 2011. 'Telomerase reactivation reverses tissue degeneration in aged telomerase deficient mice'. *Nature*, 6, 469 [7328]; 102-6.

Jaskelioff, M et al., 2011. 'Telomerase Reactivation Reverses Tissue Degeneration in Aged Telomerase-Deficient Mice'. *Nature*, 469, 102-6.

Johnson, S.A et al., 2015. 'Daily blueberry consumption improves blood pressure and arterial stiffness in postmenopausal women with pre- and stage 1-hypertension: a randomized, double-blind, placebo-controlled clinical trial'. Journal of the Academy of Nutrition and Dietetics, 115 (3): 369-77.

Jurgens, T.M, Whelan, A.M, Killian, L, Douchette, S, Kirk, S and Foy, E, 2012. 'Green tea for weight loss and weight maintenance in overweight or obese adults'. *Cochrane Metabolic and Endocrine Disorders Group*.

Khalesi, Saman et al., 2014. 'Green tea catechins and blood pressure: a systematic review and meta-analysis of randomised controlled trials'. European Journal of Nutrition, volume 53, issue 6, 1299-1311.

Khan, K.M, Cook, J.L, Kannus, P, Maffulli, N and Bonar, S.F, 2002. 'Time to abandon the "tendinitis" myth: Painful, overuse tendon conditions have a non-inflammatory pathology'. British Medical Journal, 324 (7338): 626–7.

Khaw, K-T, Wareham, N, Bingham, S, Welch, A, Luben, R and Day, N, 2008. 'Combined Impact of Health Behaviours and Mortality in Men and Women: The EPIC-Norfolk Prospective Population Study'. PLOS Medicine, 5: e12.

Kibler, B.W, 1998. 'The role of the scapula in athletic shoulder function'. The American Journal of Sports Medicine, 26 (2), 325-337.

Kim, A et al., 2011. 'Green tea catechins decrease total and low-density lipoprotein cholesterol: a systematic review and meta-analysis'. American Dietetic Association, 111 (11): 1720-9.

Kim, J.Y and Kwon, O, 2009. 'Garlic intake and cancer risk: an analysis using the Food and Drug Administration's evidence-based review system for the scientific evaluation of health claims'. American Journal of Clinical Nutrition, 89 (1): 257-64.

Koester, M.C, George, M.S, Kuhn, J.E, 2005. 'Shoulder impingement syndrome'. American Journal of Medicine, 118 (5): 452–5.

Lipton, Bruce. The Biology of Belief. Cygnus, 2005.

Little, M.P, Hoel, D.G, Molitor, J, Boice, J.D, Wakeford, R and Muirhead, CR, 2008. 'New models for evaluation of radiation-induced lifetime cancer risk and its uncertainty employed in the UNSCEAR 2006 report'. Radiation Research, 169(6): 660–76.

Lissimen, Eliz, Bashale, Alice and Cohen, Marc, 2012. 'Garlic for the common cold'. *Cochrane Acute Respiratory Infections Group.*

Maffulli, N, Ewen, S.W, Waterston, S.W, Reaper, J and Barrass, V, 2000. 'Tenocytes from ruptured and tendinopathic achilles tendons produce greater quantities of type III collagen than tenocytes from normal achilles tendons. An in vitro model of human tendon healing'. *American Journal of Sports Medicine*, 28 (4): 499–505.

Magee, David J, Zachazewski, James E and Quillen, William S. *Pathology and intervention in musculoskeletal rehabilitation*. Saunders, 2008.

Marawaha, R.K, 2014. 'Pomegranate and its derivatives can improve bone health through decreased inflammation and oxidative stress in an animal model of postmenopausal osteoporosis'. *European Journal of Nutrition*, issue 5, 1155-1164.

Marreez, Y.M, Forman, M.D and Brown, S.R, 2003. 'Physical examination of the shoulder joint-Part I: Supraspinatus rotator cuff muscle clinical testing'. *Osteopathic Family Physician*, 5 (3): 128–134.

Marsolais, D, Duchesne, E, Côté, C.H and Frenette, J, 2007. 'Inflammatory cells do not decrease the ultimate tensile strength of intact tendons in vivo and in vitro: protective role of mechanical loading'. *Journal of Applied Physiology*, 102 (1): 3–4.

McShane, J.M, Nazarian, L.N and Harwood, M.I, 2006. 'Sonographically guided percutaneous needle tenotomy for treatment of common extensor tendinosis in the elbow'. *Journal of Ultrasound Medicine*, 25 (10): 1281–9.

Mosley, Michael. *The Fast Diet*. Short Books, 2014.

Mosley, Michael. *Fast Exercise*. Short Books, 2013.

Muggeridge, D.J et al., 2014. 'A single dose of beetroot juice enhances cycling performance in simulated altitude'. *Medicine & Science in Sports & Exercise*, 46 (1): 143-50.

Murrell, G.A, 2002. 'Understanding tendinopathies'. *British Journal of Sports Medicine*, 36 (6): 392-3.

Neer, C. S, 1983. 'Impingement lesions'. *Clinical Orthopaedics and Related Research*, 173, 70-77.

Nirschl, R.P, 1992. 'Elbow tendinosis/tennis elbow'. *Clinical Sports Medicine*, 11 (4): 851–70.

Nirschl, R.P and Ashman, E.S, 2004. 'Tennis elbow tendinosis (epicondylitis)'. *Instructional Course Lectures*, 53: 587–98.

Northrup, Christiane. *Goddesses Never Age*. Hay House, 2015.

Office for National Statistics. Interim Life Tables, 2008-2010.

Oh, J.H, Kim, S.H, Kim, K.H, Oh, C.H and Gong, H.S, 2010. 'Modified impingement test can predict the level of pain reduction after rotator cuff repair'. *American Journal of Sports Medicine*, 38 (7): 1383–8.

Okello, E.J, McDougall, G.J, Kumara, S and Seal, C.J, 2010. 'In vitro protective effects of colon-available extract of Camellia sinensis (tea) against hydrogen peroxide and beta-amyloid ($A\beta(1-42)$) induced cytotoxicity in differentiated PC12 cells'. *Phytomedicine.*

Pan, A, Sun, Q, Bernstein, A.M, Schulze, M.B, Manson, J.E and Stampfer, M.J, et al., 2012. 'Red Meat Consumption and Mortality: Results From 2 Prospective Cohort Studies'. *Archives of Internal Medicine*, 172: 555-63.

Pantuck, A.J et al., 2006. 'Phase II study of pomegranate juice for men with rising prostate-specific antigen following surgery or radiation for prostate cancer'. *Clinical Cancer Research*, 12 (13): 4018-26.

Parkes, G, Greenhalgh, T, Griffin, M, and Dent, R, 2008. 'Effect on smoking quit rate of telling patients their lung age: the Step2quit randomised controlled trial'. *The BMJ*, 15; 336(7644): 598–600.

Patten, Marguerite and Ewin, Jeanette. *Eat to Beat Arthritis*. Thorsons, 2001.

Pingel, J, Lu, Y, Starborg, T, Fredberg, U, Langberg, H and Nedergaard, A et al., 2014. '3-D ultrastructure and collagen composition of healthy and overloaded human tendon: evidence of tenocyte and matrix buckling'. *Journal of Anatomy*, 224 (5): 548–55.

Plasencia, M.A, Ortiz, C, Vazquez, B, San Roman, J, Lopez-Bravo, A and Lopez-Alonso, A, 1999. 'Resorbable polyacrylic hydrogels derived from vitamin E and their application in the healing of tendons'. *Journal of Materials Science: Materials in Medicine*, 10 (10/11): 641–8.

Polizzi, Nick. *The Sacred Cook Book*. Three Seed Productions, 2013.

Presley, T.D, Morgan, A.R and Bechtold, E *et al.*, 2010. 'Acute effect of a high nitrate diet on brain perfusion in older adults'. *Nitric Oxide*.

Prospective Studies Collaboration, 2009. 'Body-mass index and cause specific mortality in 900,000 adults: collaborative analyses of 57 prospective studies'. The Lancet, 373: 1083–96.

Ray, K.K, Seshasai, S.R.K, Erqou, S, Sever, P, Jukema, J.W and Ford, I, et al., 201. 'Statins and all-cause mortality in high-risk primary prevention: a meta-analysis of 11 randomized controlled trials involving 65,229 participants'. *Archives of Internal Medicine*, 170: 1024-31.

Reinhart, K.M, Taliti, R, White, C.M, Coleman, C.L, 2009. 'The impact of garlic on lipid parameters: a systematic review and meta-analysis'. *Nutrition Research Reviews*, 22(1):39-48.

Rodriguez-Mateos, Ana et al., 2013. 'Intake and time dependence of blueberry flavonoid–induced improvements in vascular function: a randomized, controlled, double-blind, crossover intervention study with mechanistic insights into biological activity'. *The American Journal of Clinical Nutrition*, 1-3.

Rompe, J.D, Nafe, B, Furia, J.P and Maffulli, N, 2007. 'Eccentric loading, shock-wave treatment, or a wait-and-see policy for tendinopathy of the main body of tendo Achillis: a randomized controlled trial'. *American Journal of Sports Medicine*, 3 (35): 374–83.

Rosy, Sirisha Neturi et al., 2014. 'Effects of Green Tea on *Streptococcus mutans* Counts-A Randomised Control Trial'. Journal of Clinical and Diagnostic Research, Vol-8 (11): ZC128-ZC130.

Saladin, Kenneth S. *Anatomy & Physiology: The Unity of Form and Function*. McGraw-Hill Education, 2014.

Sandmark, Helene, 2000. 'Musculoskeletal dysfunction in P.E teachers'. *Occupational Environment Medicine*, 57, 673-677.

Sharkey, Neil A, Marder, Richard A and Hanson, Peter B, 1994. 'The entire rotator cuff contributes to elevation of the arm'. *Journal of Orthopaedic Research*, 12 (5): 699-708.

Shaw, M, Mitchell, R, Dorling, D, 2000. 'Time for a smoke? One cigarette reduces your life by 11 minutes'. *The BMJ*, 320(7226): 53.

Shealy, Norman C. *Life Beyond 100*. Penguin, 2006.

Siervo, M et al., 2013. 'Inorganic nitrate and beetroot juice supplementation reduces blood pressure in adults: a systematic review and meta-analysis.' *Journal of Nutrition*, 143 (6): 818-26.

Spiegelhalter, David. BBC Future: Microlives: A lesson in risk taking (Popular explanation of micromorts and microlives).

Spiegelhalter, David. Popular explanation, with derivations for some values and more mathematical detail.

Spiegelhalter, David, 2012. Using speed of ageing and microlives to communicate the effects of lifetime habits and environment'. *The BMJ*, 345.

Stabler, S.N, Tejani, A.M, Huynh, F and Fowkes, C, 2012. 'Garlic for the prevention of cardiovascular morbidity and mortality in hypertensive patients'. *The Cochrane Database of Systemic Reviews.*

Stull, A.J et al., 2015. 'Blueberries improve endothelial function, but not blood pressure in adults with metabolic syndrome: a randomized, double-blind, placebo-controlled clinical trial'. *Nutrients*, 27; 7 (6): 4107-23.

Sumner, M.D, 2005. 'Effects of pomegranate juice consumption on myocardial perfusion in patients with coronary heart disease'. *American Journal of Cardiology*, 96 (6): 810-4.

Swenor, B.K, Bressler, S, Caulfield, L and West, S.K, 2010. 'The Impact of Fish and Shellfish Consumption on Age-Related Macular Degeneration'. *Opthalmology.*

Sydenham, Emma, Dangour, Alan D and Lim, Wee-Shiong, 2012. 'Omega 3 fatty acid for the prevention of cognitive decline and dementia'. *Cochrane Dementia and Cognitive Improvement.*

Thomazeau, H, Duval, J.M, Darnault, P and Dréano, T, 1996. 'Anatomical relationships and scapular attachments of the supraspinatus muscle'. *Surgical and Radiologic Anatomy*, 18 (3): 221–5.

Van Linge, B and Mulder, J.D, 1963. 'Function of the Supraspinatus Muscle and Its Relation to the Supraspinatus Syndrome. An Experimental Study in Man'. *The Journal of Bone and Joint Surgery*, 45 (4): 750-4.

Villoldo, Alberto. *One Spirit Medicine*. Hay House U.K. Ltd, 2015.

Wen, C.P, Wai, J.P.M, Tsai, M.K, Yang, Y.C, Cheng, T.Y.D and Lee, M-C, et al., 2011. 'Minimum amount of physical activity for reduced mortality and extended life expectancy: a prospective cohort study'. *The Lancet*, 378: 1244-53.

Whang, Sang. *Reverse Aging*. Twenty-second Printing, 2010.

'What treatments are there for elbow pain?' Arthritis Research UK.

White, I.R, Altmann, D.R, Nanchahal, K, 2002. 'Alcohol consumption and mortality: modelling risks for men and women at different ages'. *The BMJ*, 27; 325(7357): 191.

Wijndaele, K, Brage, S, Besson, H, Khaw, K-T, Sharp, S.J, and Luben, R, et al., 2011. 'Television viewing time independently predicts all-cause and cardiovascular mortality: the EPIC Norfolk Study'. *International Journal of Epidemiology*, 40: 150–9.

Wilson, J.J and Best, T.M, 2005. 'Common overuse tendon problems: A review and recommendations for treatment'. *American Family Physician (American Academy of Family Physicians)*, 72 (5): 811–8.

Woodcock, J, Franco, O.H, Orsini, N and Roberts, I, 2011. 'Non vigorous physical activity and all cause mortality systematic review and meta analysis of cohort studies'. *International Journal of Epidemiology*, 40, 121-38.

Woodward, Ella. *Deliciously Ella Every Day*. Yellow Kite, 2016.

Xia, W, Szomor, Z, Wang, Y and Murrell, G.A, 2006. 'Nitric oxide enhances collagen synthesis in cultured human tendon cells'. *Journal of Orthopaedic Research*, 24 (2).

Xue, M, Qian, Q and Antonysunil, A et al.m 2008. 'Activation of NF-E2-related factor-2 reverses biochemical dysfunction of endothelial cells induced by hyperglycemia linked to vascular disease'. *Diabetes*.

Yang, W.G and Cao, G.W, 1994. 'Observation of the effects of LAK/IL-2 therapy combining with Lycium barbarum polysaccharides in the treatment of 75 cancer patients'. *Zhonghua Zhong Liu Za Zhi*, 16 (6): 428-31 (Article in Chinese).

Zeisig, Eva; Öhberg, Lars and Alfredson, Håkan, 2006. 'Sclerosing polidocanol injections in chronic painful tennis elbow-promising results in a pilot study'. *Knee Surgery, Sports Traumatology, Arthroscopy*, 14 (11): 1218–1224.

www.jamieoliver.com/news-and-features/features/jamies-plan-to-combat-childhood-obesity

www.physiospot.com/2016/02/23/regenerative-medicine-takes-a-leap-forward-with-3-d-printed-living-body-parts/#sthash

www.SimonMoyes.com – 'What is Subacromial Impingement?'

CHAPTER SIX

Allison, G.T, Godfrey, P and Robinson, G, 1996. 'EMG signal amplitude assessment during abdominal bracing and hollowing'. *Journal of Electromyography and Kinesiology*, 8: 51-57.

Aultman, C.D, Scannell, J and McGill, S.M, 2005. 'Predicting the direction of nucleus tracking in porcine spine motion segments subjected to repetitive flexion and simultaneous lateral bend'. *Clinical Biomechanics*, 20: 126-129.

Axler, C and McGill, S.M, 1997. 'Low back loads over a variety of abdominal exercises: Searching for the safest abdominal challenge'. *Medicine & Science in Sports & Exercise,* 29 (6): 804-811.

Batmanghelidj, F. *Your Body's Many Cries for Water*. CD Version, 2012.

Briggs, A.M and Buchbinder, R, 2009. 'Back pain: a national health priority area in Australia'. *Medical Journal of Australia*, 190 (9), 499-502.

Briggs, A.M, Greig, A.M, Wark, J.D, Fazzalari, N.L and Bennell, K.L, 2004. 'A review of anatomical and mechanical factors affecting vertebral body integrity'. *International Journal of Medical Sciences*, 1 (3): 170-180.

Brooks, C.M, 2012. 'On rethinking core stability exercise programs'. *Australasian Musculoskeletal Medicine*, June: 9-14.

Callaghan, J.P, Gunning, J.L and McGill, S.M, 1998. 'Relationship between lumbar spine load and muscle activity during extensor exercises'. *Physical Therapy*, 78 (1): 8-18.

Callaghan, J.P and McGill, S.M, 2001. 'Intervertebral disc herniation: Studies on a porcine model exposed to highly repetitive flexion/extension motion with compressive force'. *Clinical Biomechanics*, 16 (1): 28-37.

Caraffa, A.G, Cerulli, M, Projetti, G, and Rizzu, A, 1996. 'Prevention of anterior cruciate ligament injuries in soccer: A prospective controlled study of proprioceptive training'. *Knee Surery, Sports Traumatology, Arthroscopy*, 4:19–21.

Comerford, MJ. and Mottram, S.L. *Kinetic Control: The Management of Uncontrolled Movement*. Churchill Livingstone, 2012.

Dreyer, Danny. *Chi Running*. Simon and Schuster, 2008.

Drysdale, C.L, Earl, J.E and Hertel, J, 2004. 'Surface Electromyographic Activity of the Abdominal Muscles During Pelvic-Tilt and Abdominal-Hollowing Exercises'. *Journal of Athletic Training*, 39: 32–36.

Dunstan, D.W et al., 2012. 'Breaking up prolonged sitting reduces post prandial glucose and insulin responses'. *Diabetes Care*, May 35 [5] 976-83.

Faries, M.D and Greenwood, M, 2007. ' Core Training: stabilizing the confusion'. *Strength and Conditioning Journal*, 29, 10-25.

Fiennes, Maya. *Yoga For Real Life*. Atlantic Books, 2012.

Fitzgerald, G.K, Ake, M.J and Snyder-Mackler, L, 2000. 'The efficacy of perturbation training in nonoperative anterior cruciate ligament rehabilitation programs for physically active individuals'. *Physical Therapy*, 80: 128– 140.

Griffin, L.Y, Albohm, M.J, Arendt, E et al., 2006. ' Understanding and preventing noncontact anterior cruciate ligament injuries: a review of the Hunt Valley II meeting, January 2005'. *American Journal of Sports Medicine*, 34 (9): 1512–1532.

Hicks, G.E, Fritz, J.M, Delitto, A and McGill, S.M, 2005. 'Preliminary development of a clinical prediction rule for determining which patients with low back pain will respond to a stabilization exercise program'. *Archives of Physical Medicine and Rehabilitation*, 86 (9): 1753-1762.

Hodges, P.W and Moseley, G.L, 2003. 'Pain and motor control of the lumbopelvic region: effect and possible mechanisms'. *Journal of Electromyography and Kinesiology*, 13, 361–370.

Hodges, P.W and Richardson, C.A, 1996. 'Inefficient muscular stabilisation of the lumbar spine associated with low back pain: a motor control evaluation of transversus abdominis'. *Spine*, 21:2640-2650.

Karavirta, L, 2011, 'Individual responses to combined endurance and strength training in older adults'. *Medicine & Science in Sports & Exercise*, Mar 43 [3] 484-90.

Kavic, N, Grenier, S and McGill, S.M, 2004. 'Determining the stabilizing role of individual torso muscles during rehabilitation exercises'. *Spine*, 29: 1254- 1265.

Kavcic, N, Grenier, S.G and McGill, S.M, 2004. 'Determining tissue loads and spine stability while performing commonly prescribed stabilization exercises'. *Spine*, 29 (11): 1254-1265.

Kibler, W.B, Press, J and Sciascia, A, 2006. 'The Role of Core Stability in Athletic Function'. *Sports Medicine*, 36 (3): 189-198.

Koumantakis, G.A, Watson, P.J and Oldham, J.A, 2005. 'Trunk muscle stabilization training plus general exercise versus general exercise only: Randomized controlled trial with patients with recurrent low back pain'. *Physical Therapy*, 85 (3): 209-225.

Kujala, U.M, Makinen, V.P, Heinonen, I, Soininen, P, Kangas, A.J and Leskinen, T.H et al., 2013. 'Long-term leisure-time physical activity and serum metabolome'. *Circulation*, 22; 127 (3): 340-348.

Lederman, E, 2010. 'The myth of core stability'. *Journal of Bodywork & Movement Therapies*, 14, 84-98.

Lessard, S.J, Rivas, D.A, Alves-Wagner, A.B, Hirshman, M.F, Gallagher, I.J and Constantin-Teodosiu, D et al., 2013. 'Resistance to aerobic exercise training causes metabolic dysfunction and reveals novel exercise-regulated signaling networks'. *Diabetes*, 62 (8): 2717-2727.

Marshall, L.W and McGill, S.M, 2010. 'The role of axial torque in disc herniation'. *Clinical Biomechanics*, 25 (1): 6-9.

McGill, Stuart. *Back Mechanic*. Backfitpro Inc., 2015.

McGill, S, 2010. 'Core training: Evidence translating to better performance and injury prevention'. *Strength & Conditioning Journal*, 32 (3), 33-46.

McGill, Stuart. *Low Back Disorders*. Human Kinetics Europe, 2016.

McGill, S.M, 1998. 'Low back exercises: Evidence for improving exercise regimens'. *Physical Therapy*, 78 (7): 754-765.

McGill, S.M, 2001. 'Low back stability: From formal description to issues for performance and rehabilitation'. *Exercise Sport Science Review*, 29, 26–31.

McGill, S.M, Grenier, S, Kavcic, N and Cholewicki, J, 2003. 'Coordination of muscle activity to assure stability of the lumbar spine'. *Journal of Electromyography and Kinesiology*, 13: 353–359.

McGill, S.M. *The Ultimate Back: Assessment and Therapeutic exercise*. DVD, 2007. www.backfitpro.com.

McNair, Peter, 2004. *Sport Medicine Stretching and Injury Prevention*, June 2004, volume 34, Issue7, 443-449.

Meyer, P, Gayda, Juneau M and Nigam, A, 2012, 'Cardiovascular risk of high versus moderate-intensity aerobic exercise in coronary heart disease.' *Circulation*, 18, 126 [12] 1436-40.

Mipha, Sakyong. *Running with the Mind of Meditation*. Harmony Books, 2012.

Mosley, Michael. *Fast Exercise*. Short Books, 2013.

Myer, G.D, Ford, K.R and Hewett, T.E, 2004. 'Methodological approaches and rationale for training to prevent anterior cruciate ligament injuries in female athletes'. *Scandinavian Journal of Medicine & Science in Sports*, 14:275–285.

Panjabi, M.M, 1992. 'The stabilizing system of the spine. Part I. Function, dysfunction, adaptation, and enhancement'. *Journal of Spinal Disorders*, 5 (4), 383–389.

Paterno, M.V, Myer, G.D, Ford, K.R. and Hewett, T.E, 2004. 'Neuromuscular training improves single-limb stability in young female athletes'. *Journal of Orthopaedic & Sports Physical Therapy*, 34: 305–316.

Reed, C.A, Ford, K.R, Myer, G.D and Hewett, T.E, 2012. 'The effects of isolated and integrated 'core stability' training on athletic performance measures: a systematic review'. *Sports Medicine*, 1; 42: 697-706.

Ressel, O.J, 1989. 'Disc Regeneration; Reversibity is possible in Spinal Osteoarthritis'. *International Review of Chiropractic*, March-April.

Reeves, N.P and Cholewicki, J, 2003. 'Modeling the human lumbar spine for assessing spinal loads, stability, and risk of injury'. *Critical Reviews in Biomedical Engineering*, 31: 73–139.

Reeves, N.P, Narendrac, K.S and Cholewickia, J, 2007. 'Spine stability: the six blind men and the elephant'. *Clinical Biomechanics*, 22: 266–274.

Rottensteiner, M et al., 2014. 'Physical Activity, Fitness, Glucose Homeostasis, and Brain Morphology in Twins'. *Medicine & Science in Sports & Exercise*, Jul 7.

Roussel, N.A, Nijs, J, Mottram, S, van Moorsel, A, Truijen, S and Stassijns, G, 2008. 'Altered lumbopelvic movement control but not generalised joint hypermobility is associated with increased injury in dancers. A prospective study'. *Manual Therapy (online)*.

Sahrmann, S. *Diagnosis and Treatment of Movement Impairment Syndromes.* Mosby, 2002.

Sandmark, Helene, 2000. 'Musculoskeletal dysfunction in P.E teachers'. *Occupational Environment Medicine*, 57, 673-677.

Saner, J, Kool, J, de Bie, R.A, Sieben, J.M and Luomajoki, H, 2011.' Movement control exercise versus general exercise to reduce disability in patients with low back pain and movement control impairment. A randomised controlled trial'. *BMC Musculoskeletal Disorders*, 12: 207.

Scaravelli, Vanda. *Awakening The Spine*. Pinter and Martin Ltd, 2012.

Shrier, Ian, 2005. *Physician and Sports Medicine,* vol 33, No.3, March.

Thacker, S.B, Gilchrist, J, Stroup, D.F and Kimsey, C.D, 2002. 'The prevention of shin splints in sports: a systematic review of literature'. *Medicine & Science in Sports & Exercise*, 34 (1): 32– 40.

Thacker, S.B, Stroup, D.F, Branche, C.M, Gilchrist, J, Goodman, R.A and Porter Kelling, E, 2003. 'Prevention of knee injuries in sports. A systematic review of the literature'. *Journal of Sports Medicine & Physical Fitness*, 43: 165–79.

Thacker, S.B, Stroup, D.F, Branche, C.M, Gilchrist, J, Goodman, R.A and Weitman, E.A, 1999. 'The prevention of ankle sprains in sports. A systematic review of the literature'. *American Journal of Sports Medicine*, 27 (6): 753– 760.

Tsao, H, Galea, M.P and Hodges, P.W, 2008. 'Reorganization of the motor cortex is associated with postural control deficits in recurrent low back pain'. *Brain*, 131, 2161-2171.

Verhagen, E.A, van Mechelen, W and de Vente, W, 2000. 'The effect of preventive measures on the incidence of ankle sprains'. *Clinical Journal of Sport Medicine*, 10 (4): 291– 296.

Wand, B.M et al., 2011. 'Cortical changes in chronic low back pain: Current state of the art and implications for clinical practice'. *Manual Therapy*, 16, 15-20.

Watson, Burton. *The Complete Works of Chuang Tzu*. Columbia University Press, 1968.

White, A.A and Panjabi, M. *Clinical biomechanics of the spine*. J.B. Lippincott Company, 1978.

Willardson, J.M, 2007. 'Core stability training: applications to sports conditioning programs'. *Journal of Strength & Conditioning Research*, 21: 979-985.

Yeung, E.W and Yeung, S.S, 2001. 'Asystematic review of interventions to prevent lower limb soft tissue running injuries'. *British Journal of Sports Medicine*, 35 (6): 383–389.

Zazulak, B.T, Hewett, T.E, Reeves, N.P, Goldberg, B and Cholewicki, J, 2007. 'Deficits in neuromuscular control of the trunk predict knee injury risk: a prospective biomechanical-epidemiologic study'. *American Journal of Sports Medicine*, 35, 1123-1130.

SUMMARY

Liu, K, Daviglus, M.L, Loria, C.M, Colangelo, L.A, Spring, B, Moller, A.C and Lloyd-Jones, D.M, 2012. 'Healthy Lifestyle Through Young Adulthood and the Presence of Low Cardiovascular Disease Risk Profile in Middle Age: The Coronary Artery Risk Development in (Young) Adults (CARDIA) Study'. *Circulation*, 125 (8): 996.

Loprinzi, Paul D, Branscum, Adam, Hanks, June and Smit, Ellen, 2016. 'Healthy Lifestyle Characteristics and Their Joint Association With Cardiovascular Disease Biomarkers in US Adults'. *Mayo Clinic Proceedings*.

Mozaffarian, Dariush et al., 2009. 'Lifestyle Risk Factors and New-Onset Diabetes Mellitus in Older Adults: The Cardiovascular Health Study'. *Archives of Internal Medicine*, 169 (8): 798.

Seguin, Rebecca A et al., 2002. 'Stronger growing older'. *John Hancock Center for Physical Activity and Nutrition*.

Stallworth, J, 2003. 'An Interview with Dr. Lester Breslow'. *American Journal of Public Health*, 93 (11): 1803–1805.

University of California - Los Angeles, 2013. 'Study suggests focus on lifestyle changes, not weight loss, is key to kids' health'. *Science*, 22 August.

APPENDICES

Aliyev, R.M, 2012. 'Better functional results of conservative treatment in fresh lateral ligament injuries of the ankle with additional deep oscillation'. *Physikalische Medizin, Rehabilitationsmedizin*.

Aliyev, R, 2009. 'Clinical effects of the therapy method deep oscillation in treatment of sports injuries'. *Sportschaden: Organ der Gesellschaft fur Orthopadisch*.

Arne, Nyholm Gam and Johannsen, Finn, 1994. 'Ultrasound therapy in musculoskeletal disorders: a meta-analysis'. *Pain*.

Auerbach, B, Yacoub, A and Melzer, C, 2005. 'Prospective Study over a period of 1 Year in respect to the effectiveness of the MBST Nuclear Magnetic Resonance Therapy as used during the conservative therapy of Gonarthrosis'. *1st Joing Congress for Orthopaedic Medicine and Trauma Surgery, Berlin*.

Bisset, L, Coombes, B and Vicenzino, B, 2011. 'Tennis elbow'. *BMJ Clinical Evidence*, Jun 27, 1117.

Bjordal, J.M; Couppé, C, Chow, R.T, Tunér, J and Ljunggren, E.A, 2003. 'A systematic review of low level laser therapy with location-specific doses for pain from chronic joint disorders'. *The Australian Journal of Physiotherapy*, 49 (2): 107–16.

Brosseau, L et al., 2005. 'Low level laser therapy (Classes I, II and III) for treating rheumatoid arthritis'. *Cochrane Database of Systematic Reviews*.

Diegel, I et al., 2007. 'Decrease in Extracellular Collagen Crosslinking after NMR Field Application in Skin Fibroblasts'. *Medical & Biological Engineering & Computing*.

Favejee, M.M, Huisstede, B.M and Koes, B.W, 2011. 'Frozen shoulder: the effectiveness of conservative and surgical interventions--systematic review'. *British Journal of Sports Medicine*, Jan; 45(1): 49-56.

Gerold, R et al., 1999. 'Ultrasound Therapy for Calcific Tendinitis of the

Shoulder'. *New England Journal of Medicine*, 340:1533-1538.

Handschuh, Thomas and Melzer, Christian, 2008. 'The treatment of Osteoporosis with MBST Magnetic Resonance Therapy'. *Orthodoc*.

Hurley, Deirdre A et al., 2004. 'A randomized clinical trial of manipulative therapy and interferential therapy for acute low back pain'. *Spine*, vol 29, issue 20, 2207-2216.

Hurley, D.A, Minder, M, McDonough, S.M, Walsch, D.M, Moore, A.P and Baxter, D.G, 2001. 'Interferential therapy electrode placement technique in acute low back pain: A preliminary investigation'. *Physical Medicine and Rehabilitation*, Volume 82, Issue 4, 485–493.

Jahr, S et al., 2008. 'Effect of treatment with low-intensity and extremely low-frequency electrostatic fields (DEEP OSCILLATION®) on breast tissue and pain in patients with secondary breast lymphoedema'. *Ingentaconnect.com*.

Krosche, Martha and Breitgraf, Gisela, 2003. 'Long Term Evaluation of MBST'. *A Treatment for Cartilage Regeneration*.

Krpan, Dalibor, Stritzinger, Barbara, Lukenda, Ivan, Overbeck, Joakim and Kullich, Werner, 2015. 'Non-pharmacological treatment of osteoporosis with Nuclear Magnetic Resonance Therapy (NMR-Therapy)'. *Periodicum Biologorum*, 57: 61, vol 117, no 1, 161-165.

Kudo, P, Dainty, K and Clarfield, M et al., 2006. 'Randomized, placebo⊠ controlled, double-blind clinical trial evaluating the treatment of plantar fasciitis with an extracoporeal shockwave therapy (ESWT) device: A North American confirmatory study'. Journal of Orthopaedic Research, Feb, 24 (2): 115-23.

Kullich, W et al., 2006. 'Additional Outcome Improvement in the Rehabilitation of Chronic Low Back Pain after Nuclear Resonance Therapy'. *Rheumatologia*.

Kullich, W, 2008. 'Functional improvement in finger joint osteoarthritis with therapeutic use of nuclear magnetic resonance'. *Orthopadische Praxis*.

Kullich, W et al., 2006. 'The effect of MBST® Nuclear Magnetic Resonance Therapy Using a Complex 3-Dimensional Electromagnetic Nuclear Resonance Field on Patients with Low Back Pain'. *International Journal of Back and Musculoskeletal Rehabilitation*.

Kullich, W.C, Schwann, H and Boltzmann, Ludwig. 'MBST Nuclear Magnetic Resonance Therapy Improves Rehabilitation Outcome in Patients with Low Back Pain'. *Annals of the Rheumatic Diseases*.

Luben, R, 1997. 'Effects of microwave radiation on signal transduction processes of cells in vitro'. *Non Thermal Effects of RF Electromagnetic Fields*, ICNIRP.

Marks, R and van Nguyen, J, 2005. 'Pulsed electromagnetic field therapy and osteoarthritis of the knee: Synthesis of the literature'. *International Journal of Therapy and Rehabilitation*, 12 (8): 347-354.

Ogden, R, Alverez, J and Marlow, M, 2014. 'Shockwave Therapy for Chronic Proximal Plantar Fasciitis: A Meta-Analysis'. *Presented at the 4th annual meeting of the International Society for Musculoskeletal shockwave Therapy, Berlin, Germany, May 2001.*

Sanservino, E, (1980). 'Membrane phenomena & cellular processes under action of pulsating magnetic fields'. *Lecture at 2nd Int. Congress Magneto Medicine. Rome, November.*

Seiger, C and Draper, D, 2006. 'Use of pulsed shortwave diathermy and joint mobilization to increase ankle range of motion in the presence of surgical implanted metal: A case series'. *Journal of Orthopaedic & Sports Physical Therapy*, 36 (9): 669-77.

Shields, N et al., 2005. 'Physiotherapist's perception of risk from electromagnetic fields'. *Advances in Physiotherapy*, 7: 170-175.

Steinecker-Frohnwieser, B, Weigl, L.G, Höller, C, Sipos, E, Kullich, W and Kress, H.G, 2009. 'Influence of NMR Therapy on Metabolism of Osteosarcoma- and Chondrosarcoma Cell lines'. *Bone*, vol 44, supplement 2, page s295.

Temiz-Artmann, A, Linder, P, Kayser, P, Diegel, I, Artmann, G.M and Lucker, P, 2005. 'NMR In Vitro Effects on Proliferation, Apoptosis, and Viability of Human Chondrocytes and Osteoblasts'. *Prous Science.*
Van der Windt, D.A et al., 1999. 'Ultrasound therapy for musculoskeletal disorders: a systematic review'. *Pain*, vol 18, issue 3,1 June 1999, 257–271.

Roberta T Chow
Search for articles by this author

Affiliations
- Nerve Research Foundation, Brain and Mind Research Institute, University of Sydney, Sydney, NSW, Australia

Correspondence
- Correspondence to: Dr Roberta T Chow, Honorary Research Associate, Nerve Research Foundation, Brain and Mind Research Institute, University of Sydney, 100 Mallett Street, Sydney, NSW 2050, Australia

Rodrigo AB Lopes-Martins
Search for articles by this author

Affiliations
- Institute of Biomedical Sciences, Pharmacology Department, University of São Paulo, São Paulo, Brazil

Yousefi-Nooraie, R et al., 2008. 'Low level laser therapy for nonspecific low-back pain'. *Cochrane Database of Systematic Reviews.*

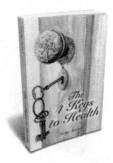

Also Available from Nicky Snazell

The 4 Keys To Health

This book is a self-help manual of preventative health. It has four chapters – mind, food, fitness, and lifestyle – with questionnaires that score you red, amber, and green in terms of health; holding 4 green keys means you are in optimum health.

This book is a result of 30 years' study in the fields of biology, psychology, physiotherapy, and pain. It is my personal insight into health, shared with my patients and audiences internationally.

You can view a YouTube video of Nicky explaining the book at:

https://www.youtube.com/watch?v=sc_i1b979XA

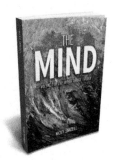

Also Available from Nicky Snazell

The Mind
(The Human Garage Part 1)

Throughout this series of books I am going to share with you
my recipes of integrated medicine for physical health, and in
this edition we focus on the mind.

The Mind is the first book in *The Human Garage* trilogy, and is
available now.

The Human Garage Part 3, The Soul, will also be available soon.
This book will explore the science and spirituality of energy
healing and the power of hands-on healing, as well as touching
on the psychic side of things.

Lightning Source UK Ltd.
Milton Keynes UK
UKOW07f0605250816

281461UK00003B/6/P